RealAge

RealAge

Are You as Young as You Can Be?

MICHAEL F. ROIZEN, M.D.

WITH

ELIZABETH ANNE STEPHENSON

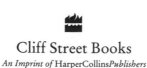

Cliff Street Books

An Imprint of HarperCollins*Publishers*

HarperCollins books may be purchased for educational, business, or sales promotional use. For information please write: Special Markets Department, HarperCollins Publishers, Inc., 10 East 53rd Street, New York, NY 10022.

FIRST EDITION

Designed by Nancy Field

Library of Congress Cataloging-in-Publication Data

Roizen, Michael F.
    RealAge : are you as young as you can be? / Michael Roizen. — 1st ed.
      p.   cm.
    Includes bibliographical references and index.
    ISBN 0-06-019134-1
    1. Aging—Computer programs. 2. RealAge. I. Title.
QP86.R565 1999
613' .0434—dc21   98-42766

99 00 01 RRD 20 19 18

To my family, for their enthusiasm for RealAge
and for their patience with the project.

They not only help me stay young
but are the reason I want to be young.

Contents

Acknowledgments

My patients inspired me to write this book, and I would like to thank them first and foremost. They encouraged me to develop RealAge and motivated me to bring this project to fruition. I hope this book helps them and the rest of the readers to live younger longer. That would be my best reward. I am especially indebted to the members of the staff and faculty of the Department of Anesthesia and Critical Care at the University of Chicago, who afforded me the time to do this project and who had the vision to understand that the best medicine happens before a patient ever gets sick.

I am grateful to the many, many other people who contributed to this book. Some deserve a specific thank you: Sukie Miller, for her consistent encouragement; Anita Shreve, for saying the book was possible and that the chapters were just what she wanted to read ("send me more"); Candice Fuhrman, for making it happen; Elsa Dixon, for making it clearer; the many gerontologists and internists who read sections of the book for accuracy; Jack Rowe and Charles Hennekins, for performing invaluable research, and for personal advice that helped make the science in this book better; Gary Becker and Robert Fogel, whose discussions made the text better and typify what makes being a faculty member at the University of Chicago fun—the opportunity to learn from giants; Dave Summerell, who taught me the value of the computer; the many anesthesiologists who encouraged me about the importance of this endeavor to our specialty; Kelle Martin, for her endless patience and good humor in producing the graphs and charts; Charise Petrovitch, for help in improving the slides; Jaimee Huth, who worked late into the night, tirelessly and enthusiastically, to produce the final copies of the manuscript; Anne-Marie Ruthrauff, for doing so much so well and doing it so calmly in the midst of a constant storm; Julia Serebrinsky, Susan Muller, and William Germino, who each made this a better book than it would have been; Tate Erlinger, Linda Van Horne, Arline McDonald, Jeremiah Stamler, Mark Rudberg, Mike

Parzen, and especially Keith Roach and Axel Goetz—the scientific partners in the process of evaluating the data and scientific content of RealAge; Sidney Unobskey and Martin Rom, who inspired the process and named it; Charlie Silver, who funded the research and assembled the innovative RealAge team that continually evaluates and updates RealAge and its Web site; my father, for being my biggest fan and most inspiring example; and especially Diane Reverand, whose faith in the work was inspiring and who not only believed in this book but improved it. Pauline Snider's contributions have been so significant as to be beyond comment. Any mistakes are in spite of her best advice.

I should leave the next space blank because words cannot express my appreciation to Elizabeth Stephenson for her work on this book. Special thanks to those people who helped her to do her job right: Jordan Karubian, James Kimball, Anne Kimball, David Wang, Thayer Lindner, Deborah Reck, Arthur Unobskey, Maia Rigas, Rachel Pomerantz, Josefina Yanguas, and her extended family of Stephensons, O'Briens, and Glickmans. (Thanks also to Timmy, for remembering to take Pauline to the beach, and Oliver, for love and companionship. Both are daily reminders that the best way to stay young is to live life exuberantly and without apology.) Yes, I owe a special thanks to Elizabeth Stephenson, who patiently asked what I was trying to say and translated it into compelling English (what we hope is compelling for you), and then made it compelling again after I tried to put more scientific writing back into the book.

Finally, I would like to thank my wife, Nancy, for her constant love and support, and our children, Jeffrey and Jennifer, for their encouragement and patience. The book is dedicated to them.

Preface

GETTING YOUNGER:
FOR LIFE!

What would you do if I gave you a hundred dollars? Would you spend it? Or save it? Think of all the things you could do with it. You could buy tickets to a pro basketball game. Or a new pair of running shoes. You could buy an armful of flowers for someone special. Or just treat yourself to cappuccinos every morning for a month. Sure, you could do a lot with a hundred dollars, but you couldn't buy a condominium with it. Or a new car. You know exactly how far a hundred dollars goes. And that's one of the remarkable things about money.

Because money has concrete value, we can compare activities as diverse as spending a couple of hours watching hoops and paying the phone bill and then choose between them. We know that a hundred dollars will buy an evening out or a pair of shoes but not both. Money values allow us to evaluate our choices.

I'm not going to give you a hundred dollars. Instead, I'm going to give you something better: years of life. I'm going to teach you how to add years to your life—high-quality, health-filled, vibrant years. I'm going to show you how to live younger through a method that makes health decisions as easy to understand as it is to understand what that one hundred dollars is worth.

The biggest problem with understanding health care decisions is that we have no common currency for medicine. We have no way of measuring decisions as diverse as buckling our seat belts, exercising, or taking vitamins regularly. But that's about to change.

As complex as medical science can be, there are only two real questions in medicine: How long will you live? And how healthy and vigorous will your life be while you're living it? Whether the issue at hand is eating a nutritious

diet, taking calcium supplements, or wearing sunscreen, the fundamental
motivation for choosing any of these behaviors is to ensure a longer, healthier
life. Unfortunately, medical studies and news reports almost never make it
seem that simple. RealAge unifies an array of health topics by determining
exactly how they affect youth and vigor. RealAge correlates these to a common measurement—years of life.

For example, think of the neighbor who looks as if she's in her early forties,
but who's really sixty. And remember how surprised you were to learn that
your coworker, who you thought was in his fifties, was only forty-three?
Some people are young for their age: They are physiologically and mentally
as active and vibrant as someone much younger. The sixty-year-old woman
may have a RealAge—that is, a physiologic age—of only forty-five. Why?
Because she has learned how to slow the pace of aging. Your coworker, on the
other hand, has probably abused his body, causing it to age much faster than it
should. Remember your school reunion: Even though everyone was the same
chronologic age, people no longer looked the same age. Some people wore the
years well, were young and exuberant, despite the passage of time. Others
looked as if they had aged ten years more than everyone else—and they probably had.

Your RealAge is an estimation of your age in biologic terms, not chronologic years. If your RealAge is five years younger than your chronologic age,
it means that your rate of aging is such that you are in the same shape physiologically as the average person who is five years younger than you. Likewise,
if your RealAge is five years older than your chronologic age, you have aged
to the same biologic condition as someone who is five years older. RealAge
measurements allow us to quantify the age difference between our calendar
age and our biologic age. Using the latest and most sophisticated computer
technology and statistical methodology, RealAge is able to translate health
risk into years of your life.

Better yet, the RealAge program shows every single one of us just how
simple it is to become one of those people who really is younger than his or
her years. We really can slow the pace of aging—and even reverse it.
Although we've never been able to talk about "getting younger" before—time
moves in only one direction, forward—now we can. Even though you can't
change your calendar age, you can "make" your RealAge younger. That is,
you can have the health profile of someone who is chronologically younger.
Best of all, it's not that difficult to do. Slowing the pace of aging can be relatively easy and painless. That means you can start feeling more invigorated,
energetic, and healthful almost as soon as you start the RealAge program. You
won't just live longer, you'll live younger.

More of us are living longer than human beings have ever lived before. Our life expectancy is increasing, and, barring unforeseen circumstances, most of us can expect to live into ripe old age—ripe old calendar age, that is. Yet, how well you live is largely up to you. Most of us don't want to live to be ninety if the last thirty years of our lives are filled with illness, restricted ability, and dependence on our families or nursing care. We want to be able to play golf, tango, or climb a mountain right until the day we die. We want all those extra years to be quality years—years in which we write the novel we've always dreamed of writing or learn how to paint. We want those years to be years when we travel the globe, visiting the far-off places we've only read about. We want to have fun with our grandchildren and enjoy our children as adults. We don't want to give up the things that make our lives worth living.

Longer lives don't mean much if they aren't active lives. That is what RealAge is all about: making simple decisions in our day-to-day lives that will stave off the biologic aging processes that make our old age feel "old."

Every one of us was born with a potential—the potential of who we will become. Part of this potential is social—the kind of education you get, the job you take, the opportunities and happenstances that come your way. The other part of this potential is biologic. How long and how well will you live? How healthy will you be? For far too long, the medical community has written off aging as something that is purely genetic, assuming that a person's whole life is "written in the genes" with which he or she is born. The more we know about genetics, our biologic inheritance, the more we know that this assumption is not true. Studies continue to show that for most of us, lifestyle choices and behaviors have far more impact on longevity and health than does heredity. Your genes (the elements that carry inherited information) define your basic biology, but how you interact with the world around you—whether through food choices, exercise, or social connections—is how *you* control the way your genes will affect your body. Those interactions shape both the quality and quantity of your life. Most of us do not live as well or as long as our genes or our bodies would allow. We shortchange ourselves. By taking care of our bodies, we slow the pace of biologic aging and capitalize more fully on our potential.

Through the RealAge program, you will learn to understand your health care decisions in terms of the one thing that really matters: your biologic age. RealAge establishes a measurement system to calculate the relative biologic age of our bodies, so that you can learn to evaluate health care decisions as diverse as putting tomato sauce on spaghetti or taking a jog, in the same terms and then make informed decisions about each habit.

RealAge calculations provide a way to interpret different types of health information and to make informed choices about our behaviors. RealAge gives a value to each of our choices, just as the price tag on a product in a store gives a value to that product. Although some of these changes are easy and some are a bit more difficult, most are relatively painless. None of us can or will do everything possible to get younger, but because RealAge breaks these decisions down into steps, every single one of us can do some things to start getting younger. We can make health decisions that fit into our particular lifestyles and decide which aspects of healthy living would affect us the most. We can decide what really matters, what's worth the effort, and what we may want to postpone. Once we understand the multiple, often unrelated, factors on which the totality of our health depends, we can start living healthier one step at a time. You make the choices about how you want to age—or *not*.

1

Getting Younger— Just the Facts

IT'S EASIER THAN YOU THINK

As a doctor, I have often felt I was fighting an uphill battle. My job is to cure people after they are *already* sick. But preventing illness in the first place is *always* the best cure. Practicing my specialty of cardiovascular anesthesiology has meant that I have spent much of my working life with patients who are among the sickest of the sick, people who need bypass surgery or emergency operations to fix potentially fatal aneurysms. After spending so much time in the operating room with patients who were so severely sick, I was frustrated by not being able to do more for them. I was grateful that I really *could* save lives, but at the same time, I was mad as heck. So many of these patients were sick because they had mistreated their bodies over time. Moreover, every single one of them knew better. They knew that they should exercise more, eat healthier foods, and take care of themselves, but they just weren't doing it. That seemed to me a true tragedy, not to mention a national health care crisis. Why were so many people—smart, educated, thoughtful people—not paying attention to the reports of studies that correlated good health behaviors with long, healthy lives? It would have been easy to blame it on the patients. *But it wasn't their fault.* Clearly, the medical community was failing to communicate its message effectively.

In my internal medicine practice and my anesthesia preoperative clinic, I told my patients again and again how they could live healthier. I told them how they could lengthen—and strengthen—their lives and how they could increase the quantity and the quality of their years. But the tide of patients coming into my office and into the operating room with entirely preventable illnesses did not stem. I felt as if all my talk was for nothing. Why did they persist in habits that were harmful to their health, even though they knew better? What could I do—what could all doctors do—to explain health better? Good health is an attainable goal, but my patients weren't listening.

REALAGE:
THE BEGINNING OF AN IDEA

One day, a friend said to me, "Health is so confusing. One day the papers are telling you to do one thing, and the next day they're telling you to do the opposite. There's just so much information. I don't know what to do with it all." I empathized, but I didn't know exactly how to change things. How could people measure one alternative against another?

When another friend, Simon Z., developed a severe illness, it all came together. For some reason, stepping out of my role as a doctor and into my role as a friend made the idea flash in my head: Health *is* like money. It has an exchange value. Health decisions and behavioral choices that you make today are capital toward living younger tomorrow. What we were missing was a common currency for health.

Simon, who was forty-nine, was afflicted with severe arterial disease. He had a terrible circulatory problem that made it nearly impossible for him to walk more than a quarter of a block without terrible pain, and he needed a major operation. His lifelong smoking habit wasn't helping any. Even though he was relatively young, his body was in the condition of someone much older. I was afraid that he might not be my friend for much longer.

Simon was a tough cookie—and an even tougher patient. A self-made man, he had a drive and determination that was hard to match. He had worked hard for everything he had ever gotten in his life, and, with a wonderful family, good friends, and a booming career, his was an American success story. Yet he was a heart attack away from losing it all. As a doctor, I wanted to cure him. As a friend, I didn't want to lose him. For all Simon's attention to detail in his job, family, and friendships, he had overlooked the one thing that made it all possible: himself.

Telling him to quit smoking didn't work. (Quite literally, I called him every single day for years to ask him if he had quit yet. The answer was always "no.")

"Simon," I said one day when he was in for a checkup, "how old are you?"

"Mike, please," he grumbled. "You *know* I'm forty-nine."

"Simon, this isn't a joke," I replied. "How old are you *really*?"

"What are you getting at?" he said, eyeing me suspiciously.

"Did you know that all that smoking has made you older?" I asked him. "Eight years older. Right now, you may be forty-nine. But your body is as old as someone who is fifty-seven, maybe more. For all practical purposes, your age *is* fifty-seven."

"I can't be fifty-seven," he said.

"Why not?" I asked.

"Because no man in my family has ever lived to the age of fifty-eight."

The message hit home. Simon quit smoking. He began exercising and eating right. He reduced his RealAge and began celebrating "year-younger" parties, rather than his usual "one-more-year-over-the-hill" birthday parties. Over time, he became younger.

Fundamental to economics is the concept of "net present value." Net present value is used by economists to determine the current value of investments that have future payoffs. The RealAge concept allows us to calculate the value of different types of health behaviors and choices. In biologic terms, the difference between your calendar age and your RealAge is a calculation of the net present value of your health behaviors; it is the estimate of what age you are physiologically when compared with the rest of the population. For example, when I say someone's RealAge is forty-five compared with his or her chronological age of fifty, it means that the person has the health profile of the average forty-five-year-old. In terms of age, his or her net present value is five years younger. Each behavior has a net present value and alters your RealAge by a specific number of years. Instead of considering health decisions as something that will pay off thirty years down the road, you will be able to see just how each choice is paying off in the present.

Has this been demonstrated? Is it real? Yes. The rest of the book gives you the net present value, or RealAge change, for each choice. It also examines how and why that choice affects you.

A QUESTION OF AGE: WHAT DOES IT MEAN TO GET OLD?

No matter who you are, no matter what else happens in your life, one thing is guaranteed: You will get older—each and every day. It's one of life's promises, and there's no stopping it.

At least, not until now. Now we know that slowing the process of aging, reversing aging, is the best thing we can do to promote health. "Younger" and "healthier" are almost always one and the same. Most of the major diseases we confront—cancer, arthritis, heart disease—rarely occur until our bodies begin to show the signs of aging. Indeed, these diseases are, far too often, the hallmarks of aging, their onset defining the moment when we first feel old.

Surprisingly, no one knows *why* we age. Even though aging is one of the most clearly visible biological processes—a process that's been written about as long as anyone has written about biology—there is no good scientific explanation for aging, except to say that our bodies were designed to grow older. Aging is built right into us, and no one can say exactly why. Scientists have at least seven major theories about why we age, and all of them have some credibility. Some scientists believe that our bodies are programmed to die—that our genes program our cells to divide a certain number of times and that once division has reached that maximum number, our bodies begin to fail. This is known as the telomere theory. (Telomeres are genetic elements that control the number of allowable cell divisions.) Others argue that there is a general degradation of neuroendocrine stimuli—that is, the neurologic and hormonal systems that regulate the organism finally wear out, making us more susceptible to a variety of diseases. A third hypothesis is the "wear-and-tear" theory, that living itself makes us old. A fourth theory is that our bodies eventually build up so many toxins and other waste products that our systems begin to shut down. In a further elaboration of this hypothesis, many scientists believe that this waste buildup can even affect the structure of our genes. You may know this fifth theory as the free-radical theory of aging: Our bodies build up free radical "oxidants" that damage our organs and our DNA, causing us to age. A corollary to this theory is the glucose toxicity theory, which also has to do with waste buildup in our bodies. The final theory of aging derives from the law of entropy: In the universe there is a continual movement from order to disorder, and in our bodies, that movement is marked as aging.

Although no one knows exactly *why* we age, we do know, at least in part, *what* ages. Aging is not one thing but many things. And that's the key to RealAge. Aging is the catchall term for all sorts of processes—everything from getting wrinkles to wearing out our hearts. Aging doesn't happen as some mysterious metaphysical phenomenon. Aging happens in the particulars. That is, your arteries get clogged. Arthritis flares up. Your parts start to wear down, and you don't heal as quickly as you used to. With RealAge, we go to the source; we get down to the details. We all know people who look younger than their age. And we all know people who look like they're older. The question is, How can you turn yourself into one of those people who look, feel, and—in physiologic terms—*are* younger than their age?

First, stop thinking about health as the prevention of disease and start thinking about it as the prevention of aging. The chance of any of us being afflicted by any one disease in any one year is pretty slim. We read that 3 in 1,000 women will get a certain kind of cancer or that 2 in 100 men will die from a specific variety of stroke. These kinds of data aren't enough to convince us that we should really eat that salad instead of a burger and fries. These events seem too remote.

However, eating that hamburger will make you older tomorrow than if you ate that salad today. And you will be younger tomorrow if you exercise today. The better condition you are in—that is, the younger you stay—the better prepared you will be to fight the factors that age you. When you take care of your body, time slows down. You will have *more* time—time to be what you want to be and to do what you want to do. By quantifying how different behaviors affect the rate of aging, RealAge lets you understand the relative value of your health choices.

UNTANGLING AGING:
BEHAVIOR, GENETICS, AND
THE AGING PROCESS

As recently as twenty years ago, doctors largely believed that as soon as we understood genetics, we would solve many of the basic medical problems that eluded us. The overwhelming belief was that youth, health, and longevity were determined from birth and that there was nothing to be done about it. "It's all in the genes you're born with" was the word of the day. Almost everyone, including the scientific community, believed that a person's life span was largely a matter of fate.

For diseases as diverse as diabetes, Alzheimer's, many cancers, and cardiovascular disease, we've long known that genetic components are involved in many cases. Some of us are more prone to weight gain, and some of us are more prone to high cholesterol. Those tendencies can increase the likelihood of certain kinds of diseases and aging. Surprisingly, the more scientists have learned about genetics, the more they have learned just how much the environment, and our interactions with it, matter. We largely control how our genes affect us. We all have the genes we were born with, but how we age is primarily up to us.

Despite commonly held beliefs that aging is mostly out of your control, inherited genetics account for less than 30 percent of all aging effects, and the importance of genetic inheritance matters less and less the older your calendar age. By the age of eighty, behavioral choices account almost entirely for a person's overall health and longevity. People who are still able to live young even when their calendar age is old weren't necessarily born with "good" genes nearly so much as they have made "good" choices. They exercise, eat lots of fruits and vegetables, keep their minds engaged, and do many of the things that this book advocates to keep themselves young.

Although we tend to imbue our genes with mystery, when it comes right down to it, genes direct our bodies to make proteins. They provide information about what proteins our cells should and shouldn't produce, how much, and when. The fact that you made it into the world at all means that all your essential genes are working just fine. To develop from an egg to a fetus requires incredible genetic coordination. Simply being born means that everything pretty much went right. Since most people with severe genetic illnesses suffer in childhood, growing up to adulthood means that even more went right. For the most part, when we discuss aging and genetics, we are talking about subtle differences. (For further information on genetics and aging, see Chapter 5 on cancer genetics and Chapter 12 on evaluating hereditary risks.)

Separating biology and behavior is difficult, if not impossible: Children inherit not just genes from their parents but also behaviors. Those behaviors can have biologic effects, including the rate at which the children age. For example, children who eat a lot of saturated fats when they are young are more likely to die of arterial disease when they get old (or, as it may be, not so old). The behaviors learned and ingrained in youth can affect your whole life, including the rate at which you age.

Cardiovascular disease provides an excellent example of the way biologic predispositions and social behaviors interrelate. Some people are *biologically* predisposed to the early onset of arterial aging. They have inherited a tendency toward high blood pressure, high cholesterol, or weight gain. Others are *culturally* predisposed to the disease because they are far more likely to develop such habits as eating foods high in saturated fat that can accelerate arterial aging. Finally, we know that there is often, *if not usually*, a combination of both: The bad habits interact with the biologic predisposition, and cardiovascular aging is accelerated.

By starting with good behaviors, you live as long—and as young—as your genes will allow.

AGE BUSTERS:
THE THREE MOST IMPORTANT
FACTORS THAT AFFECT AGING

So, exactly what are those behavioral changes that will help keep you young? Essentially everything you do contributes to or prevents aging. Eating a diet low in saturated fats, exercising, and quitting smoking are probably lifestyle choices you already know are good for you and, although you may never have thought about it exactly this way, prevent aging. But did you know that flossing your teeth nightly can make a big difference in how fast you age? Flossing regularly can make your RealAge as much as 6.4 years younger (see Chapter 5). And did you know that folate can help your arteries stay young? Folate reduces arterial aging and can make a person's RealAge as much as three years younger (see Chapter 7). Many of the choices that help prevent aging are easy and simple to do. Learn to think about the wide variety of choices in your life as they relate to your health currency—your RealAge. Through RealAge, you are able to weigh the relative values of each and decide which changes are worth it for you. Best of all, it is much less work than you think.

Aging of the Arteries

In no uncertain terms, you are as young as your arteries. Aging of the arteries is the most important factor in the overall process of aging. When your arteries are not taken care of properly, they get clogged with fatty buildup, diminishing the amount of oxygen and nutrients that can get to your cells. When this happens, not only your cardiovascular system, but your entire body, ages more quickly. Cardiovascular disease is the leading killer of adult Americans, killing more than 40 percent of us and seriously afflicting more than half of us. Having high blood pressure (a blood pressure reading over 140/90 mm Hg) can make a person's RealAge more than twenty-five years older than having low blood pressure (a blood pressure reading of 115/76 or below). The better you take care of your arteries and the younger *they* are, the younger *you* will be. This book lists a whole range of things for each individual to do—everything from taking folic acid supplements to flossing your teeth—that will make your arteries younger and healthier, and *that* will make you feel stronger and livelier.

Aging of the Immune System

Don't let your immune system make you old. As you age, your immune system begins to get sloppy, ignoring important warning signals and becoming negligent. You can end up with cancer or another disorder caused by a malfunction of your immune system. For example, when you are young—except in relatively rare cases—genetic controls in your cells protect your cells from becoming cancerous. If one of these cellular controls slips up, your larger immune system identifies precancerous cells in the body and eliminates them. Thus, your body has a double block against cancer, one on the cellular level and one on the organism-wide level. As you age, both the cell-based genetic controls and your immune system become more likely to malfunction, and you are more likely to develop a cancerous tumor. Many types of arthritis are examples of a breakdown of the immune system, which is why arthritis is a disease associated with aging. By keeping your immune system fit, you do your best to avoid such diseases and prevent premature aging. This book tells you which vitamins (and at what doses) help protect your genetic control systems and immune system. The program also describes ways to reduce the stresses in your life that can upset the balance of your immune system, and such practices as strengthening exercises that will help keep your immune system running young.

Social and Environmental Factors

How we react to our environment biologically, psychologically, and socially has a lot to do with how young we stay. The environment in which we live, the substances we put into our bodies, the risks we take, and the stresses we undergo can all contribute to aging. Breathing secondhand smoke, eating foods high in saturated fats, working in an unsafe environment, or using a cell phone while driving can all increase the likelihood that our lives will be shorter or more ridden with illness than they would be otherwise. When we think only about disease, we forget about other factors that are outside our bodies that can make us healthy. Some choices—for example, becoming a lifelong learner by enrolling in classes, reading, or otherwise stimulating your mind—can help keep you younger longer. Having fun with your friends can do the same. In subsequent chapters, I detail the impact of these choices and show you how interacting with your environment in a particular way can keep you young.

FROM SCIENCE TO YOU:
LIVING YOUNG

RealAge is a way of measuring the pace of aging. By adopting the suggestions in this book, you are slowing the rate of aging and sometimes even reversing it. In Chapter 2, I explain how we are able to calculate RealAge and discuss the science behind the numbers. I give you two options for calculating your own RealAge (using the charts provided in this book or, for a more accurate calculation, using the computerized survey on the RealAge Web site, www.RealAge.com). Both options not only provide you with an individual calculation that distinguishes you from everyone else around you, but also compare you with the health and youth average for your age group. Your RealAge calculation will weigh the risks you face against the health-related behaviors you choose. The end product is a RealAge that is uniquely descriptive of *you*. As you adopt behaviors that change your RealAge (for example, eating breakfast every day), you can recalculate your RealAge. With each new calculation, you can chart your progress and watch the years disappear.

How young can you become? When I told one fifty-year-old friend of mine all the things she could do to reduce her rate of aging, she asked me, "Mike, if I did all of those things, I could have a RealAge of twelve, couldn't I?" Well, for those of us who don't want to relive our teenage years, fortunately, no. In this book, all of the chapters use calculations that reflect the greatest possible effect of each behavior when no other mediating factors are considered. Both the worksheets in Chapter 2 and the RealAge computer program use a multi-variable equation that balances each factor in relation to all the other RealAge factors. This equation evaluates how all these factors interrelate.

The more Age Reduction™ habits you adopt (the specific plan is described in Chapter 3), the less likely you will be to gain the maximum effect from adopting any single practice by itself. But the more good habits you adopt, the better your across-the-board protection from aging will be, and that advantage will have a cumulative effect over time. Although none of us can be twelve again, it is relatively easy for individuals in their mid-fifties or mid-sixties to reduce their RealAge by five to eight years and only somewhat more difficult for them to reduce it by fifteen or sixteen years. The maximum amount a person can reduce his or her RealAge below his or her calendar age is about twenty-five years over an entire lifetime. And remember, the effect magnifies with age: At fifty, you may have a RealAge of forty-five, but by seventy-five, if you continue on the RealAge program, your RealAge may be only fifty-five. That means that in twenty-five years, your body may have aged as little as most people's do in ten.

Clearly, RealAge is not a guarantee of longevity. In health, there are never guarantees. But RealAge is an accurate reading of your risk. The lower your RealAge, the better the odds that you will have more years left—not to mention a younger, healthier, and more energetic life. The calculation of risk is the best approximation we have of the body beneath: The lower the risk, the younger the body. Think of your RealAge as your aging speedometer; it is a reading of how fast you're going. With aging, *faster is not better*. By making simple decisions, you can take your foot off the gas pedal and slow down your rate of aging. How you age is largely controlled by you.

GETTING YOUNGER ALL THE TIME

Since I developed the RealAge concept, I haven't been able to keep quiet. I talk about RealAge to doctors and others all over the country. I have encouraged patients to take the RealAge computer program and have seen them make the decision to take their aging into their own hands. I have joined people as they have celebrated "year-younger" birthday parties and observed them becoming younger in front of my very eyes. While the response has been, for the most part, overwhelmingly positive, there have been a few naysayers. On occasion, after presenting a talk about RealAge, I have heard people grumble, "We Americans just don't have any respect for old age. It's just youth, youth, youth." These criticisms leave me dismayed, not to mention disappointed in myself, for not communicating the essence of RealAge so that everyone in my audience understood.

The whole point of RealAge is to *promote* old age. Healthy, vibrant, and *young* old age. RealAge shows you how you can live at eighty with all the energy and vigor of a fifty-five-year-old, how you can be the ninety-year-old who still lives on your own, travels, and forcefully expresses feisty opinions—the person who leaves the "kids" marveling, "How does she do it?" Having respect for old age means wanting to end the suffering that so often goes along with it. No one wants to be bedridden, afflicted with heart disease, or undergoing cancer treatment. Everyone wants to be able to do all the things he or she has always done and *more*. And that means staying young biologically, even as you get older chronologically. The data from the Fries Study of University of Pennsylvania alumni, the MacArthur–Mount Sinai study on differences in aging between twins, and Fogel's study of longevity statistics in national health databases show that people who live healthier live longer and with less disease and disability. Those who adopted healthier behaviors not only lived seven years longer on average, but also did not suffer the onset of old-age disability until five to seven years closer to death. In other words, the period of disease and disability was shortened.

What science shows us is that enjoying a healthy and vibrant old age depends on taking the proper steps to take care of yourself all along the way. Until RealAge, health recommendations were more like promissory notes or junk bonds—something that might have a payoff in the distant future but with little or no guarantee. And who was convinced? Certainly not the 85 percent of Americans who don't get enough physical activity even though they know better. When you take steps to change a behavior now—taking the right vitamins, learning to relax, or taking up exercise—the payoff is not just that you will live longer, but that you will live younger. You slow the rate at which your body ages. The payoff is not thirty years down the line, but now. Why get old when you can stay young?

2

Calculating RealAge

TAKE THE REALAGE TEST: WHAT'S YOUR REALAGE?

How old are you now? How young could you be? Learn how to calculate your RealAge.[1] You can do it either by using the charts provided in this book, which will give you a good approximation of your RealAge, or by going on-line to the RealAge Web site and calculating your biologic age more accurately using the RealAge computer database. By answering easy questions about 125 health factors, habits, and behaviors, you can determine whether you are aging more quickly or more slowly than your contemporaries. Once you know your RealAge, you will have the information you need to start getting younger. By choosing from the recommendations in this book or in your computer printout, you can develop a step-by-step Age Reduction Plan customized to your needs and lifestyle.

Now that you understand the principle of RealAge—that you can get younger—you may be wondering how you can calculate a number that accurately describes your "true" physiologic age. How can I say that some people

---

[1] The RealAge effects specified in all chapters other than this chapter calculate the effects of the factor being considered *individually*. Let's take the example of blood pressure. Many factors contribute to your blood pressure reading, such as sodium intake and potassium levels, so that some of the effects attributed to blood pressure are attributable to other things as well. For example, exercise lowers blood pressure: three of the twelve years difference in RealAge between a fifty-year-old man who has the ideal blood pressure of 115/76 and one who has a high blood pressure of 140/90 is attributable to the stamina exercise component. The changes in RealAge described in all chapters except this chapter do not take into account the covariance or interaction between factors. Please refer to the tables in this chapter or the RealAge Web site at www.RealAge.com.

are younger and others are older when their calendar ages are the same? People are so different from each other. For all those who get cancer from smoking, there is always one diehard who has smoked a pack a day since he was twelve and is going strong at ninety. So, how can I say that quitting a pack-a-day smoking habit will make you seven years younger? Or that taking an aspirin a day can make you not fifty-five, but fifty-three and a half?

For a long time, researchers saw aging as a linear and roughly equal process. Most researchers considered all seventy-year-olds to be the same. This assumption was good for census bureau statisticians, but made for an inaccurate representation of reality. When you look at the population, it is apparent that all seventy-years-olds are not alike. Many are mobile, full of life, and living as young as fifty-year-olds. Others are homebound, bedridden, or suffering from a wide range of health complications. Not everyone ages equally.

THE NUTS AND BOLTS OF REALAGE: THE SCIENCE BEHIND THE NUMBERS

If you chart the health, longevity, and, ultimately, *youth* of a "population age cohort," a group of people all born in the same year, you will find that with few exceptions, people age at a similar rate until they reach their late twenties or mid-thirties. With the exception of those who have inherited rare genetic disorders or have been in serious accidents, everyone is basically healthy and able. Men reach the peak of their performance curve in their late twenties, and women, in their mid-thirties. Our bodies have fully matured, and we are at our strongest and most mentally acute. Then, somewhere between twenty-eight and thirty-six years of age, most people reach a turning point—a transition from "growing" into "aging."

If you examine the population as a whole and track any one biologic function—whether kidney function or cognitive ability—performance declines as we age. In general, each biologic function decreases 3–6 percent per decade after age thirty-five. That decrease is a measure of the *average* for the population as a whole. Although these types of measurements have been the standards used by scientists to calculate the rate of aging, these averages don't take into account the variation *among* individuals. For older populations, the variation is so great that it is often meaningless to calculate an average at all because averages are statistically meaningful only if the people or things being measured actually congregate around a midpoint. With aging, this does not happen. In fact, if you really look at the numbers, there is so much variation among individuals that the "average" obscures more than it shows. Rather than gathering around a mean (the center), there are people in every age group who fit into every category of function—some showing dramatic decline, others showing virtually none.

The variations in the ability to function cover the entire range of possibility. For every seventy-year-old who's debilitated from cardiovascular disease, there's another who's running road races or traveling the globe. You can see this variation in Figure 2.1. If a horizontal line were drawn across the three lines representing the rapid, average, and slow rates of aging, you would find that people of different calendar ages fall at the same place on the curve representing aging.

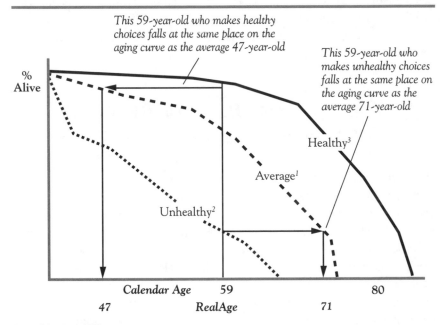

This 59-year-old who makes healthy choices falls at the same place on the aging curve as the average 47-year-old

This 59-year-old who makes unhealthy choices falls at the same place on the aging curve as the average 71-year-old

% Alive

Healthy[3]

Average[1]

Unhealthy[2]

Calendar Age   59

47   RealAge   71

80

Possible Aging Trajectories:
Consider the possible aging trajectories of a 59-year-old.
[1]This 59-year-old who makes "average" choices will be the physiological equivalent of the average 59-year-old.
[2]This 59-year-old who makes "unhealthy" choices will be the physiological equivalent of the average 71-year-old.
[3]This 59-year-old who makes "healthy" choices will be the physiological equivalent of the average 47-year-old.

In fact, for certain functions, such as mental acuity and IQ, some people show almost no decline and even improve as they progress from calendar age thirty-five to seventy-five. The question is how can *you* be one of those people who stay at the top of the curve, as young at seventy-five as you were at thirty-five? And that means not just living longer, but living better, suffering less illness and disability. Studies have repeatedly shown that making your RealAge younger means that you live longer *and* healthier.

To understand how the numbers work, consider a real-life example—the impact of smoking on life expectancy. Statistics show that the average life expectancy is seventy-seven years for men and eighty-three years for women. These numbers include everyone who dies prematurely from smoking. If you eliminate the data for smokers from the data for the general population, life expectancy goes up substantially. Thus, we can say that smokers have shorter lives and more medical problems than nonsmokers. We can also say that non-smokers have longer lives. In our equations, the RealAge team calculate a person's RealAge with respect to smoking by contrasting the ten-year survival rate, a calculation of life expectancy, of the smoker to that of the nonsmoker. By calculating the degree of risk and prorating it to the average ten-year survival rate for that person's chronologic age group, we found the number of years that smoking can subtract from one's life and that *not* smoking can add to one's life. We apply this process to a whole range of behaviors and conditions, using a complex routine of statistical techniques to blend them and arrive at a number that reflects your biologic age.

A fifty-two-year-old woman who smokes twenty-four cigarettes a day has an 88 percent probability of living for the next ten years. Likewise, the sixty-year-old woman who doesn't smoke also has an 88 percent probability of living ten years. Although eight calendar years separate these two individuals, their risk of dying within the next ten years is exactly the same: 12 percent. In other words, the smoker is the same physiologic "age" as the nonsmoker who is eight calendar years older. RealAge is a calculation of *your* relative risk of dying versus that of the population as a whole, based on the law of averages. If your relative risk matches that of the average person who is ten years younger, that is the same thing as saying that your RealAge is ten years younger. You are at the same risk of suffering severe aging or a major health problem as someone that much younger. Physiologically, you are equal.

This risk-analysis calculation is the clearest measure we have for determining the rate at which you are aging. We draw data from clinical studies calculating the risk of death for a variety of factors and integrate them into survival-table analyses (Kaplan-Meier curves). We have derived these curves to evaluate individual conditions, habits, and other factors that tend to affect physiologic age. Our computer-based equations use the most up-to-date and reliable medical information available, which is then modeled by statisticians using the best and most subtle statistical formulations for multivariate equations.

In our calculations, we start with the most general statistic: average life expectancy for American men and women. We then break each category into smaller and smaller categories. For example, we consider weight-to-height ratios.

We calculate the long-term effects of smoking. We evaluate the benefit that people get from taking aspirin regularly, exercising, or managing health problems effectively. Each breakdown allows us to refine our measurement and to consider how much of an impact each action has on the aging process. Finally, we consider all these categories together, calculating a multivariable equation in which we are able to weigh these multiple and diverse factors together and develop a unique RealAge calculation especially tailored to each person. We integrate the risk calculations for 125 factors and arrive at a number uniquely descriptive of *you*.

Sounds complicated? It is. But don't worry. To participate, all you have to do is answer a set of questions that allows us to calculate your RealAge. We do the rest.

THE STUDIES THAT PROVIDE THE DATA: WHERE DO THE NUMBERS COME FROM?

RealAge is an information system. Instead of providing new scientific data, it is a way of reinterpreting already published results. We use data from the most up-to-date studies done by the leaders in each field of medical research, so you are getting the best information the medical community has to offer. What we do is unify all that information: We are able to integrate specific recommendations from hundreds of studies into a general framework, so you can understand how the recommendations relate to you. Whereas most medical researchers have calculated their statistics in relation to "risk of disease," we have used their data and recalculated them to determine "risk of aging." RealAge translates currently available research into information you can use—something you can integrate into your own life.

I, in conjunction with the four other medical experts who form the RealAge scientific advisory team, have pored over more than 25,000 medical studies, evaluating what they tell us about aging, and, more important, what they tell us about the *prevention of aging.* Our calculations are based on data from more than 800 of the 25,000 studies and have been checked against a very large proprietary database. Our formulas are constantly being updated as new research becomes available. As statistics relating to these and other factors change, we recalculate our equations to accommodate the change. (Our on-line computerized RealAge program is updated whenever new and important research appears. For example, because Americans are becoming progressively heavier, we have modified our weight-to-height ratios to reflect these expanding waistlines.)

Although my colleagues and I rely on all kinds of scientific information for our calculations, let me describe our major sources of data. We predominately use clinical studies of two types: large-scale, risk-factor epidemiology studies and smaller-scale randomized trials. The large-scale studies look at many people, sometimes more than 100,000 individuals, and in one instance (the Mr. FIT study), as many as 350,000. The researchers who coordinate these studies track huge populations for a certain period, looking at one behavior or testable factor, such as blood pressure, and evaluate risks associated with that behavior or factor. These studies give statistics for a large population, more accurately reflecting variations within the study sample. The drawback is that these studies do not provide very detailed information and are not controlled studies. The researchers are not able to regulate with any kind of reliability who takes a specific drug or engages in a specific behavior. That is why scientists also do smaller controlled studies. In a randomized controlled study, a study population of a few hundred to 10,000 people is randomly divided, and each group is assigned a certain task. For example, half the group may be told to take the vitamin folic acid and half may be told to take placebos (harmless sugar pills). Each participant is then tracked for a long period, and his or her health conditions are recorded. At the end of the study, the researchers compare the groups and evaluate the effect of a particular behavior or condition on the overall health of the groups.

We select only factors that have been shown to make a quantifiable difference in the profile of risk (in other words, aging) in at least three peer-reviewed studies. We integrate and compare the various studies that have pertained to a certain issue; calculate what each study tells us about aging; and, finally, come up with a RealAge number that tells you in one easy-to-understand number — years—what the impact of each behavior is on *you*.

WHAT'S YOUR REALAGE?

There are two ways you can estimate your RealAge: by taking the RealAge survey on computer or by using the charts included in this chapter. The computer program is customized to you, whereas the charts provide accurate but more general approximations of your RealAge. In the RealAge questionnaire—both the one offered here and the on-line version—we ask you detailed questions about a variety of behaviors that are known to relate to aging. What do you eat? How often do you exercise? Do you floss your teeth? Do you own a dog? How many close relationships do you have? How long did your parents live? Indeed, we ask you questions about 125 factors that affect your health and your youth. Your answers to these questions are the raw data needed to calculate your RealAge.

Your RealAge by Computer

If you have access to a computer with an internet connection, you can take the RealAge quiz on-line. To get to the RealAge Web site, open your Web browser and go to the RealAge page. The Web page address is www.RealAge.com. Once you connect to the page, follow the instructions for answering the survey to calculate your RealAge.

There is no charge for this service (the company promises this service will be free for at least one year from the release date of this book). Your account stores RealAge information about you that can be accessed as many times as you like. All information you provide is completely confidential and accessible only to you through a password you choose. As you adopt new Age Reduction strategies (the plan in Chapter 3), you can chart your progress and literally watch the years disappear.

The computer survey is the easiest and most accurate way of calculating your RealAge. The computer test takes about thirty-five minutes to complete and provides a readout of your current RealAge as soon as you finish answering all the questions. You'll need to know your blood pressure, heart rate, weight, height, cholesterol values (both total cholesterol and high-density lipoprotein cholesterol), and the amounts of any vitamins or other supplements you take. (If you do not know these values, the average for your gender and age will be used until you provide your values.) The final calculation rarely takes more than two minutes to tabulate. After the calculation, the computer presents you with a list of Age Reduction suggestions tailored to your health and behavior profile. These suggestions are a list of possible choices you can make to make your RealAge younger, showing how much each one affects your age. Using your computer mouse, select the suggestions that you would consider incorporating into your life. The computer then recalculates your RealAge, showing you what your RealAge would be if you adopted these behaviors. That way, you can know how much of a difference each choice would make to you. The computer then helps you to set goals, showing you calculations for what your RealAge would be in three months, one year, and three years if you follow your plan.

Vary your choices to see which combinations will help you get younger sooner. You can then make informed choices about your health. You can choose which Age Reduction strategies you want to integrate into your life and in which order. You can develop a strategy for Age Reduction that suits you. The resulting Age Reduction plan is then stored in the computer, and you can access your account as often as you wish. Rather than just hoping that your new exercise routine will help you twenty years from now, you can see how much of a difference it is making right now.

Your RealAge by the Charts

The second way to calculate your RealAge is by filling out the charts included in this chapter. You simply respond to the questions asked, choose which answer best describes you, and fill in the corresponding Tally column. Because of the complexity of the mathematics involved in calculating RealAge, the charts provide a less accurate reading than the computer program. In fact, RealAge has become possible only because we now have the calculating power of super-computers that can rapidly make subtle statistical differentiations, accounting for the covariance between factors and drawing from a huge database of information. The charts you fill in by hand provide a relatively accurate reflection of your RealAge. They are modified to account for many interactions, and have been tested on more than one thousand individuals and on countless hypothetical cases, so that they represent the best possible approximation.

When filling out the charts, you will be asked to respond to a list of questions. Possible answers to each question lie to the right of the list. Choose the box that best describes you. For example, you will be asked if you currently smoke or have ever smoked. The answers range from "less than five cigarettes in life" to "more than twenty pack years" (a pack year is one pack per day for one year). Mark the one that describes you best. Then look at the number at the top of the column. It will read, depending on your answer, something like "years younger –3" or "years older +3." Write the number that corresponds to your answer in the right-hand Tally column, making sure to retain the positive or the negative sign. When you have completed the questionnaire, add all the numbers. Remember that a negative number should be subtracted; for example, $(+2) + (–3) = (–1)$. When you have added all your answers, you will get a total tally number. Multiply that number by the "multiplier," an age-conversion factor that is provided at the bottom of Chart 2.1, to get your net RealAge change. If that number is a positive number, then your RealAge is that much older than your calendar age. If you get a negative number, then your RealAge is that much younger than your calendar age. For example, if you are now fifty but get a final number of +4, then your RealAge is fifty-four. Likewise, if the final number is –4, then your RealAge is forty-six. The calculation is simple and easy, and taking the quiz and tabulating should not take more than forty-five minutes.

After you have finished computing your RealAge, look back over your answers. Any place that you have marked a "plus" number, you have marked a behavior that is causing you to age prematurely. Write those behaviors down. Then read about them in this book to learn how and why those behaviors are causing you to age. Next, you will want to develop your own Age Reduction plan, as described in the next chapter.

CHART 2.1

Your Current RealAge:
How Old Are You...Really?

Completing this chart produces a rough approximation of the more exact calculations provided by the RealAge computer program. These charts apply to people who are 25 to 100 years old who do not have acute or chronic illness.

Health Factor	Years Younger −3.0	Years Younger −2.5	Years Younger −2.0	Years Younger −1.5	Years Younger −1.0	Years Younger −0.5
Patrolling Your Own Health						
My health status, compared with that of others					Excellent	
Habits and Conditions						
Blood pressure (systolic/diastolic, mm Hg)	90/65 to 120/81		Less than 90/65; no heart disease		121/82 to 129/85	
Immunization status						
Cigarette smoking (in pack-years)	Smoked fewer than 5 cigarettes in life		Ex-smoker; no cigarettes for more than 5 yr		Ex-smoker; no cigarettes for 3-5 yr	
Exposure to secondhand smoke						
Cigar smoking						
Pipe smoking (p/s)						

Instructions: Begin by filling out the chart as best you can. (Explanations of the abbreviations, units, and footnotes can be found at the end of the chart). Go down each row, selecting the best answer and writing its corresponding "years-younger" or "years-older" number in the "Tally" box at the end of each row. (If you have no idea what the best answer would be, skip that item or estimate the answer.) Add up all the "Tally" numbers. Place that total in the appropriate box on the last page of this chart. Multiply that number by "Multiplier M," a number that can be found, for your particular age, in a nearby table. The result is your net RealAge change, in years. This can be a minus number or a positive number. Add your chronological age. The result is your RealAge, in years.

No Change	Years Older +0.5	Years Older +1.0	Years Older +1.5	Years Older +2.0	Years Older +2.5	Years Older +3.0	Tally
Very good or fair						Poor or bad	
130/86	Women, 131/67 to 140/90	Men, 131/87 to 140/90	Women, 141/91 to 150/95	Men, 141/91 to 150/95	Women, higher than 151/96	Men, higher than 151/96	
Current	Not current for diphtheria and tetanus, hepatitis B, measles, influenza, pneumo-coccal disease						
Ex-smoker; no cigarettes for 1–3 yr		Ex-smoker; no cigarettes for 5 mos to a year	Ex-smoker; no cigarettes for 2–5 mos	Smoker; 0–20 pack-years		Smoker; more than 20 pack-years	
None		0–1 hr a day		1–3 hr a day		More than 3 hr a day	
None	Ex-cigar smoker;no cigars for 3 yr	Cigar smoker; fewer than 4/wk	Cigar smoker; 4–8/wk	Cigar smoker; 9–18/wk	Cigar smoker; more than 18/wk		
None	Ex-pipe smoker; no pipe smoking for 3 yr	Pipe smoker; fewer than 4 times/wk	Pipe smoker; 4–8 times/wk	Pipe smoker; 9–18 times/wk	Pipe smoker; more than 18 times/wk		

Health Factor	Years Younger −3.0	Years Younger −2.5	Years Younger −2.0	Years Younger −1.5	Years Younger −1.0	Years Younger −0.5
Use of chewing or other nonsmoking tobacco						
Use of aspirin or other NSAIDs such as ibuprofen (Advil, Motrin, etc.)						Women over 50 and men over 40 who take 1 tablet or pill/day, if no contra-indication
Breakfast						More than 5 times a week
Number of days per week snacking occurs between meals						Rarely, or snack is fruit only
Average sleep time per day					Women, 6.5 to 7.4 hr	Men, 7.5 to 8.4 hr
Total physical activity performed for at least the last three years (give yourself most positive category)				More than 90 min of any exercise (ex: walking) per day, for more than 3 yr	More than 60 min of any exercise (ex: walking) per day, for more than 3 yr	More than 20 min of any exercise (ex: walking) per day, for more than 3 yr
Amount of stamina exercise (heart rate over 70% of maximal)[1]					More than 60 min/wk	40 to 60 min/wk
Amount of strength-building exercise (must exercise at least 4 of 8 major muscle groups)[2]					More than 30 min/wk	20 to 30 min/wk
Heart rate					Lower than 76 beats/min; does less than 30 min of stamina exercise/wk; does not have heart disease	
Vehicle driven most often						Large car

No Change	Years Older +0.5	Years Older +1.0	Years Older +1.5	Years Older +2.0	Years Older +2.5	Years Older +3.0	Tally
None	Has *not* used either for 3 yr	*Has* used either for 3 yr	*Has* used either for over 3 yr				
Takes no NSAIDs							
4 or 5 times a week	2 or 3 times a week	Less than 2 times a week					
Occasionally and not usually fruit	3 to 5 days a week, and snack is usually not fruit	Almost every day, and snack is usually not fruit					
Women, 7.5 to 8.4 hr	Men, 6.5 to 7.4 hr	Less than 6.4 hr	More than 8.4 hr				
More than 10 min of any exercise (ex: walking) per day, for more than 3 yr	More than 5 min of any exercise (ex: walking) per day, for more than 3 yr	More than 5 min of any exercise (ex: walking) per day, for less than 3 yr	None				
20 to 40 min/wk	10 to 20 min/wk	Less than 10 min/wk					
10 to 20 min/wk	5 to 10 min/wk	Less than 5 min/wk					
Lower than 76 beats/min; does more than 30 min of stamina exercise/wk; does not have heart disease	76 to 91 beats/min; does less than 30 min of stamina exercise/wk; does not have heart disease	76 to 83 beats/min; does more than 30 min of stamina exercise/wk	83 to 91 beats/min; does more than 30 min of stamina exercise/wk; OR higher than 91 beats/min; does less than 30 min of stamina exercise/wk	Higher than 91 beats/min; does more than 30 min of stamina exercise/wk			
Mid-sized car	Small car		Motorcycle				

Health Factor	Years Younger −3.0	Years Younger −2.5	Years Younger −2.0	Years Younger −1.5	Years Younger −1.0	Years Younger −0.5
Wearing of seat belts and presence of air bags, in last 10 trips in a car						Seat belts were worn 10 of 10 times, AND car had air bags 10 of 10 times
Riding on a motorcyle within the last month						
Use a a helmet when on a motorcycle or bicycle						
Miles driven per year						
Usual speed driven						
Use of cellular phone while driving						
Driving after drinking alcohol						
Alcohol consumption on average day (one drink is 4 oz wine, 12 oz beer, or 2 oz spirits)					Men over age 40, 1 to 2 drinks a day	Men over age 40 and women over age 50, 1/2 to 1 drink a day
Highest alcohol consumption in one day within the last year						
Educational level of spouse						Higher than 12th grade
Total cholesterol level					Under age 70, lower than 160 mg/dl, if no chronic disease	Age 70 or older, lower than 160 mg/dl

No Change	Years Older +0.5	Years Older +1.0	Years Older +1.5	Years Older +2.0	Years Older +2.5	Years Older +3.0	Tally
Seat belts were worn 7–9 of 10 times, and car had air bags at least 6 of 10 times	Seat belts were worn fewer than 7 of 10 times, and car had air bags fewer than 6 of 10 times						
No	Sometimes						
Always	More than 50% of the time	Sometimes (between 25% and 50% of the time)			Never, or less than 25% of time		
Less than 30,000	More than 30,000						
Less than 5 mph over speed limit	5 to 14 mph over speed limit		More than 14 mph over speed limit				
Fewer than two callls a day	More than four calls a day						
Never	Less than once a month			More than once a month	More than twice a month		
Men over age 40, none to 1/2 drink OR more than 2 but less than 3 drinks a day. Women over 50, none to 1/2 OR more than 1 but less than 3 drinks a day		Men under age 40, none to 1/2 drink OR more than 2 but less than 3 drinks a day. Women under age50, none to 1/2 OR more than 1 but less than 3 drinks a day	More than 3 drinks a day				
3 drinks or less	4 drinks or less	5 drinks or less	More than 5 drinks				
	12th grade or lower						
Under age 70, 161 to 200 mg/dl; OR age 70 or older, 161 to 240 mg/dl	Age 70 or older, 241 to 280 mg/dl	Under age 70, 201 to 240 mg/dl	Over age 70, higher than 280 mg/dl	Under age 70, 241 to 280 mg/dl		Under age 70, higher than 280 mg/dl	

Health Factor	Years Younger −3.0	Years Younger −2.5	Years Younger −2.0	Years Younger −1.5	Years Younger −1.0	Years Younger −0.5
HDL (healthy) cholesterol					Men, or women age 50 or over, higher than 55 mg/dl	Women under age 50, higher than 55 mg/dl
Fasting triglyceride levels (mg/dl)						Lower than 89.3
Kidney disease						
Pills and tablets of all sizes and kinds taken per day with or without a prescription. Do not include vitamins.						0 to 4
Adherence to instructions regarding taking of medications						
Dental disease			None			
Sun exposure						
Presence of firearms in home						
Presence of smoke detectors in home						
Diet						
Fat in diet						20% to 30%
Saturated fat in diet				Less than 6.7%		6.7% to 10%

No Change	Years Older +0.5	Years Older +1.0	Years Older +1.5	Years Older +2.0	Years Older +2.5	Years Older +3.0	Tally
45 to 54 mg/dl	Women under age 50, 40 to 44 mg/dl	Men, or women age 50 or older, 40 to 44 mg/dl	Women under age 50, 30 to 40 mg/dl	Men, or women age 50 or older, 30 to 40 mg/dl	Women under age 50, lower than 30 mg/dl	Men, or women over age 50, lower than 30 mg/dl	
89.3 to 208.8	Higher than 208.8						
None			Creatinine, 1.5 to 1.69 mg/dl	Creatinine, 1.70 to 1.99 mg/dl		Creatinine higher than 2 mg/dl	
5 to 7	More than 7						
Perfect or near perfect adherence to instructions	Not perfect or near perfect adherence to instructions			Poor adherence; often stops or starts medications without talking to doctor			
	Gingivitis only			Periodontitis			
Less than 20 min/day; no blisters before age 20	More than 20 min/day and/or blisters before age 20						
RealAge effect is less than 0.5 yr for women with no history of family violence				If female and also in abusive relationship			
RealAge effect is less than 0.5 yr if no one smokes in the home			If device is not installed for each floor and tested, and smoking occurs in the home				
31% to 40% OR less than 20%			More than 40%				
10.1% to 13.3%			More than 13.3%				

Health Factor	Years Younger −3.0	Years Younger −2.5	Years Younger −2.0	Years Younger −1.5	Years Younger −1.0	Years Younger −0.5
Trans fat in diet						Less than 1.5%
Polyunsaturated fat in diet					More than 5.85%	
Fruits (servings/day)					4 or more	
Vegetables (servings/day)					5 or more	
Flavonoids (mg/day)[3]					High amount: more than 30 mg/day	Moderate amount: 19–29.9 mg/day
Diversity of diet: How many different food groups does your daily diet usually contain? Food groups = milk or milk products; protein (meat, fish, poultry, or plant protein); fruits; grains; and vegetables						
Fiber in diet (grams/day)				Over 21.1	15.2 to 21.1	
Nutrients in Diet or Taken as Supplement						
Vitamin C (amount in food and supplements)					Men over age 40 and women over age 50, more than 1,000 mg/day	Men over age 40 and women over age 50, 160 to 1,000 mg/day. Men age 40 and under, and women age 50 and under, more than 1,000 mg/day
Vitamin D (amount in food and supplements)						400 to 2,000 IU or 10 min of sun a day
Vitamin E (amount in food and supplements)					Women over age 50 and men over age 40, more than 400 IU/day as a supplement	Women under age 50 and men under age 40, more than 400 IU/day as a supplement

No Change	Years Older +0.5	Years Older +1.0	Years Older +1.5	Years Older +2.0	Years Older +2.5	Years Older +3.0	Tally
1.5% to 2.64%	More than 2.64%						
4.26% to 5.85%		Less than 4.25%					
		None					
		None					
		Low amount: less than 19 mg/day					
More than two varieties, on average, a day		Two or fewer varieties, on average, a day					
9.2 to 15.1		3.2 to 9.1	Less than 3.2				
Men age 40 and under, and women age 50 and under, 160 to 1,000 mg/day	Less than 160 mg/day						
	Less than 400 IU and less than 5 min of sun a day						
	No supplement taken every day						

Health Factor	Years Younger −3.0	Years Younger −2.5	Years Younger −2.0	Years Younger −1.5	Years Younger −1.0	Years Younger −0.5
Folate, or folic acid, a B vitamin (amount in food and supplements)						More than 700 mcg/day
Vitamin B$_6$ (amount in food and supplements)						More than 6 mg/day
Fish, excluding shellfish (portions/wk)[4]					More than 2 portions/wk	
Percentage of food prepared without fat or sauces containing a lot of fat, or food that is not fried						
Iron (amount in supplements)						
Vitamin A (amount in food and supplements)						
Calcium (amount in food and supplements)						More than 1,200 mg/day
Vitamin B$_{12}$ (amount in food and supplements)						
Multivitamins						
Selenium (amount in food and supplements)						

No Change	Years Older +0.5	Years Older +1.0	Years Older +1.5	Years Older +2.0	Years Older +2.5	Years Older +3.0	Tally
224 to 700 mcg/day	Less than 224 mcg/day						
1.5 to 6 mg/day	Less than 1 mg/day						
Some fish eaten, but less than 2 portions/wk			None				
No known RealAge effects other than those for saturated fat or fat in diet							
	Any amount of iron as a supplement if you are not iron-deficient						
	More than 15,000 IU/day	More than 25,000 IU/day					
800 to 1,200 mg/day	500 to 800 mg/day	Less than 500 mg/day					
	If you do not eat meat or get less than 18 mcg/wk as a supplement, OR 175 mcg/wk if you have gastritis or are over age 64						
1 or more a week if you do not eat a diverse diet							
No known RealAge effect as yet proven (data expected within 3 yr)							

Health Factor	Years Younger −3.0	Years Younger −2.5	Years Younger −2.0	Years Younger −1.5	Years Younger −1.0	Years Younger −0.5
Eating of meat					Never, or less than once a week	
Potassium in diet						
Servings of tomato paste (ex: tomato paste, pizza, marinara sauce) eaten per week					Men, more than 10 servings/wk	Men, 7–10 servings/wk
Green tea consumption						
Weight						
Body mass index (see Table 8.4)[5]						In the absence of acute or chronic disease, 19 kg/m² or lower
Changes in weight (women)						
Weight gain (since age 18)						
Diabetes						
Diabetes and control of blood sugar						
Cardiac Disease						
Coronary artery disease (CAD), but no heart attack yet (as diagnosed by symptoms or scan tests)						

No Change	Years Older +0.5	Years Older +1.0	Years Older +1.5	Years Older +2.0	Years Older +2.5	Years Older +3.0	Tally
Once a week	More than once a week						
More than 76 mmol/day	60 to 76 mmol/day	Less than 59 mmol/day					
Women, no known RealAge effect; men, retards aging from prostate cancer and may retard arterial aging	Men, fewer than 2 servings/wk						
Women, no known RealAge effect; men, may retard aging from prostate cancer							
19.1 to 26.9 kg/m²				27 to 31.9 kg/m²		32 kg/m² or higher	
Weight changes of no more than 5% in any 5 years		Weight changes of no more than 10% in any 5 years		Weight changes of more than 10% in any 5 years			
Gain of less than 20 lb		Gain of 20 to 40 lb			Gain of more than 40 lb		
None	Type II (adult onset), tight control	Type II (adult onset), average control	Type II (adult onset), poor control	Type I (juvenile onset), tight control		Type I (juvenile onset), average or poor control	
			Has CAD involving 1 vessel, and on active rehab program	Has CAD involving 1 vessel, and not on active rehab program	Has CAD involving 2 or 3 vessels, and on active rehab program	Has CAD involving 2 or 3 vessels, and not on active rehab program	

Health Factor	Years Younger −3.0	Years Younger −2.5	Years Younger −2.0	Years Younger −1.5	Years Younger −1.0	Years Younger −0.5
Coronary artery bypass graft surgery (CABG)						
Angioplasty (PTCA, balloon dilation of cardiac vessels)						
Heart attacks						
Need for pacemaker						
Beta-blocker with surgery if over age 60						Makes your RealAge 1 yr younger if you need surgery and receive a beta-blocker for 2 wk surrounding surgery	
Pulmonary or Lung Disease						
Forced expiratory volume as a % of normal value						Higher than 90% of predicted
Asthma within 3 yr (answer this and topic above if you had asthma)						None, or rarely and FEV$_1$ 100% of predicted or higher
Stroke						
Mental Disorders						
Depression						
Panic Disorders						

No Change	Years Older +0.5	Years Older +1.0	Years Older +1.5	Years Older +2.0	Years Older +2.5	Years Older +3.0	Tally
			Has had CABG involving 1 vessel			Has had CABG involving 2 or more vessels	
			PTCA involving 1 vessel	PTCA involving 2 (or unknown no. of) vessels		PTCA involving 3 or more vessels	
					Had heart attack involving inferior or posterior part of heart	Had heart attack involving anterior part of heart	
None					Yes, required		
No RealAge effect if you do not need surgery OR have calendar age of less than 60							
Unknown	75% to 90% of predicted		65% to 75% of predicted		Lower than 65% of predicted		
	FEV_1 80% to 99% of predicted		FEV_1 70% to 90% of predicted		FEV_1 lower than 70%		
None			Ischemic stroke (inadequate blood flow to brain)			Hemor-rhagic stroke (bleeding into brain)	
	Yes, slight			Yes, serious		Yes, severe	
None	Present but controlled			Uncontrolled			

Health Factor	Years Younger −3.0	Years Younger −2.5	Years Younger −2.0	Years Younger −1.5	Years Younger −1.0	Years Younger −0.5
Suicide Attempts						
Musculoskeletal Disorders						
Low back pain						
Osteoarthritis						
Osteoporosis						Absent
Air Pollution: Respond to One of the Next Two Lines						
Level of sulfate in the atmosphere (mg/m³) at usual residence						Less than 5 mg/m³
or						
Level (in mg/m³) of fine particulates (smaller than 2.5 μm in diameter) in atmosphere at usual residence						Less than 10 mg/m³
Heredity and Other Factors						
Use of hormone replacement therapy (HRT) for post-menopausal women with no history of breast cancer and no 1st-degree relative who had breast cancer befor age 50	Had HRT for 7–12 yr in the first 7–12 yr of menopause	Had HRT for 5–7 yr in the first 5–7 yr of menopause	Had HRT for 13–20 yr in the first 13–20 yr of menopause	Had HRT for 1–4 yr in the first 1–4 yr of menopause and is now more than 20 yr into menopause	Had HRT for 50% of years since menopause	Had HRT for 25% of years since menopause
Age of parents at time of death				Both lived past age 75	Only mother lived past age 75	Only father lived past age 75
Age of grandparents at time of death					All four lived past age 75	Three lived past age 75
Divorce of parents						Not divorced prior to your 21st birthday

No Change	Years Older +0.5	Years Older +1.0	Years Older +1.5	Years Older +2.0	Years Older +2.5	Years Older +3.0	Tally
None				Yes, but not within last 5 yr		Yes, and within last 5 yr	
No RealAge effect proven by itself							
No RealAge effect proven by itself							
	Present						
5 to 14.9 mg/m³	15 mg/m³ or more						
10 to 24.4 mg/m³	more than 24.4 mg/m³						
Had HRT for less than 25% of years since menopause	Had HRT for no more than 12 yr after menopause and more than 20 yr into menopause	Never had HRT and is now 3–4 yr after menopause	Never had HRT and is now 5–12 yr after menopause				
						Neither lived past age 75	
One or two lived past age 75			None lived past age 75				
		Separated but not divorced prior to your 21st birthday				Divorced prior to your 21st birthday	

Health Factor	Years Younger −3.0	Years Younger −2.5	Years Younger −2.0	Years Younger −1.5	Years Younger −1.0	Years Younger −0.5
Parents/Immediate Family (Brothers, Sisters, Parents, Grandparents, Children)						
Colon cancer (c/c)						
History of heart disease before age 50						
Stress, Social Connections, Relaxation Therapy						
Major disruptive life events in the last 12 months[6]						
Social groups, friends, relatives seen more than once a month[7]				6	3, 4, or 5	2
Relaxation or other stress-relieving therapy						
Sense of humor						Yes
Positive outlook on life						
Marriage status				Happily married man		Happily married woman
Highest educational level completed						Higher than grade 16 (college graduate)
Yearly salary					Higher than $150,000	$60,001 to 150,000

No Change	Years Older +0.5	Years Older +1.0	Years Older +1.5	Years Older +2.0	Years Older +2.5	Years Older +3.0	Tally
No known RealAge effect if one 1st-degree relative had c/c prior to age 40, if an aspirin/day is taken, or if colonoscopy is performed regularly			Not getting yearly colonoscopy, and two or more 1st-degree rels had c/c prior to age 40				
No RealAge effect if one or fewer 1st-degree relatives had heart disease prior to age 50						(Not proven but expected): two or more 1st-degree relatives had heart disease before age 50	
None		1		2		3	
1				None			
No determined RealAge effect yet							
	No						
No documented RealAge effect							
Single woman or widowed man		Divorced man or widowed woman		Divorced woman		Single man	
Grades 12 through 15	Grades 5 through 11	Grade 4 or lower					
$30,001 to 60,000	$15,000 to $30,000	Less then $15,000					

Health Factor	Years Younger −3.0	Years Younger −2.5	Years Younger −2.0	Years Younger −1.5	Years Younger −1.0	Years Younger −0.5
Sexual Practices and Other Practices						
Mutually monogamous relationship of more than 10 yr, and partner is of opposite sex						
Orgasms (per year)	Men, 300 or more		Men, 200 to 300	Women, satisfied with quantity and happy with quality	Men, 100 to 200	Women, satisfied with quantity or quality
Regular use of condoms (for those not in a mutually monogamous relationship)						
Gender of sex partner						Sex partner is opposite gender
Sex partner uses intravenous drugs, trades sex for drugs or money, is an ex-prisoner, or has a sexually transmitted disease						
Use of marijuana						
Use of cocaine, LSD, heroin, or intravenous drugs of any type						
People in household (do not count pets)						4 to 6
Pet ownership						Dog
Total						

Abbreviations: FEV$_1$, forced expiratory volume in one second; LSD, lysergic acid diethylamide; NSAIDs, nonsteroidal anti-inflammatory drugs; and PTCA, percutaneous transluminal coronary angioplasty.

Units: IU, international units; kg/m², kilograms per meter squared; mcg/day, micrograms per day; mg/day, milligrams per day; mg/dl, milligrams per deciliter; mg/m³, milligrams per cubic meter; mm Hg, millimeters of mercury; mmol/day, millimoles per day; "pack-year," one pack of cigarettes a day for one year; and μm, micromoles.

No Change	Years Older +0.5	Years Older +1.0	Years Older +1.5	Years Older +2.0	Years Older +2.5	Years Older +3.0	Tally
Yes				No			
	Women, unsatisfied with quality and/or quantity	Men, 25 to 40		Men, 5 to 25	Men, fewer than 5		
Yes		No					
	If female and sex partner is also female					If male and sex partner is also male	
No				Unknown		Yes	
Use one time a week or less	Use more than once a week but less than daily	Use every day	Sometimes use more than three times a day				
Never			Have used, but not in last 10 yr		Have used within last 10 yr	Yes, current use	
3	2 or 7	8	1 (you) or 9 or more				
None							

Footnotes:
[1] Stamina exercise is aerobic exercise that increases heart rate to at least 70% of the maximal heart rate (calculated in beats per minute by subtracting chronological age from 220).
[2] Examples of strength-building exercises would be lifting weights, resistance exercise, and treadmill on an incline. Major muscle groups = back, biceps, abdominals, chest and triceps, hamstring, quadriceps, gastrocnemius, and foot and ankle.
[3] Flavonoids are found in onions, tea, celery, and cranberries.
[4] A portion of fish is about the size of a pack of cards and weighs aproximately 3 oz.
[5] Body mass index (in kilograms per meter squared) is the ratio of weight to height.
[6] Major life events include death of a family member, job change, relocation, divorce, lawsuit, and financial insolvency.
[7] This line pertains to those who offer support through major life events and applies only when two or more major life events have occurred in one year.

Total "Tally" Nos.
from Chart   Multiplier M   Net RealAge Change:

┌─────────────┐   ┌─────────────┐   ┌─────────────┐
│   │   X   │   │   =   │   │
│   │   │   │   │   │
└─────────────┘   └─────────────┘   └─────────────┘

                                                        +

           Multiplier M   Chronological Age:

Age	Multiplier
< 40	0.3
40 to 49	0.4
50 to 59	0.5
60 to 69	0.6
70 to 79	0.5
80 to 89	0.4
90 to 100	0.3

┌─────────────┐
│   │
│   │
└─────────────┘

        =

   Your RealAge:

┌─────────────┐
│   │
│   │
└─────────────┘

INTERPRETING THE RESULTS:
WHAT YOUR REALAGE MEANS TO YOU

Once you have calculated your RealAge, how should you interpret the results? They are as easy to understand as reading your bathroom scale. If your RealAge reads "forty-six," then you are as old physically as an average forty-six-year-old. If your RealAge is younger than your chronologic age, Congratulations! That means that you are taking steps to protect your youth and are aging more slowly than most of your peers. See what you can do to make your RealAge even younger.

If your RealAge is older, the news is not so good. You are aging faster than most of your peers. Do not be disheartened. Instead, be proactive. Now that you know what your RealAge is, what will you do to get younger? Consider what choices you can make to reduce your risk. You have the opportunity to slow your rate of aging, bring yourself back in line with your peers, and maybe even get younger.

What are those choices? They vary from simply taking a vitamin pill to initiating a full-blown exercise and weight-loss program. Although a few of these measures may be difficult—quitting smoking, for example—the vast majority are simple and much less painful than you ever imagined. Quick and easy strategies help you get younger fast (see Chart 3.1 in Chapter 3).

3

Developing an Age Reduction Plan

ARE YOU AS YOUNG AS YOU COULD BE?

Now that you have calculated your RealAge, it's time to develop your own Age Reduction Plan. Look back over the RealAge Age Reduction suggestions that the computer gave you. Or reread the charts you filled out to see what you can do to become younger. Evaluate your options. What changes are you willing to make? Which ones aren't you willing to make? (Or, at least, which ones aren't you willing to make right now?) Some choices may already be part of your life. Perhaps you already get a regular night's sleep every night, or maybe you have never had any problems with weight gain. That's great. These factors are helping to keep you young. But what else could you be doing?

You've taken the test. You've come up with a number that represents your true physiologic age. Now, it's time for the best part of RealAge. It's time to start getting younger. Look over the list of Age Reduction strategies (see Chart 3.1) and determine which ones could help you to get younger. Begin with the Quick Fixes. They're so easy there's no reason not to adopt them, and they can save you anywhere from five to eight years of aging with almost no effort. Taking the right vitamins in proper doses, taking an aspirin a day, and making sure your vaccinations are current are quick and easy ways to make your RealAge younger. Then work your way down the list, adding Age Reduction behaviors as you see fit. Always check with your physician before you initiate or stop any Age Reduction strategy.

CHART 3.1

44 Things You Can Do to Make Your RealAge Younger!

QUICK FIXES

These RealAge age busters are simple, easy things that anyone can do. You can become 5 to 8 years younger with hardly any effort at all.

1) Take an aspirin a day.

❏ I do it
❏ I will
   do it

- Take one 325-mg tablet of aspirin a day if you are a man over 40 or a woman over 50. Check with your doctor beforehand to make sure you are aspirin tolerant.

  RealAge benefit: 0.9 years younger in 90 days
                     1.9 years younger in 3 years

2) Take vitamins C and E daily for their antioxidant and antiaging power.

❏ I do it
❏ I will
   do it

- Consume food containing vitamin C three times a day. Get more than 1,200 mg a day of vitamin C in diet or supplements, spread out so that you get at least 400 mg in any 12-hour period.

- Consume 400 IU of vitamin E a day.

  RealAge benefit: Up to 6 years younger

3) Take folate daily to reduce artery-aging levels of homocysteine.

❏ I do it
❏ I will
   do it

- Consume 700 mcg of folate (folic acid) a day in diet or supplement. The usual supplement requirement is 400 mcg.

  RealAge benefit: 1.2 years younger

4) Take calcium and vitamin D daily to keep your bones young.

- Consume 1,200 mg of calcium daily in food or supplements if you are a woman or 1,000 mg daily if you are a man.

- Consume 400 IU of vitamin D in food or supplements, or get 10 minutes of sun a day.

  RealAge benefit: 1.1 years younger

5) Take vitamin B_6 daily.

❏ I do it
❏ I will
   do it

- Consume 6 mg of vitamin B_6 a day in food or supplements.

  RealAge benefit: 0.4 years younger

6) Don't take needless vitamins and supplements.

❏ I do it

❏ I will
do it

- Take a multivitamin (without iron) that contains all the other vitamins and minerals (especially C, D, E, folate, and calcium) in the correct daily amount. Do not take vitamin A as a supplement and use a multivitamin that contains less than 8,000 IU of vitamin A. Do not take iron as a supplement except under the supervision of a doctor.

  RealAge loss: 1.7 years older for taking needless vitamins or supplements

7) Floss and brush daily.

❏ I do it

❏ I will
do it

- Gingivitis and periodontal disease cause aging of the immune and arterial systems. We do not know why gum disease causes aging, but we do know that it does. For example, a 55-year-old man free of periodontal disease has a RealAge that is 2 years younger than his peer who has gingivitis and 4.2 years younger than his peer who has full-blown periodontal disease.

  RealAge benefit: As much as 6.4 years younger

8) Take proper safety precautions when driving.

❏ I do it

❏ I will
do it

- Buckle your seat belt every time you ride in a car and drive within 5 mph of the speed limit. Never use a cell phone while driving. When buying a car, buy one that is midsize or larger and make sure it has air bags. Dismantle the air bags only if you are under 5 feet, 2 inches tall or sit extremely close to the steering wheel.

  RealAge benefit: 0.6 to 3.4 years younger, depending on your present age

9) Wear a helmet when riding a bike.

❏ I do it

❏ I will
do it

- Wear a helmet every time you ride a bike, and you will protect yourself from needless head injuries. You lower your risk of head injury and related aging by as much as 80 percent.

  RealAge benefit: 1 year younger

10) Keep immunizations current.

❏ I do it

❏ I will
do it

- It probably won't save you years of aging, but it's simple to do: Keep your immunizations current. By making sure you have an annual flu shot and tetanus, measles, mumps, rubella, hepatitis B, and pneumonia vaccinations, you can help prevent illnesses that can cause you to age.

  RealAge benefit: 6 days younger

11) Take the RealAge program and develop an Age
Reduction Plan.

❏ I do it
❏ I will
do it

• Age Reduction planning is the quickest and easiest, yet most important step for keeping you young. It can make the RealAge of a 70 year old as much as 26 years younger. Achieving the first 5 to 8 years of Age Reduction is relatively easy. More than that amount requires some work. However, isn't having a RealAge of 44 to 48 when your calendar age is 70 worth some work?

RealAge benefit: As much as 26 years younger

MODERATELY EASY CHANGES

These choices will make you younger fast, and they require only a little bit more effort than the quick fixes. Some, such as hormone replacement therapy for women, are as easy as the quick fixes but require more thought before you decide to choose them. These changes can help you become 10 to 12 years younger.

12) For women: Begin hormone replacement therapy (HRT) during menopause.

❏ I do it
❏ I will
do it

• The most powerful antiaging agent for postmenopausal women is estrogen-based HRT. Determine, with your doctor, whether you are a candidate for HRT. A woman who uses an HRT regimen that is appropriate and comfortable for her can make her RealAge 8 years younger by age 70. Unfortunately, there is no scientifically proven HRT that predictably makes a man's RealAge younger.

RealAge benefit: 8 years younger at age 70

13) Get enough sun, but not too much.

❏ I do it
❏ I will
do it

• Some sun (10 to 20 minutes every day) makes your RealAge 0.9 years younger by producing active vitamin D. Wearing sunscreen when you are in the sun longer than 20 minutes, avoiding tanning salons, and taking precautions to avoid excessive sun exposure help prevent aging.

RealAge benefit: 1.7 years younger

14) For men: Eat tomato paste and drink green tea.

❏ I do it
❏ I will
do it

• Eating 10 servings of tomato paste and tomato products a week helps prevent prostate cancer. The carotenoid found in tomatoes, lycopene, when eaten in conjunction with a bit of oil, provides an immune-strengthening antioxidant that has been shown to reduce prostate cancer. Drinking green tea may also help prevent prostate cancer.

RealAge benefit: 0.8 years younger

15) Avoid exposure to passive smoke.

❏ I do it

❏ I will
do it

• Don't tolerate working or living in a smoke-filled environment. Passive smokers experience almost as much aging as real smokers.

RealAge loss: 6.9 years older for those exposed to 4 hours a day or more of passive smoking

16) Have sex.

❏ I do it

❏ I will
do it

• The more orgasms you have a year, the younger you are. The average American has sex 58 times a year. Increasing the number to 116 through mutually monogamous and safe sex is associated with a RealAge as much as 1.6 years younger (and more sex is possibly associated with a RealAge as much as 8 years younger, depending on frequency and the individual).

RealAge benefit: 1.6 years younger

17) Have safe sex.

❏ I do it

❏ I will
do it

• The major risks for consenting adults who have sex outside mutually monogamous relationships are both psychological and physical. One in five sexually active Americans has some kind of sexually transmitted disease, which can increase the rate of aging. Avoid casual sex with high-risk partners and always use condoms correctly.

RealAge loss: 5 to 8 years older for unprotected sex

18) Drink alcohol in moderation.

❏ I do it

❏ I will
do it

• Women who have one-half to one alcoholic drink a day and men who have one or two drinks a day have a younger RealAge. People who are at risk or have a family history of alcohol abuse or addiction should not follow this step.

RealAge benefit: 1.9 years younger

19) Take all necessary (and only necessary) medicines, and take them correctly.

❏ I do it

❏ I will
do it

• Adhering to the medication regimens prescribed by your doctor makes your RealAge 0.9 years younger. Avoiding drug interactions makes your RealAge 0.7 years younger. Discuss your medication with your doctor and pharmacist and always disclose all prescriptions, over-the-counter drugs, vitamins, or supplements that you take both regularly and occasionally.

RealAge loss: 1 year older for taking medicines incorrectly

20) Eat breakfast daily.

❑ I do it
❑ I will
 do it

• No one is sure why, but eating breakfast makes you younger (see Chapter 10).

RealAge benefit: 1.1 years younger

21) Laugh a lot.

❑ I do it
❑ I will
 do it

• Laughter is a whole-body stress reducer. It helps open lines of communication with others; reduces anxiety, tension, and stress; and makes your immune system younger.

RealAge benefit: 1.7 to 8 years younger

MODERATE CHANGES

These Age Reduction strategies require a little more work and commitment, but once you put your mind to it, you'll watch those needless years fade away.

22) Eat a balanced diet that is low in calories and high in nutrients.

❑ I do it
❑ I will
 do it

• Eating a diverse diet that includes four servings of fruit, five servings of vegetables, and six servings of breads and grains a day will help keep you feeling young. Eat fish twice a week and do not eat red meat more than once a week.

RealAge benefit: 4 years younger

23) Eat a diet low in fat.

❑ I do it
❑ I will
 do it

• Aim to eat less than 60 grams of fat a day and less than 20 grams of saturated or trans fat daily (see Chapter 8). When you do eat fat, eat monounsaturated fats, such as those found in olive oil and avocados.

RealAge benefit: 6 years younger

24) Get a good night's sleep regularly.

❑ I do it
❑ I will
 do it

• Sleeping regular hours can help you stay young. That means 7 hours a night for women and 8 hours a night for men.

RealAge benefit: 3 years younger

25) Own a dog, and walk it!

❑ I do it
❑ I will
 do it

• Dog owners stay young longer—presumably because they get exercise caring for their dogs.

RealAge benefit: 1 year younger

26) Become a lifelong learner.

❏ I do it

❏ I will
do it

• People with higher levels of education and those who continue to be involved in activities that stimulate their minds undergo less mental aging. The college graduate who continues his or her education has a RealAge that is 2.5 years younger than that of the high school dropout.

RealAge benefit: 2.5 years younger

27) Identify your genetic risks and use Age Reduction strategies to reduce them.

❏ I do it

❏ I will
do it

• If, for example, cardiovascular disease runs in your family, take extra precautions to prevent arterial aging. Your RealAge will be 4 years younger if both your parents (or grandparents, if your parents aren't that old yet) lived past the age of 75. f no first-degree relative (parent, brother, or sister) had breast, colon, or ovarian cancer diagnosed early, you are an additional 0.2 to 11 years younger than if a first-degree relative had those diagnoses.

RealAge benefit: 4 years younger if both parents lived past 75

MODERATELY DIFFICULT CHANGES

These Age Reduction steps require commitment and work, but the payoff is often huge in "years younger."

28) Lower your cholesterol.

❏ I do it

❏ I will
do it

• Try to keep your total cholesterol level below 240 mg/dl and aim to have your HDL ("healthy") cholesterol level at 40 or above.

RealAge benefit: 3.7 years younger

29) Exercise regularly, expending at least 3,500 kilocalories of energy a week.

❏ I do it

❏ I will
do it

• Walking the equivalent of an hour a day or doing more vigorous exercise for a shorter time can bring your level of physical activity up to the optimum Age Reduction range. Walking just half an hour a day gives you half the "years younger" that exercise can provide.

RealAge benefit: 3 to 8 years younger

30) Build stamina.

❏ I do it
❏ I will
do it

- Do stamina-building exercises that boost your heart rate and aerobic intake for at least 20 minutes three times a week. You should exercise vigorously enough to raise your heart rate to 70 percent of the maximum for your age group or to break into a sweat.

RealAge benefit: 6.4 years younger

31) Make yourself strong.

❏ I do it
❏ I will
do it

- Do strength-building exercises, such as weight lifting, three times a week for at least 10 minutes. These exercises are particularly important for women because they help maintain bone density.

RealAge benefit: 1.7 years younger

32) Avoid air pollution and environmental toxins.

❏ I do it
❏ I will
do it

- Living in an area with high air quality reduces the aging that exposure to hydrocarbons, ozone, and particulate matter can cause. Avoid jobs that expose you to pollutants or toxins.

RealAge loss: 2.8 years older

33) Patrol your own health.

❏ I do it
❏ I will
do it

- Seek high-quality medical care and be alert to any early warning signs of developing conditions. Do what you can to ensure that you are feeling healthy and do not ignore any indications that something is wrong.

RealAge benefit: As much as 12 years younger

34) Manage chronic diseases.

❏ I do it
❏ I will
do it

- Learning how to manage diseases, such as diabetes, cardiovascular disease, arthritis, and many others, can dramatically decrease the impact they can have on aging.

RealAge benefit: Depending on the disease, the effect on aging can, with proper disease management, be diminished considerably, sometimes to almost indiscernible rates.

35) Build social networks.

❏ I do it
❏ I will
do it

- Having a network of close friends and/or family members can help prevent aging from excessive stress.

RealAge benefit: 2 to 30 years younger

36) Manage your finances and live within your means.

❑ I do it
❑ I will
   do it

• Feeling out of control financially (particularly undergoing a bankruptcy) can cause unnecessary aging.

RealAge loss: 8 years older

THE MOST DIFFICULT CHANGES

These are the things that age you the most and are the hardest to fix. However, working to overcome these obstacles is one of the most important things you can do to keep your RealAge young.

37) Keep blood pressure low.

❑ I do it
❑ I will
   do it

• Keeping your blood pressure at 115/76 mm Hg or less makes you 9 years younger than if your blood pressure were 130/86. It also makes you over 25 years younger than someone with blood pressure of 160/90 or more. Reducing your blood pressure from 130/86 to 115/76 makes you 4.5 years younger in 6 months and 9 years younger in 3 years, provided you do so before any permanent structural damage occurs in the arteries. Blood pressure of 120–130/80–85 is considered normal but not ideal.

RealAge benefit: 10 to 15 years younger for blood pressure of 115/76

RealAge loss: 10 to 15 years older for blood pressure of 140/90

38) Stop smoking.

❑ I do it
❑ I will
   do it

• Smoking one pack of cigarettes a day makes you over 8 years older than a nonsmoker. Cessation of smoking makes you 1 year younger in 2 months and 7 years younger in 5 years.

RealAge loss: 8 years older for smokers

RealAge benefit: If you quit, you regain 7 of the 8 years you lost from smoking.

39) Maintain a constant desirable weight.

❑ I do it
❑ I will
   do it

• Reduce your weight gradually to what it was when you were age 18 (women) or 21 (men). Lose weight slowly and consistently, avoiding yo-yo dieting, because rapid gains and losses also cause aging. Your goal should be to reduce your total body mass index to less than 23 (see Chapter 8).

RealAge benefit: 6 years younger

40) Reduce stress.

❏ I do it   • Having three or more major life events in a one-year period
❏ I will   can create more than 30 years of aging. Having lots of friends,
   do it   strong support networks, and strategies for coping with stress
                     can minimize the effect.

                   RealAge loss: 30 to 32 years older during high-stress times for
                              people without strategies for stress reduction. As
                              little as 2 years older for people with effective
                              strategies for stress reduction.

41) Cut back on excessive consumption of alcohol.

❏ I do it   • Alcohol addiction and abuse can cause severe aging, bringing
❏ I will   about liver failure and triggering cancers. Drinking more than
   do it   two drinks a day causes you to age needlessly.

                   RealAge loss: 3 years older

42) Overcome a drug addiction.

❏ I do it   *RealAge loss:* 8 years older for drug use
❏ I will
   do it

43) Recover from a severe emotional trauma.

❏ I do it   *RealAge benefit:* 8 to 16 years younger
❏ I will
   do it

44) Not so difficult, but very important: Stick to your RealAge plan!

❏ I do it   *RealAge benefit:* Up to 26 years younger
❏ I will
   do it

YOUR PERSONAL AGE REDUCTION PLAN

Once you have identified strategies that could help you reduce your RealAge, you will want to read through the rest of this book to learn why and how the different choices will make you younger. You may reconsider your decision not to adopt an Age Reduction strategy once you see the kind of impact it can have. For example, from my clinical practice, I know that many women are hesitant to begin estrogen-replacement therapy following menopause. Once they learn the facts, many of them change their minds. The following chapters will give you the information you need to make informed decisions about the way in which you will age. They will allow you to weigh the merits and benefits of everything from owning a dog to lifting weights. This personalized plan, based on your RealAge goals, is what the book is referring to when it cites the Age Reduction Plan. Use Chart 3.2 to develop a step-by-step Age Reduction Plan. Don't try to do everything at once.

Begin by adopting just two or three strategies. Trying to do too much at once can be overwhelming. A common problem with all health initiatives— whether diets or exercise regimens—is that we take on too much at once. Then, after a few days of playing superhero, we give up on everything, never to return to the initial plan. The patients of mine who have been the most successful at age reduction have begun by choosing only two or three strategies. They followed those strategies for three months, and after they successfully incorporated them into their daily routines, they added two or three more, and so on. They frequently go back and recalculate their RealAge and modify and update their Age Reduction Plans. One patient calls me every Monday morning. "Mike," she says, "I've done such and such. What's my RealAge now?"

By adopting the steps from the Quick Fix category first, you can begin reducing your RealAge in just a few days or months with little effort. Reducing your RealAge further requires more resolve. Most of the choices are not that difficult; you just need practice. What better payoff than adding high-quality years to your life?

Losing weight, adopting a three-tiered physical activity program, quitting smoking, managing stress, managing a chronic disease, and controlling blood pressure are the decisions that require the most commitment. But the payoff is huge. The RealAge difference between two people who have the same chronologic age but different blood pressure readings (above 140/90 versus 115/76 or below) can be as much as twenty-five years (see Chapter 4). Likewise, a person who has developed strategies for stress management— including a strong support network of friends and family—can have, in times of crisis, a RealAge as much as thirty years younger than a person of the same age facing a similar crisis who does not have a support network (see Chapter 11). Remember to prioritize your plan. Which steps are easy? Which steps are difficult but important? Which are less important? Deciding that you will floss your teeth every night requires only that you buy dental floss and use it. Other decisions involve more work.

Decide what kind of a load you can handle. If you have two Age Reduction goals that are in the "most difficult" category, you probably won't want to adopt both at the same time. Pick one Age Reduction strategy and follow it, and once you have the hang of it, pick another. Don't, for example, try to quit smoking and lose weight at the same time. Choose one, and once you have succeeded with it, adopt the other.

Break a large task into parts. If you are trying to lose weight, first begin by eating a diet that is rich in fruits, vegetables, and fibers. Then work on cutting back the amount of saturated and trans fats you eat (see Chapter 8). Don't worry about watching pounds right away; start by developing healthy eating habits. You may be surprised that the pounds come off on their own. Once you have eating under control, start to cut back on calories or begin to integrate exercise into your life. The most important thing about Age Reduction strategies is not that you start them, but that you continue them. Exercise, for example, gives no benefit once you stop. To get the years-younger benefit, you have to stay physically active for the rest of your life.

Put your Age Reduction Plan somewhere where you can easily see it. Tape it to the bathroom mirror. Look at it often and remember what you can do to get younger. Recalculate your RealAge every few months, or whenever you adopt a new Age Reduction strategy. That way you'll know just how young you have become.

CHART 3.2

Personal Age Reduction Plan

My RealAge is: _____.

I want my RealAge to be: _____.

Now that I have calculated my RealAge, what behaviors could I adopt to make myself younger?

1. _____.
2. _____.
3. _____.
4. _____.
5. _____.
6. _____.
7. _____.
8. _____.

Which ones am I willing to change?

1. _____.
2. _____.
3. _____.
4. _____.
5. _____.
6. _____.

Which three are the most important?

1. _____.
2. _____.
3. _____.

Which three are the easiest?

1. _____.
2. _____.
3. _____.

Dates: _____ to _____.

In the next 3 months, I will adopt the following three Age Reduction behaviors:

1. _____.
2. _____.
3. _____.

Dates: _____ to _____.

After 3 months, I will continue the first three behaviors and also adopt the following three Age Reduction behaviors:

1. _____.
2. _____.
3. _____.

In 3 months, my RealAge will be: _____.

In 1 year, my RealAge will be: _____.

In 3 years, my RealAge will be: _____.

THE DIFFERENCE BETWEEN REALAGE MAXIMUMS AND REALAGE INTERACTIONS: THE IMPACT ON YOU

As you read this book and review the choices that will help you reduce your RealAge, remember that the RealAge numbers presented in these chapters are the *maximum possible* effects. They presume only that a single behavior is affecting age reduction and do not take into account the interactions between the effects of several behaviors. Therefore, the numbers are *not* cumulative. This method has the benefit of allowing you to compare the relative value of health choices, but has the drawback of not accounting for multiple interactions.

Let's consider an example. The chapter on vitamins states that taking vitamins C and E (in food or supplements) can make you six years younger. The impact is astounding. Is it true? Yes. Is it true for you? Not necessarily. Although a person who does nothing else to protect himself or herself from aging may well have a RealAge benefit of as much as six years simply by taking these two vitamins, most of us make many other health decisions as well. The vitamin choice is mediated by other choices, such as exercising, smoking, and eating a vegetable- and fruit-laden diet.

Indeed, none of us has only one factor affecting his or her rate of aging. We all have multiple factors. You cannot simply add up all the years of benefits that certain behaviors provide and subtract those from your calendar age. Let's say you floss your teeth regularly (6.4 years younger), have low blood pressure (12 years younger), own a dog (1 year younger), exercise (9 years younger), and have a low weight (8 years younger). You cannot simply total these years and subtract them, to say you are 36.4 years younger than your calendar age. The RealAge concept would be meaningless as you worked your way back into childhood, even into negative years! Rather, the beauty of the RealAge calculation process on the Web, and to a lesser extent from Chart 2.1 in Chapter 2, is that it is able to consider the interrelationship between the range of behaviors and determine the impact of these interactions for you.

When you calculate your RealAge, the effect of any one behavior will depend on the other health behaviors and choices you follow. These involve complex equations and complex mathematics, which is why modern computers are required. But these complex calculations are now possible and can inform you of the relative and absolute value of your choices. This is what makes RealAge so revolutionary: It gives us the ability to calculate the effect of complex and multiple behaviors on aging all at once. It places a value on the effects that different behaviors will have on you, providing the information you need to make informed choices about the way in which you are going to age.

REALAGE MEANS INFORMED CHOICES

Read the rest of the book to find out why and how behaviors as diverse as taking vitamin E and enrolling in a continuing education class can help you make your RealAge younger. I will go over the studies and discuss the biologic impact of forty-four health and behavior choices. I will show you which ones help keep you young longer and provide suggestions and strategies for incorporating these changes into your life. I begin with the big three: aging of the arteries, aging of the immune system, and environmental aging, showing how each one contributes to the overall aging equation. In subsequent chapters, I explain how specific factors, such as taking the right vitamins in the proper doses, diet and weight management, physical activity and exercise, healthy everyday habits, proper medical management, and stress reduction can help you become and stay younger.

By keeping your RealAge young, you help to keep your calendar age from making you feel "old." What could be better than making it all the way to ninety with the youth and vigor of someone twenty-five years younger? This book gives you the value system for understanding your health choices, teaching you how to live more high-quality years with as little aging of your mind or body as possible. I give you the information you need. You make the choices about how you want to grow old. Or stay young.

4

Arterial Aging

KEEPING THE ROADWAYS CLEAR

Preventing arterial aging is the most important thing you can do to reduce your RealAge. Heart attacks, strokes, and vascular disease are all caused by aging of the arteries. Not taking care of your cardiovascular system can make your RealAge as much as twenty years older than your chronologic age. The good news is that you can easily and measurably slow arterial aging.

- The most important marker for arterial aging is blood pressure. By keeping blood pressure at the ideal level of 115/76 mm Hg, you can make your RealAge as much as ten years younger than if your blood pressure were at the national median of 129/86 and as much as twenty years younger than if your blood pressure were 140/90 or more. And virtually all of us can attain a blood pressure of 115/76.

  Difficulty rating: Most difficult

- Atherosclerosis—the buildup of fats along the arterial wall—is the second leading cause of arterial aging, just behind high blood pressure. The two conditions reinforce one another. Reducing the amount of lipid plaques along the walls of your arteries will help keep your arteries young.

  Difficulty rating: Most difficult

- Taking an aspirin (325 mg) a day can make your RealAge 1.9 years younger by the time you reach fifty and 2.6 years younger by the time you hit seventy. Aspirin helps keep your arteries free from lipid buildup.

  Difficulty rating: Quick fix

- Hormone replacement therapy in the form of estrogen and progesterone can make the average postmenopausal woman as much as eight years younger, depending on her particular history. Unfortunately, DHEA, advertised as the "hormone replacement therapy for men," has no such effect.

  Difficulty rating: Moderately easy

It's this simple: Nothing ages you faster than mistreating your heart and arteries. *And* nothing keeps you younger than keeping your cardiovascular system healthy. More Americans—both men and women—die from cardiovascular disease than from any other cause. Current statistics predict that 50 percent of us will be seriously afflicted by cardiovascular disease and more than 40 percent of us will die from it. Heart attacks, strokes, many types of kidney disease, and even Alzheimer's disease are largely caused by aging of the circulatory system.

Most of the premature aging your arterial system undergoes is self-inflicted. You age yourself by not taking proper care of yourself. The bad news is that most of us are not motivated enough to change our behaviors to protect ourselves from arterial aging. The good news is that you can start right now.

Your cardiovascular system is the primary system that ties your body together. Because arteries connect to every cell in the body, their health affects your health. Although we hear a lot about heart attacks and strokes, these are only the most dramatic manifestations of arterial disease. By the time a heart attack or stroke occurs, a person's arteries are almost always severely damaged; that is, they've gotten old.

Think of the cardiovascular system as a highway system. If roadways are the infrastructure of the city, the conduits that get us from here to there, then our circulatory system is the infrastructure of our bodies. Our blood vessels carry nutrients and oxygen to our cells and then carry carbon dioxide and other by-products away from our cells. Our arteries, just like streets and highways, wear down. They become clogged with fatty buildup, called plaque, or narrowed from swelling and inflammation. The older and more congested our arteries get, the more subject they are to the body's version of traffic jams— blood clots. This reduction in blood flow means that our cells are not getting the nutrients they need and suffer buildup of metabolic by-products. The heart has to work harder to get the blood where it's supposed to go, increasing blood pressure and stressing the arteries even more. Indeed, just as a major traffic jam can affect a whole city, cardiovascular disease can stress your whole body.

If you look at blood under a microscope, you will see that it consists of not just liquid, but many different kinds of cells—red cells, white cells, and platelets. It is the platelets—and sometimes white cells—that we have to watch out for when it comes to cardiovascular disease. Platelets are covered by an enzyme that, when activated, causes them to stick to other platelets and form a clot. Generally, clotting is a good thing; it is an important function that prevents excessive bleeding. As you age, however, you can develop blood clots where you don't want them—namely, on the walls of your arteries. Over the years, fat builds up on the walls of your arteries, slowing the flow of blood and causing platelet pileups—blood-vessel traffic jams— that further slow the flow of blood. These platelet pileups can form small clots in the arteries. If a clot gets too big, it can fill the entire artery, and blood can't get through at all, causing the tissue supplied by that artery to be at risk of dying. Likewise, when your arterial system comes under stress, the walls of your arteries can become inflamed and swollen, again closing off the flow of blood. In this case, oxygen and essential nutrients don't get to your organs as they used to, causing them to age more rapidly.

How can you prevent arterial aging? You probably know quite a few good habits that make a difference: eating a diet low in saturated fat, exercising, and avoiding stress. Conversely, bad behaviors, like being sedentary, can cause our cardiovascular system to age unnecessarily, and bad habits tend to reinforce each other. The worse our food choices, the more likely we are to be overweight. The more overweight we are, the less likely we are to exercise, and so on. Even mild forms of cardiovascular disease can slow us down and make us feel old fast.

The most important step in your antiaging plan is to protect your heart and arteries. That is why almost every chapter in this book addresses the problem of arterial aging. In this chapter, I show you the basics. I show you how to think about cardiac health as a conglomerate of health decisions that intersect with every aspect of your life. You will need to learn to think of cardiac health holistically: Everything you do contributes to or detracts from it. For example, simple things like taking an aspirin a day, drinking a glass of red wine with dinner, and taking the right vitamins in the proper amounts are quick, easy, and painless ways to make your cardiovascular system healthier.

BLOOD PRESSURE: LOWER IT!

Blood pressure readings are measurements of the overall health and well-being of our hearts and arteries. That is why monitoring your blood pressure is one of the best ways of gauging your RealAge. For example, the difference between having low blood pressure rather than high blood pressure can mean a RealAge difference of more than twenty years!

Do you know how high your blood pressure is? Chances are it's too high. Eighty-nine percent of Americans have blood pressure higher than the ideal for preventing aging—115/76 mm Hg (millimeters of mercury). Nearly a quarter of all Americans (58 million) have blood pressure above the American Heart Association's danger zone of 140/90. Even the old standard that many consider ideal—120/80—is too high for optimal health (and youth). More to the point, high blood pressure, also called hypertension, is one of the leading causes of heart attack, stroke, heart failure, and kidney failure. High blood pressure has no symptoms. Most of us live with it and feel fine. As a result, it is hard for patients to take high blood pressure seriously or to see it as an indicator of a serious health risk.

In fact, I have patients who, even though they know about the devastating effects of high blood pressure, do almost anything to avoid taking their medication. Here's one story. Roger V., a longtime associate at the University of Chicago, had, over the years, asked me for medical advice. One day, he called me about his father-in-law, Jake. Jake had just retired from a lifetime career as an engineer. A World War II veteran, and proud of the fact that he'd never been sick a day in his life, he was never one to go to the doctor. When Jake had his retirement physical, it was the first time he had seen a doctor since leaving the service some forty years earlier in 1946. Jake reported that his doctor told him he had a "touch" of high blood pressure—160/90, more than a "touch" by anyone's standards. But Jake steadfastly refused to go on any medicine or even to return to the doctor.

Jake and his wife, Sara, bought a motor home. For three years, they took trips, went to art museums and cultural events, and meandered around the country just enjoying their free time. After forty years of working hard, they were finally reaping the benefits. Jake called it the "great life." He told Roger and his daughter, Joyce (Roger's wife), "Don't worry about my blood pressure. Now that I'm not working, I'm not under any stress. My blood pressure's sure to have dropped."

Since nothing "seemed" wrong, no one paid too much attention. Then it happened. Jake had a stroke. The stroke left him partially paralyzed and impaired his speech. He needed a walker to get around. In a matter of minutes, he had lost the "great life" he had worked all his life to enjoy.

Despite all the medical care Jake received after the stroke, he still refused to take his blood pressure medication. Finally, his kidneys started to fail, a side effect of hypertension. Roger and Joyce brought him to see me.

Giving him the "cold, hard facts," I finally convinced Jake to accept blood pressure treatment. With medication, his blood pressure dropped and his kidney function improved. Indeed, he managed to live a fairly good life, remaining relatively independent for another decade, until his kidneys finally gave out entirely. Although his poststroke life was adequate and he made the best of it, it was not the life he had dreamed about. And it didn't have to happen.

But that's not the end of the story. Several years ago, Jake's daughter, Joyce, was also diagnosed as having high blood pressure. Just like her father, she refused to go on medication. Roger pushed her to take the medicine, but she still refused.

"Joyce," I asked her, "are you *nuts?*"

She replied, "I just don't like taking medications."

"Joyce," I told her, "you just watched what happened to your father. Think how hard it was on him and your mother. It broke your heart to watch him suffer. It broke all our hearts. And now you're telling me that you are going to risk *exactly* the same thing?"

I explained how and why high blood pressure is a silent killer—and a silent ager. After showing her that lowering her blood pressure could make a twenty-year difference in her RealAge, I finally convinced her of the importance of taking blood pressure medicine. But her resistance remained strong. She was concerned about side effects. I told her that although blood pressure medication could have side effects, most of them could be counteracted.

When taking some blood pressure-controlling drugs, some people feel dizzy when they exercise, a symptom of dehydration. They just need to drink plenty of fluids. A small percentage of people have lower potassium levels, but most need only to add a banana a day to their diets. In rare cases, side effects can include gout as well as impotence for men and a change in sexual pleasure for women. With a little adjustment of the medication and dosages, these side effects can usually be eliminated. There are a number of different blood pressure drugs, and some of them work better for some people than others. Sometimes side effects are the most important clues for figuring out what's going on in your body.

Luckily, Joyce was finally convinced. By taking the medication, she reduced her blood pressure to 125/85, making her RealAge younger by eight years, and she suffered only minimal side effects.

The most crucial thing is not to go off the medication without a physician's consent. Discontinuing these medications abruptly puts enormous stress on your body and causes all kinds of unnecessary aging. It can be life threatening.

Because high blood pressure causes aging without overt symptoms, it can be difficult to focus on keeping it low. Keeping your blood pressure at 115/76 can make your RealAge as much as ten years younger than if your blood pressure were the national median of 129/86. In contrast, having blood pressure higher than 140/90 can make your RealAge six to ten years older than if you had the national average (see Table 4.1). In certain population groups—African Americans, for example—the aging effect for high blood pressure is even greater.

What Is Blood Pressure, and How Is It Measured?

Most of us have had our blood pressure taken every single time we've visited a doctor since we were children. But what exactly does blood pressure measure? What does blood pressure tell us about our overall health?

Blood pressure is the amount of force exerted by blood on the walls of the arteries as blood flows through them. The higher your blood pressure, the more stress and strain you are putting on your body. In RealAge terms, you are burning away years faster than you need to.

The only way to measure your blood pressure is to perform a quick, painless test using an instrument called a sphygmomanometer—the rubber cuff and gauge that they strap on you the minute you walk into a doctor's office. When your blood pressure is measured, make sure to ask what it is and to write it down. Keep track of your blood pressure and how it varies over time. Your blood pressure is not always at the same level. It is often elevated when you are anxious, upset, or in a hurry. Just being in a doctor's office can raise your blood pressure ("white-coat hypertension"). When your blood pressure is measured, make sure you've had enough time to calm down, are sitting and relaxed, and aren't talking to someone about an issue you feel passionately about. If your blood pressure is high or higher than you'd like, go to your local pharmacist and buy a sphygmomanometer. Either your doctor or the pharmacist can show you how to use it. Monitor your blood pressure regularly, keeping track of any fluctuations. You will keep far more vigilant watch over your own blood pressure than anyone else will. After all, it's your body, and you have the most to lose.

Blood pressure is always presented as a fraction. For example, 129/86 mm Hg is the median blood pressure for Americans in their mid-to-late forties and early fifties. The top number in the fraction is called the systolic blood pressure, the pressure exerted on the artery walls when the heart beats. The bottom number, the diastolic blood pressure, is the pressure exerted when the heart is at rest, between beats. As mentioned, the ideal blood pressure for maintaining youth and vigor is 115/76. As a general guideline, every increase of two points in the systolic number or three points in the diastolic number increases your RealAge an average of 1.5 years.

As you age, systolic blood pressure (and sometimes also diastolic blood pressure) tends to increase. Why? As you age, the walls of your arteries become atherosclerotic—less elastic and clogged with buildup from fats and lipids. This arterial hardening forces the heart to work harder. The heart becomes enlarged, and the arteries become scarred and damaged. It is a vicious cycle: The more damaged the arteries become, the harder the heart has

TABLE 4.1

THE REALAGE BENEFIT OF LOW BLOOD PRESSURE

Having a blood pressure of 115/76 mm Hg (the ideal) as opposed to 129/86 (the national median) means

Men would be, physiologically:

- 5.5 years younger at 35
- 7.0 years younger at 55
- 12 years younger at 70

Women would be, physiologically:

- 5.0 years younger at 35
- 7.5 years younger at 55
- 10 years younger at 70

THE REALAGE LOSS OF HIGH BLOOD PRESSURE

Having a high blood pressure of 140/90 as opposed to 129/86 (the national median) means

Men would be, physiologically:

- 11.6 years older at 35
- 16.5 years older at 55
- 20.2 years older at 70

Women would be, physiologically:

- 5.5 years older at 35
- 7.5 years older at 55
- 9.0 years older at 70

to work, causing it to enlarge even more and creating more scarring. Arterial plaques can form, then enlarge, and heart attacks and strokes are more likely to occur. One and a half million Americans suffer heart attacks every year, and more than a third of those people (550,000) die. Half a million Americans have strokes every year, and 150,000 die from them and their side effects annually.

In less than 5 percent of these cases is high blood pressure caused by some underlying medical condition. In these instances, when the root cause is corrected, blood pressure returns to normal. In more than 95 percent of the cases, there is no specific cause of high blood pressure; many times it is the result of the poor care we've given our arteries over the years.

How Do You Achieve Ideal Blood Pressure?

What should you do if your blood pressure is higher than the ideal of 115/76?

- Eat a more nutritious diet that is low in saturated fat.

- Get more exercise.

- Lose weight.

- Stop smoking.

- Cut your sodium intake to less than 1,600 mg a day.

- Increase your potassium, calcium, and magnesium intake.

- Avoid stress and consider strategies to reduce stress, such as increasing social connections or using relaxation therapy, biofeedback methods, or yoga.

- If your blood pressure is close to or higher than 140/90, talk to your doctor about taking medicine to reduce hypertension.

Because nutrition, exercise, and stress reduction are important components of aging, this book has chapters devoted to each (see Chapters 8, 9, and 11). If you have higher-than-ideal blood pressure, pay special attention to the recommendations in these chapters. If your family has a history of cardiovascular disease, pay *extra* attention. These chapters show you how easy it is to incorporate heart-healthy eating and exercise habits into your life. Lowering your blood pressure is *not* an impossible task.

Talk to your doctor. He or she can help you formulate a blood pressure-reduction plan that fits you, with special consideration for your particular needs and concerns. Your doctor can help you decide if you should be on medicine for hypertension. If so, he or she can work with you to choose the medication that works best for you. Remember, there are several kinds of treatments, and some may suit you better than others, so you should ask about all of them. If you experience side effects or don't feel as good as you think you should, don't discontinue your medicine—doing so can provoke a heart attack or stroke. Talk to your doctor about possible alternative treatments.

In addition, your doctor can tell you whether your high blood pressure is "sodium sensitive." Many people are sensitive to sodium; that is, their blood pressure responds to the amount of sodium they ingest. If you think that you are salt sensitive, you should cut back on foods containing salt (see the section on sodium in Chapter 7). And if you think that getting rid of your salt shaker will do it, think again. Most of the sodium we ingest comes not from salt we add to foods, but from sodium added by manufacturers to packaged foods. There are high levels of sodium in everything from soda pop to most breakfast cereals. Learn to be a label reader. Eat fresh fruits and vegetables instead of processed food to avoid sodium.

Reducing blood pressure requires *more* commitment than most of the RealAge Age Reduction strategies that we talk about in this book. When you start to think it's too much work, remember that your RealAge will become 1.5 years younger for every two-point drop in systolic blood pressure and every three-point drop in diastolic blood pressure. What could be better than that?

STOPPING ATHEROSCLEROSIS: OPEN UP YOUR ARTERIES!

The second most significant sign of arterial aging is atherosclerosis, the buildup of fats and lipids along the walls of the arteries. This narrowing of the arteries can lead to the formation of clots, which can, in extreme cases, cause heart attacks and strokes. Indeed, atherosclerosis is a primary *cause* of high blood pressure. High blood pressure is often the first sign that the arteries are starting to harden. The higher blood pressure rises, the more quickly fats build up, causing even more atherosclerotic aging, and so on. It's a vicious cycle.

What causes fats to build up? We're not sure. Scientists postulate that either inflammation of the blood vessel walls or an excessive and accelerated bombardment of blood against the arterial walls—the very same conditions high blood pressure causes—triggers this process. Moreover, the higher your total blood cholesterol—specifically, the higher your LDL cholesterol—the worse the problem becomes. There are two common types of cholesterol, low-density lipoproteins (LDL) and high-density lipoproteins (HDL). I always remember "L" for "lousy" and "H" for "healthy" because LDL cholesterol accelerates fatty buildup in the arteries, whereas HDL cholesterol actually helps inhibit such buildup. That's why you want to have a low LDL reading and a high HDL reading. If you have a high total cholesterol reading, have your doctor determine the levels of each. (See Chapter 8 for more information on cholesterol.)

Men are more likely to suffer from arterial aging than women and at an earlier age. Women usually don't undergo arterial aging until after menopause, and then it can be deferred even longer by taking hormone supplements (discussed later in this chapter). Also, some population groups and families are more prone to arterial aging than others. For example, if you are a man and a number of close relatives (a father, a brother, or an uncle) have had heart attacks or strokes, especially under age sixty-five, you, too, could be at risk of atherosclerosis at an early age. You will need to pay particular attention to arterial aging. The same would be true of people who are significantly overweight; those who have high LDL cholesterol readings; and, of course, those who have high blood pressure.

All of us can do simple things that will help keep our arteries young. The following sections of this chapter show that taking an aspirin a day is a quick, easy step toward arterial youth that almost all of us can incorporate into their lives. In Chapter 7, learn how vitamins C and E protect your arteries. Taking both of these substances in the recommended doses can reduce your RealAge by more than six years. Be sure to read the section on folate (Chapter 7) because taking folate regularly will help keep lipids from building up in your arteries. Note in the section on aging of the immune system (Chapter 5) that you should be careful to brush and floss your teeth to avoid periodontal disease. The bacteria that cause periodontal disease are believed to trigger an immune response that, in turn, causes inflammation, or swelling, of the arteries. An area can then form along the arterial wall, creating a niche in which fats can accumulate, causing the arteries to become atherosclerotic.

When it comes to arterial youth, there are the additional big three: nutrition, exercise, and stress. These are so important that a chapter is devoted to each. Think of them as being interrelated. By eating a diet that is rich in nutrients and low in saturated fats, you will be able to reduce your RealAge by more than ten years. By exercising regularly (it's not that hard!), you can reduce your RealAge by more than eight years. Pay particular attention to Chapter 11, which gives tips for managing stress, because stress and emotional upheaval can cause significant arterial aging.

Now let us consider two factors that can specifically keep your arteries free from clots—taking an aspirin a day and hormone replacement therapy.

AN ASPIRIN A DAY
KEEPS THE DOCTOR AWAY

Why Not Lower Your Age Today?

If I were asked to name the one drug that is the hands-down winner for the most useful drug of the century, I would say, as most doctors would, aspirin. Aspirin is the basic cure-all medicine. Got a headache? Take an aspirin. Got a fever? Take an aspirin. And now, feeling old? Take an aspirin.

The fact that aspirin works to quell pain, fever, and swelling is not news. But how can it slow the aging process? Taking an aspirin, or even half an aspirin, a day will help keep your arteries free of buildup. Moreover, aspirin therapy reduces the incidence of certain kinds of colon cancer and other cancers in the gastrointestinal tract. Taking an aspirin a day (325 mg) can have the long-term benefit of reducing your RealAge by as much as 1.9 years when you are at calendar age fifty-five and by as much as 2.6 years by the time you reach seventy.

Aspirin helps keep your arteries free from clots by inhibiting the prostaglandin system—an enzyme system that causes platelets to stick together. Aspirin seems to prevent the aging of blood vessels in other ways, too—in ways that we are still trying to understand. For example, some theorize that aspirin may help the body build auxiliary blood vessels, so that if and when clots do develop, the body has alternate routes for blood to flow around the clots. Aspirin may help decrease inflammation in the walls of the blood vessels, caused by infections elsewhere in the body, and thus prevent turbulent blood flow that can lead to fatty buildup.

Better yet, the most recent studies on aspirin and aspirin-related drugs show a decrease in the incidence of strokes, especially the practically undetectable small-scale strokes that are often associated with memory loss. Aspirin and chemically similar drugs, such as ibuprofen (for example Motrin and Advil), are called nonsteroidal anti-inflammatory drugs, or NSAIDs. All NSAIDs appear to have this antistroke effect. Best of all, the sustained use of aspirin or other NSAIDs has even been shown to reduce the incidence of Alzheimer's disease, presumably because it helps keep the arteries in the brain young. Although we don't know all the ways aspirin may help blood vessels, we do know that it has a significant impact.

If you are a man over forty or a woman just reaching menopause, you can decrease arterial aging by beginning an aspirin-a-day therapy. Many studies have documented the benefits of aspirin in preventing cardiovascular disease. Some have been small-scale studies and some have been large-scale studies, but all have indicated that aspirin helped reduce the incidence of heart attacks. In the most highly controlled of all these studies, the effect of aspirin was quite dramatic: Aspirin reduced the incidence of heart attack by as much as 44 percent.

Approximately ten thousand physicians were recruited to be guinea pigs for this research. All these doctors regularly took pills that were supplied to them by the study coordinators. Some of the participants were given real aspirin, and the others were given placebos. In the seven years of this study, the physicians who took aspirin had 44 percent fewer heart attacks than those who took the placebos. In fact, the results were so dramatic that the National Institutes of Health (NIH) panel overseeing the study halted it in midstream, deciding that the participants who had not been taking aspirin, but who were at risk of heart attack, should receive the benefits of aspirin.

The benefits of aspirin are achieved over a long period. The risk factors in these studies are calculated presuming at least a ten-year period of aspirin therapy. I estimate that a patient would need to be on this therapy for at least three years to get the full benefit. Keep in mind that benefits are lost once you stop taking aspirin regularly. So if you are a man over forty or a woman starting menopause, you should take an aspirin a day for the rest of your life. (Remember to check with your physician before initiating or stopping any Age Reduction strategy.) Remember, too, that there are gender differences. Women probably benefit less from aspirin than men because women usually don't develop cardiovascular disease until menopause, usually after age fifty. Unfortunately, most of the aspirin studies have not provided specific data on women. Since there is no significant difference in the cardiovascular systems of men and women, and on the basis of what we know about women's health and aging in general, I feel comfortable urging women to start taking an aspirin a day around the time of menopause.

Aspirin and the Risk of Cancer: An Added Benefit

More good news: Besides helping to prevent arterial aging, an aspirin a day seems to reduce the incidence of certain kinds of colon cancer. So far, the studies are suggestive, not conclusive, and we still don't know how aspirin helps to decrease the risk of cancer. We just know that it does. While conducting a study of people who were at a high risk of a hereditary kind of colon cancer called familial polyposis, researchers accidentally discovered that patients who took aspirin and other NSAIDs (for example, Advil or Motrin) had significantly lower rates of colon cancer than their family histories would have predicted. Further studies confirmed this decreased risk. Then a major study coordinated by the American Cancer Society, involving about 635,000 people, found that those who took aspirin or other NSAIDs regularly over a ten-year period had a significantly lower rate of cancer in the gastrointestinal track. In another study of 121,000 nurses, those who took aspirin regularly over a ten-year period had a 44 percent lower incidence of colon cancer. Aspirin has been linked to a decreased incidence of other cancers, too.

Does Aspirin Therapy Have Side Effects?

Aspirin is one of the oldest and safest drugs. Its main ingredient, acetylsalicylic acid, is found in willow bark, which has been used as a home remedy for headaches for more than three hundred years. Aspirin, as we now know it, was discovered more than a hundred years ago by the German scientist Hermann Dresser, who isolated it in its chemical form. Since then, those powdery white pills have been a staple of the family medicine cabinet.

For the same reason that aspirin is good for the arteries, it can be harmful if you have ulcers or other abdominal pain. Since aspirin inhibits the enzyme system that causes clotting and is itself acidic, too much aspirin can cause ulcers to bleed more than normally and to heal more slowly. Sometimes aspirin can even cause ulcers. If you are prone to such problems, you should talk to your doctor. He or she may recommend a coated aspirin that does not dissolve in the stomach directly. Taking aspirin with a glass of warm water one or two hours after eating helps dilute the aspirin and reduces any acidic effect that might cause stomach troubles. Alka-Seltzer is another way to ingest aspirin without causing stomach problems, but its sodium content is extremely high, so it can create a problem for people with high blood pressure or other heart problems.

As mentioned, aspirin "thins" the blood by inhibiting clotting. Do you have to worry about thinning it too much? Not usually. Aspirin works in two different ways. To combat pain and swelling, aspirin has an inhibitory effect that lasts only a few hours. Its effect on the blood platelet system is different. Aspirin disarms the clotting function of a platelet for the life of that platelet. Platelets regenerate every seven to ten days, and you need to constrain six-sevenths of the platelets to receive this benefit to the arteries. In general, one aspirin a day is not enough to inhibit clotting seriously, so don't let fears about cuts not healing stop you from taking it. The one-a-day dosage keeps the clotting of platelets at a constant low, usually without affecting normal clotting when you need it. If you are about to undergo major surgery, your doctor may recommend that you stop taking aspirin two or three days ahead of time, just to make sure your platelet system will be adequate for clotting.

"Designer Aspirin" and Other NSAIDS: Can Aspirin Really Be Improved?

Aspirin is clearly a wonder drug, but it and the other nonsteroidal anti-inflammatory drugs, in addition to reducing pain, can eat away at the stomach lining (causing bleeding and ulcers), inhibit clotting, and in rare cases damage the kidneys.

The problem with aspirin and its cousins, such as ibuprofen, is that they aren't "specific": that is, their effects have more than one target. Their beneficial effects come from the ability to block cyclooxygenase-2 (COX-2), an enzyme that promotes inflammation, pain, and fevers. Unfortunately, the drugs are even more effective at inhibiting COX-1, a related enzyme essential for the health of the stomach lining and the kidneys. It might be beneficial to create compounds that selectively inhibit COX-2 but don't have any effect on COX-1. New drugs that do exactly this may be in drugstores within the next two years.

Over the past decade, epidemiologic data have indicated that aspirin and other nonsteroidal anti-inflammatory drugs can protect against certain cancers, Alzheimer's disease, and arterial aging. Inhibition of COX-2 seems to be the key to the ability of these drugs to reduce aging. These new aspirin-like compounds should be able to provide pain relief, and may also slow the development of cancer and Alzheimer's disease without stomach or kidney damage. Thus, designer aspirin may really be a better aspirin, providing youth-promoting benefits for the arterial and immune systems without the aging side effects.

Also, if you have diabetes, asthma, kidney problems, or blood pressure that is either too high or too low, be sure to talk to your doctor before starting this regimen. Aspirin seems to lower blood pressure and can inhibit kidney function in individuals with diabetes or kidney problems. And sometimes aspirin can trigger an asthmatic effect. You shouldn't take aspirin if you have either chicken pox or the flu because of the very rare possibility of getting Reye's syndrome, a toxic reaction to aspirin that affects children almost exclusively, but can occasionally affect an adult. The chances of any problems occurring from taking just one aspirin a day for Age Reduction are slim. If you do fall into any of the categories mentioned, there are some alternatives your doctor can recommend.

Since many of these studies have shown that aspirin and other NSAIDs are advantageous, does it matter if you take aspirin or the aspirin-like NSAIDs, such as ibuprofen? I prefer aspirin. We know much more about aspirin than the other NSAIDs, so we know how safe it is. Aspirin has clearly been shown to have a significant Age Reducing effect. Aspirin was the first NSAID we ever had; it is the prototype. Since some people couldn't take, or didn't want to take, aspirin, chemists invented aspirin-like drugs that were close to aspirin. The best known of these drugs is ibuprofen, but there are many others. These drugs approximate the effect of aspirin but have different side effects and benefits. For example, for many people, they provide better pain relief. When it comes to deactivating the enzyme system that causes blood platelets to stick together, newer versions of aspirin just don't work as well as the original. The reason is that aspirin deactivates the system for the life of the platelet, but most other NSAIDs do so only temporarily. The effectiveness of aspirin and some other NSAIDs in reducing the risk of cancer seems to be the same, however. Never take aspirin and other NSAIDs together, except under supervision of a doctor, and talk to your doctor before starting either treatment.

An even newer generation of NSAIDs will probably be on the market soon, with all the Age Reduction benefits and none of the side effects. But don't wait.

Aspirin has stood the test of time. Taking an aspirin a day is one quick and easy step to prevent arterial aging. Another, at least for women, is hormone replacement therapy.

HORMONE REPLACEMENT THERAPY: FEELING LIKE A KID AGAIN

Hormones? We usually associate them with the onset of puberty, the chemicals that turned our sweet children into temperamental teenagers. As we grow older, a decrease in the levels of hormones, especially the sex hormones, promotes arterial aging. For those of us concerned about staying young, reversing that process may be one of the mainstays in preventing arterial aging.

Hormones cause us to grow, to metabolize food, to flee in the face of danger. They are produced by such glands as the adrenal and the thyroid, and are largely directed by signals from the hypothalamus in the brain. Hormones are released into the bloodstream and stimulate various physiologic activities. Adrenaline, released during fear or excitement, is a hormone. So is cortisol. Without a doubt, the most well-known hormones are the sex hormones—testosterone for men and estrogen and progesterone for women.

As we reach puberty, hormones are released into our bloodstream, and we undergo the physiologic changes that turn our childhood bodies into adult ones. During early adulthood and through our peak reproductive years, these hormones remain at a high level in our bloodstream. As we reach our fifties and sixties, production of these hormones decreases dramatically. By our eighties and nineties, these hormones are almost nonexistent in our bloodstream. That leads to the question, Will we stay younger longer if our hormone levels remain high?

This question is not an easy one to answer. I believe that a decrease in hormone levels is one of the factors that make us age. Correspondingly, hormone replacement therapy works to keep us younger. This assertion is definitely true regarding estrogen and progesterone therapy for women, and I heartily recommend this treatment for most women, unless they have an unusually high chance of getting breast or uterine cancer. Some new but highly controversial evidence has shown that it might be true for DHEA replacement in men. That, however, has not been proved.

The problem with hormone treatments is that many of the hormones that might be used as supplements—with the exception of estrogen and progesterone—either have not been very well studied or are known to have serious side effects. For example, anabolic steroids, the kind of hormones athletes are barred from taking, do add muscle mass but also cause all kinds of other problems—everything from skeletal deterioration to psychosis. Some hormone replacement therapies can even cause cancer. Hormone systems are "level sensitive," so taking more than your body is designed to handle is bad for you. Unlike money, low-fat guacamole, or summer vacations, more is not necessarily better. Indeed, most hormone systems have associated with them a disease that comes from having too little of the hormone in the bloodstream and another disease that comes from having too much.

No matter what you think about aging, it is best not to put something into your body that might be harmful. Hormone replacement therapy is an evolving treatment. Studies will show us more over time. In this chapter, I review the data for two hormone replacement treatments: one for women (progesterone-estrogen treatment), which I recommend, and one for men (DHEA treatment), which I cannot recommend—at least not yet.

Hormone Replacement for Women: Estrogen and Progesterone Therapy

Heart disease is not common for women until after menopause. Even so, 40 percent of all women die from arterial and coronary problems—that's *ten times* the number of women who die from breast cancer. More than thirty-five studies have shown that hormone replacement therapy helps protect the body against deterioration of the arteries. Hormone treatment decreases the risk of cardiovascular diseases by up to 35 percent in the first ten years after menopause and decreases the risk of death by 20 percent even after twenty years of use.

We still do not know why estrogen and progesterone have these effects, but they do. These hormones appear to help keep the tissue lining of the blood vessels healthy. When these tissues are healthy, they secrete substances (vasodilators) that help prevent the buildup of harmful kinds of cholesterol on the walls of the arteries, thus decreasing the kind of arterial blockages that can lead to heart attacks, strokes, and heart failure. In addition, estrogen helps prevent the buildup of fibrinogen, a chemical that causes blood clotting.

For the same reasons that hormone therapy helps your heart, hormone therapy helps your mind. It keeps the blood vessels in the brain supple and free from blockages. Alzheimer's disease is a frightening disease, a slow and frustrating descent into confusion. Alzheimer's affects women disproportionately: half the women over age eighty-five are afflicted by it. Although we still do not know much about preventing the disease, one of the factors clearly implicated in the onset of Alzheimer's is arterial aging. A series of studies published between 1994 and 1998 show that for women taking estrogen replacement therapy, the incidence of Alzheimer's disease was reduced by as much as 50 percent. These women have better mental function, less confusion, and fewer memory problems.

The third benefit of hormone replacement therapy is that it helps prevent the deossification of bone—the loss of calcium in the bones that can cause osteoporosis. Although osteoporosis can affect both men and women, the condition is far more common in women. And although all women should be sure to get enough calcium, hormone replacement therapy further helps slow this process (see Chapter 7 on calcium).

Hormone Replacement Therapy and the Risk of Cancer

On the downside, hormone replacement therapy has been specifically implicated in breast, ovarian, and uterine cancers. Why? Hormones work as chemical signals: The body produces hormones in a gland, such as the pituitary gland, and sends them into the bloodstream to give instructions to other parts of the body. For these other parts of the body to "hear" the signal, they must have a specifically attuned instrument called a receptor, a place where the chemical signal is able to attach and transmit its message. Just as important as estrogen are the estrogen receptors. Without them, the body wouldn't be able to respond to the signal.

Three types of estrogen receptors have been identified so far. E1 (estrogen-1) receptors are located in breast and uterine tissue and are linked to the development of female traits, such as enlarged breasts, menstruation, and a high-pitched voice. The interaction between estrogen and the E1 receptors appears to promote breast, ovarian, and uterine cancers, apparently by initiating tissue growth. E2 receptors are linked to the cardiovascular system and allow estrogen to have a protective cardiovascular effect. Finally, E3 receptors allow bones to strengthen.

Taking estrogen supplements after the body has quit producing high levels of estrogen extends the period of exposure to estrogen, increasing the risk of cancer. Even though hormone replacement therapy does increase the risk of cancer, that risk is still low except in high-risk groups. In fact, a new study showed that estrogen therapy is associated with a 35 percent reduction in colorectal cancers, meaning that estrogen can protect you from certain types of cancer as well. Members of high-risk categories for breast and uterine cancers include women who are overweight by 40 percent or more, are either childless or were over age twenty-nine at the time of the birth of their first child, and have one or two direct family members (a mother, sister, or daughter) who had breast cancer before age forty. For these women, the Age Reduction effects of estrogen are diminished, making the RealAge effect of hormone replacement therapy only one or two years younger at age seventy. For women not in these high-risk categories, the Age Reducing effects of hormone replacement are even more than the median eight years.

For most women, most of the time, hormone replacement therapy is a good thing. Talk it over with your doctor. Weigh your risk of cancer against your risk of other possible diseases—osteoporosis, coronary disease, and Alzheimer's disease. Make an informed choice. For women who have not had hysterectomies, I generally recommend the combination estrogen-progesterone therapy, because progesterone does not increase the risk of uterine cancers and the combination seems to cause fewer side effects than therapy with estrogen alone. See how it works for you. If you notice side effects—more headaches, high blood pressure, moodiness—talk to your doctor about reducing the dosage or readjusting the balance between estrogen and progesterone.

Also, ask your doctor to let you know when any of the new "designer" estrogen replacement drugs becomes available. These estrogen-like compounds promise to retard bone loss and arterial aging, but won't pose a risk of uterine or breast cancer. These new drugs will target the E2 and E3 receptors, providing both cardiovascular and bone-strengthening benefits, but will overlook the E1 receptors, preventing the kind of overexposure to estrogen that increases the risk of cancer. Since these drugs will not cause the development of breast tissue or have other "feminizing" effects, men may also be able to take them.

Synthetic estrogens are similar to native estrogens in that their structure causes them to interact and bind with specific receptors. However, the synthetics do not interact in the same way with estrogen receptors as do native estrogens. This difference—not interacting in the same way with all types of estrogen receptors (E1 versus E2 versus E3)—is one of the great promises of modern biotechnology. Imagine a synthetic "designer" estrogen that would antagonize E1 receptors (stopping the development or growth of breast cancer) and would not cause feminization, but would stimulate E2 and E3 receptors to retard arterial aging and strengthen bones. The first of these so-called designer estrogens has been released: Evista by Eli Lilly, which at present seems to decrease the risk of breast cancer and retard skeletal aging by strengthening bones. Does Evista delay arterial aging? Does it work for men? Only further research will answer these questions, but there will probably be a breakthrough with this drug or an alternate designer estrogen in the near future.

In the meantime, work with your doctor to formulate a traditional estrogen treatment that works best for your body. As always, make sure you get annual gynecological examinations, mammograms, and Pap smears so that precancerous conditions and early cancers can be detected and stopped early.

Estrogen-progesterone treatment keeps you young. It protects your arteries, helps protect your bones from the loss of calcium, can reduce your risk of colorectal cancer, and can offset the discomfort of menopause.

Men, Hormone Replacement, and the Case for DHEA

Unfortunately, there is no such good news about hormone therapy for men. Dehydroepiandrosterone (DHEA), a hormone secreted by the adrenal cortex, has received a lot of attention lately. It has been hailed as the hormone treatment for men. A few feature articles about DHEA appeared in the health pages of the local newspaper, then a couple of news stories aired on TV, and suddenly my office was full of converts to DHEA. But DHEA has not been proved to improve arterial health, or any other kind of health, for that matter. It even has potential risks.

The news stories claimed that DHEA made men feel great. DHEA is a steroid, and all steroids make you feel great. For the short term. Over the long term, though, they can do a lot of harm. Certain steroids can cause cancer, weaken the immune system, and pose other serious health risks.

DHEA is a hormone that is a precursor to androgens and estrogen. The body breaks DHEA down into the sex hormones. Since DHEA is considered a food supplement instead of a drug, it can be bought without a prescription. The dosage levels in different brands can vary widely, and no rigorous medical studies have been conducted on the long-term effects of taking DHEA. More important, almost all the studies that have monitored DHEA for more than a year have evaluated the effects of variations in *naturally* occurring levels of the hormone in the bloodstream and have not considered the role of supplements.

Men who take DHEA report increased energy, improved moods, and the return of that holy grail of male youth, bursting libidos. "I feel like I'm twenty again," says one sixty-year-old convert. "My wife has that sparkle back in her eye," says another, with that "you-know-what-I-mean" grin. Unfortunately, these reports are more anecdotal than scientific, and a feeling of well-being does not mean that DHEA can't cause real damage. We know all sorts of drugs (cocaine, for example) that make you feel good, but that aren't good for you. DHEA might make you feel younger now, but might also make your RealAge older in the long run.

In the most significant study on the effects of DHEA on aging, the so-called Rancho-Bernardo study, researchers found that over a twelve-year period, men whose naturally occurring DHEA levels remained high had a somewhat lower risk of heart disease and arterial aging. In some cases, the incidence of these diseases was as much as 40 percent lower. Despite this initially promising evidence, the follow-up study, over a nineteen-year period, showed that the benefit of having an elevated DHEA level had been reduced, so the risk was only 14 percent less. In RealAge terms, the benefit of DHEA would be only about 1¹/₂ years at most.

People have also speculated that DHEA might improve the immune response. This effect would be in direct contrast to the effect of the stress hormones, the corticosteroids. Doctors sometimes prescribe corticosteroids to organ transplant patients to suppress the immune system. Whether and how much DHEA can improve immune response remain subject to speculation. Significant benefits have been shown in animal studies, but these studies have largely been on rodents, a group of mammals that do not produce DHEA naturally. Thus, these studies do not provide a good basis for assumptions about human beings. Although the human studies have indicated that DHEA might help, they were not controlled studies and used very small sample sizes. So we still don't know.

I have outlined the possible benefits, but what are the possible drawbacks? A study at Johns Hopkins found that women who had high levels of male hormones, such as DHEA and its derivatives (androgens), had higher incidences of ovarian cancer. That raised a red flag. Doctors worried that DHEA might be tied to other kinds of cancers as well. Other indicators show that DHEA puts a strain on the liver. If, despite my warnings, you decide to take DHEA, make sure you take it in conjunction with such antioxidants as vitamins C and E, which will help reduce the strain on the liver.

In addition, DHEA is the precursor to androgens, and high levels of androgens have been linked to prostate cancer. DHEA may also increase tumors of the pituitary gland. Since DHEA functions as a growth hormone under certain conditions, it may cause isolated precancerous cells to transform into rapidly growing tumors. Greater androgen levels can also increase the problem of male pattern baldness—not dangerous, but certainly something that will make you look, if not feel, older.

If you take DHEA, you first need to have a complete physical, including a measurement of your current DHEA levels. You might be one of those people with a naturally high level, anyway. And you will need to have screenings every six months for prostate cancer, as well as to have regular checks of your DHEA levels to make sure that they are in the right range. That's a lot of hassle for a drug with no confirmed powers of age reduction.

DHEA seems to play no role in heart disease. It doesn't seem to retard aging of the blood vessels, although long-term studies haven't been done yet. As for the sexual powers attributed to DHEA, in the one controlled study on the use of supplements, there was no indication that DHEA improved libido or sexual desire. As for other claims that have been made for DHEA—that it increases muscle mass, helps one lose weight, and improves one's mood— they are more cases of wishful thinking than proven scientific results.

Many studies are being done on DHEA right now. In the next five years, we should know if it has any benefits or serious risks. We will have a much better sense of what the proper dosage should be and if there really are Age Reduction effects. Until then, I recommend the use of other Age Reduction methods, and not taking DHEA.

So, the scoop on hormone replacement therapy is: *yes* for women and *no* for men. Or, at least, *not yet* for men. Under no conditions should you take anabolic steroids unless they are specifically prescribed by a doctor. They are extremely dangerous, causing everything from cancer to extreme psychosis. If you take Age Reduction seriously, you should be especially careful to stay away from steroids because they add years—*many years*—to your RealAge. Most of all, when it comes to hormones, be an informed consumer. If a new treatment comes out and you're interested, ask your doctor if it's the right treatment for you.

THE ARTERIAL SYSTEM: THE ROAD TO YOUTH

The health of your arterial system is the most important gauge of your RealAge. Luckily, a wide variety of health choices can help you keep your arteries young. Reducing your blood pressure and preventing atherosclerotic build-up are essential for preventing arterial aging. Eating a diet low in saturated fats and rich in fruits and vegetables, exercising, reducing stress, taking the right vitamins, taking an aspirin a day, and, if you are a woman, working with your physician to find comfortable hormone replacement therapy are choices you can make to keep your heart and arteries young.

5

Immune to the Years

SLOWING AGING OF THE IMMUNE SYSTEM AND PREVENTING CANCER

As you age, so does your immune system, the system that protects you from diseases. Keeping your immune system young and strong helps keep cancer at bay. Cancer is the second leading killer in the United States and may soon surpass heart disease as number one. It is far easier to prevent cancer than to cure it. This chapter explains how cancer works and discusses strategies for prevention. A normally functioning immune system also helps prevent arthritis and even heart disease. Protecting your immune system can make your RealAge as much as six years younger.

- Prostate cancer kills more men than anything but heart disease and lung cancer: 250,000 new cases are diagnosed a year, and 40,000 men die from prostate cancer annually. Yet, in the war against prostate cancer, tomato paste—yes, that red stuff on pizza and pasta—and green tea may be a winning combination. These two simple substances can make your RealAge as much as 0.8 years younger.

  Difficulty rating: Moderately easy

- Although we read all the time about the risk of cancer from sun exposure, that doesn't mean we should avoid the sun altogether. To produce an adequate amount of vitamin D, we need to spend some time catching rays (or, as suggested in Chapter 7, taking vitamin D as a supplement). Vitamin D appears to strengthen the immune response and helps prevent certain kinds of cancers. Learn how to strike a balance between too much sun and not enough. Just taking simple precautions can make your RealAge 1.7 years younger.

  Difficulty rating: Moderately easy

• If you thought taking care of your teeth was just cosmetic, think again. By avoiding periodontal disease, you can make your RealAge 6.4 years younger. In contrast, people with acute periodontal disease are 3.4 years older than their chronologic age. Why? Because the bacteria that cause periodontal disease appear to trigger an immune response that causes inflammation throughout the body. A side effect seems to be inflammation of the arteries, a major precursor to heart disease. Although the exact cause and effect are not well understood yet, people who floss may live younger longer.

Difficulty rating: Quick fix

Now that you've read about how to prevent arterial aging, I know the next question you're going to ask. I hear it every time I give a lecture. "If we prevent arterial aging and lower our risk of heart attacks, strokes, and other forms of cardiovascular disease, won't we just die from something worse? 'The Big C'? Cancer? We've all got to die from something, don't we?"

Yes. We will all die sometime. But then again, why invite it? Although most of us feel that we are helpless in the face of cancer, just remember that 80 to 90 percent of cancers are linked to environmental causes. That means cancer isn't just fate, but something you can do a lot to prevent. How? By controlling your environment. Despite the recent stir about cancer genes, fewer than 10 percent of all cancers are linked to genetic inheritance. Although I can't say that 80 to 90 percent of cancer can be prevented, I can guarantee that by making yourself younger, you can stave off your risk of cancer by as much as twenty RealAge years. By controlling your environment, you can minimize the aging of the immune system, making your RealAge younger. Think of it this way: Although all of us have to die of something, there is no reason *not* to reduce your risk of getting cancer at calendar age fifty to that of the typical forty-year-old. You can choose to keep your immune system youthful and, by doing so, greatly reduce your risk of getting a life-threatening cancer or other disorder of the immune system.

If the cardiovascular system is the body's transportation system, the immune system is its security system. The immune system protects the body from outside invasion by locating and destroying potentially harmful bacteria and viruses. It protects the body against insurrection from within by rooting out cells that have become abnormal or malignant. As we age, our immune system begins to fail us. There are two fundamental ways in which your immune system can fail. It can become negligent, allowing abnormal cells— either infectious agents or cancer cells—to grow unchecked. Or it can become overzealous, turning on the body and attacking normal tissues, as occurs in such autoimmune diseases as many forms of arthritis, connective tissue diseases, and allergies. Since the immune system is so complex, it can go in both directions at once. Your immune system can be negligent—as in cancer—and overactive—as in arthritis—at the same time.

Protecting our cardiovascular system is relatively straightforward, but keeping our immune system in working order is more complex. The immune system is made up of millions of free-floating cells that roam the body in search of abnormalities. All these cells need to coordinate with each other to provide adequate protection. And the state of our immune system—the youth of our immune system—depends greatly on how well we care for it.

For example, we know that people who exercise have higher concentrations of certain immune system cells that identify and destroy potentially hazardous toxins and invading organisms. We know that taking antioxidants, such as vitamin C and vitamin E, helps improve the immune response. We also know that hazardous chemicals, too much sun, and radioactivity can age your immune system and increase your risk of cancer. Stress clearly weakens our immune response—the death of a loved one, for example, measurably decreases the number of T cells in a person's bloodstream for as long as a year after the event. And, of course, there is AIDS (acquired immunodeficiency syndrome), a disease that directly attacks the immune system. Throughout the following chapters, there will be sections that address aging of the immune system. Pay attention to the sections on this subject in the chapters on environmental hazards (Chapter 6), vitamins and supplements (Chapter 7), food and nutrition (Chapter 8), exercise (Chapter 9), and stress (Chapter 11) and learn how to make your RealAge younger by keeping your immune system younger.

CANCER: AN OUNCE OF PREVENTION IS BETTER THAN A WHOLE LOT OF CURE

Cancer is the most ironic of diseases. Except in rare cases, it is not caused by an invasion of some external agent, such as a bacterium or virus. Nor is it caused by wear and tear on the body or by parts breaking down. Rather, it is a disease of one's own body gone awry. Cancer begins with one cell that, instead of keeping in line with the cells around it, suddenly begins growing, dividing, and dividing again, forming a mass of malignant cells—a tumor. If the tumor gets large enough or spreads (metastasizes), it can be fatal. Cells are usually subsumed to the good of the organism, but when a cancer appears, the organism becomes subsumed to the cell.

Cancer is the second leading cause of death in the United States, accounting for 22 percent of all mortalities annually. More than a million Americans are diagnosed with cancer each year, and more than half a million die from cancer. Another 800,000 develop small *in situ* (noninvading) cancers and various mild kinds of skin cancers; both types, for the most part, do not spread and can be easily removed. These *in situ* cancers are not generally counted in the annual cancer statistics, but are cancers nonetheless. For women aged thirty-five to seventy-four, cancer is the leading cause of death. For men of the same age range, cancer is second only to cardiovascular disease as the leading cause of death. Despite the high incidence of cancer and the enormous amount of effort put into fighting it, cancer remains one of the most pernicious human diseases.

Even though newfound cancer genes have been the subject of much speculation, most cancers arise from our interactions with the world around us. Astoundingly, almost one-third of all cancers diagnosed in Europe and in the United States can be linked to tobacco use and account for more than 150,000 deaths in the United States each year. Food choices are thought to contribute to another third of cancers, especially stomach and colon cancers. People who eat diets that are low in saturated fats and rich in nutrients have a significantly lower incidence of cancer. Thinner people are at lower risk of breast, prostate, and uterine cancer, perhaps because such cancers are linked—at least some scientists postulate—to high exposure to the sex hormones estrogen and testosterone, and these hormones are stored in fat. People who drink excessively have higher levels of mouth and liver cancer. And people who have spent too much time in the sun, especially before age thirty, are more likely to develop skin cancer. Occupational hazards—exposure to such toxins in the workplace as asbestos and formaldehyde—account for about 5 percent of all cancers.

In the early 1970s, President Nixon announced a "War on Cancer," hoping that a big monetary investment and a redoubled effort by America's scientists would lead to the cure. Twenty-five years later, we are still not much closer to that cure. If a tumor is found early and can be removed surgically, it will not regrow in about 50 percent of the cases. Much of the time, treatment delays the spread of a cancer. Once a cancer has metastasized, the likelihood that radiation or chemotherapy will actually stop the disease is only about 10 percent—not especially promising. Although several new gene-targeting drugs and drugs targeted to stop the blood vessel growth that is necessary for the growth of tumors appear promising in stopping the spread of cancer, they are still in development and years away from being a standard treatment procedure. Indeed, the key words in cancer therapy today are *avoidance* and *early detection.* And "early detection" by no means compares with "cancer-free." Although someday there may actually be a cure that works, at present, the best way to fight cancer is to avoid getting it in the first place.

How are we to keep cancer at bay? There are two ways. First, by avoiding exposure to known cancer-causing agents, you can reduce the odds that a cancer will ever develop. Second, by taking steps to strengthen your immune system, you can better prepare your body to fight off any early cancer that does develop, destroying it before it even gets started.

Understanding Cancer: What It Is and How It Works

One of the reasons scientists haven't yet found a cure for cancer is that the causes are often extremely complex. In fact, the term *cancer* describes the phenomenon—the growth of tumors—and defines a general category that contains a broad range of diseases. Cancers can be caused by radiation, viruses, carcinogens, random mistakes in the cell cycle, an inherited genetic predisposition, or just plain chance. In many cases, cancers can develop because of a combination of factors. For example, although no one doubts that smoking increases the incidence of lung cancer—nearly 90 percent of lung cancers are linked to cigarette smoking—some smokers appear to be even more susceptible to cancer than other smokers. Some people appear to produce higher levels of the enzyme that makes smoke carcinogenic; thus, their genetic predisposition, combined with their behavioral choices, contributes to an even greater risk of lung cancer. This effect is a good example of how cancers can be caused by both environmental factors and inherited tendencies.

The risk posed by smoking can be compounded by other factors as well. For example, asbestos and radon are known carcinogens (cancer-causing agents). Smoking greatly amplifies the risk of either, since smokers have significantly higher sensitivity levels than nonsmokers to these carcinogens. Although nonsmokers exposed to asbestos are five times more likely to develop lung cancer, smokers exposed to asbestos are *ninety times* more likely to develop lung cancer! Cigarettes and heavy drinking are another volatile combination, causing more cancers and more aging when used together than either cause alone.

Now that I have told you that most cancers are brought about by environmental causes, I am going to seem to contradict that statement: *All cancers are genetic.* When I say that, I do not mean that they are hereditary, although they sometimes are. Five to 10 percent of all cancers are thought to stem from a strong predisposition to the disease inherited in our genes. The other 90 percent are caused by genetic *mistakes* that develop spontaneously over the course of a lifetime. Although a person can inherit a genetic tendency for a specific kind of cancer, the vast majority of cancers occur because of mutations in our DNA (deoxyribonucleic acid) that occur *after we are born*. We do not inherit these mutations, we accumulate them.

Cancer is a disease of our DNA, the substance that regulates the growth of the body, and that is contained in every cell we have. Think of DNA as your body's instruction book. It contains information that guides all your growth and physiologic changes from the time you are born until the day you die. Your DNA determines what color eyes you will have, how tall you will be, that you will have an arm where you are supposed to have an arm, and even that you will have arms instead of wings. You inherit your initial set of DNA from your parents—half from your mother and half from your father—when the egg and sperm fuse. Since each of our cells contains an identical set of DNA, as we grow, this DNA is duplicated with every single cell division. Each of us starts out as a single cell, but by the time we are adults, our bodies contain 75 trillion cells. That means trillions and trillions of cell divisions during your lifetime.

Cells fall into one of two basic types: germ line cells and somatic cells. Germ line cells are our reproductive cells—eggs in the female and sperm in the male. All the other cells in the body are somatic cells, which form more than 99 percent of the body. The somatic cells are living, changing cells; they grow, divide, die. As long as you are alive, your body replaces these cells continuously. During your lifetime, you replace virtually all the somatic cells in your body, except brain and nerve cells, thousands, if not hundreds of thousands of times. Your stomach lining, for example, is in an almost continual state of cell division, making new cells every day. Most cancers stem from mutations of somatic cells.

When a cell divides, the DNA in that cell is copied and passed on to the new cell. But the DNA in any one cell can become damaged. Pieces of the instructions on the genes can get knocked out or changed—mutated. If the mutation occurs in the wrong place—in an active gene, for instance—it can disrupt the function of the cell, causing it to die. Or it can cause the cell to begin dividing wildly, becoming a cancer.

We get mutations in two ways. First, mutations can arise through mistakes in the cell-division process. Second, mutations can occur when the DNA in a cell is damaged by an irritant like radiation or free radicals. In either case, these mutations, if they do not kill the cell, get passed on when a cell divides. How many of these mutations will you undergo in your lifetime? Probably millions.

If you consider the vast number of divisions necessary to maintain 75 trillion living cells, the chances are that sometime, somewhere, something will go wrong. And it does. Sometimes the DNA contained in each cell, which must replicate itself completely before each cell division, becomes damaged. Sometimes it doesn't copy correctly. When the cell divides, the new daughter cells can contain this error, a mutation.

Luckily, most of these mutations do not matter. They do not occur in sections of the DNA in which there are active genes or do not disturb the action of a gene. The body doesn't even notice them. In contrast, lethal mutations are so significant that they kill the cell right away, at which point the mutation disappears and is not passed on. Probably 99.9 percent of all the mutations you undergo belong to one of these two classes.

Between the harmless and the lethal mutations is a third class of mutations, a tumor-causing mutation. These are the rare cancer-causing mutations that tell the cell to begin growing and dividing uncontrollably. Your body has a regulatory system that keeps the number of cells in your body at a more or less constant level. The genes that regulate this process are known as cell-cycle genes because they tell the cell when to divide, to grow, and to divide again. Some of these cell-cycle genes are known as "proofreader" genes: they scan the DNA when it replicates, ensuring that no mutations have been acquired. If a mutation has occurred, the proofreaders either fix it or kill the cell. A few of these cell-cycle and proofreader genes are also known as oncogenes (cancer genes) because mutations in these genes are tied to the development of cancers. If a gene that is supposed to tell a cell to stop growing stops working—that is, mutates—then the cell grows uncontrollably, dividing faster than it should. Moreover, its daughter cells also inherit the mutation and grow out of control themselves. The effect multiplies, and soon there is a mass of rapidly dividing, quickly growing cells, a tumor, "the Big C."

Generally, your body is able to recognize abnormal cells and destroy them before they cause harm. By means of the proofreader genes and other anti-cancer genes, most abnormal cells are rooted out and excised. The general immune system also destroys many precancerous and early cancer cells. The exact mechanisms of this response are poorly understood: the immune system is not always able to recognize the differences between cancer cells and normal cells. However, it has long been known that people with healthier immune systems are less likely to develop cancers and that precancerous cells are often rooted out by the body. Research is increasingly showing the role that the general immune system plays in cancer prevention. Hence, your body prevents cancer by a double mechanism—one genetic, one immunologic. Cancers—the life-threatening kind—occur when a mutation develops, coupled with a failure of both protective systems, when each has "aged" too much to stop the cell from taking over as a cancer.

The longer you live—that is, the more divisions your cells undergo—the more likely it is that you will undergo a mutation in a cell-cycle gene. It's the law of averages. A mutation assaults your first line of defense—the line of defense within the cell that protects the body. By exposing your body to harmful chemicals, radiation, or the buildup of free radicals, you increase your rate of mutation exponentially. The odds that you will undergo a mutation in the wrong place increase dramatically.

As you age, your second line of defense, your immune system, tends to be less vigilant and does not as readily detect and destroy these abnormalities. The weaker your immune system, the more likely that it will not provide the necessary backup. The longer you live, the more likely that you will get improper cell divisions, the more likely that the DNA in a specific cell will contain a mutation, and the more likely that your immune system won't be there to catch a mistake. The most important thing to remember is this: You can slow, and even reverse, the rate of aging of the immune system.

The RealAge strategy for keeping your immune system young and avoiding cancer is twofold: (1) decrease your exposure to factors that increase DNA damage in your cells and (2) adopt behaviors that strengthen your immune response. You keep your RealAge young by avoiding exposure to factors that cause mutations and by boosting your immune system so it scavenges those mutations as well as possible. Doing all the things you can do to keep your immune system youthful can make your RealAge over twenty years younger.

Cancer Genes: What Do They Mean to You?

Although the vast majority of cancers are thought to stem from environmental causes, it is worth considering those people who have an inherited genetic predisposition to the disease. Almost every week a major news story reports the discovery of a new cancer gene. "Researchers have identified the breast cancer gene." "Scientists announce the discovery of the colon cancer gene." Most of these genes—or, more precisely, genetic mutations—run in families, isolated populations, or ethnic enclaves. They are mutations that lie in the germ line cells—that is, in the egg and sperm—and that get passed down from parent to child. They are often identified in populations that are endogamous, that is, in which people marry within the same group. The propensity for these specific genetic mutations occurs in such populations because the more closely related people are, the less their genetic variation. Since many of these mutations are recessive, appearing only when both parents are carriers, the trait is more likely to show up when both parents have a similar genetic background. Also, it is easier for researchers to trace genetic predisposition to a disease when they can trace a cultural and historical context, linking family histories with biologic events.

If you belong to a population that is at risk of a genetically linked cancer, the discovery of a gene can have an immediate impact. You can be tested for the gene to learn whether you have inherited it. Although this sounds ominous, and getting such tests can be frightening, there is a more positive way of thinking about it. By getting tested, you will know whether you have the gene. If you don't have it, you can quit worrying. If you do have it, you can minimize the risks *and the aging* it can cause.

If you do not belong to the group at risk, the news about cancer genes is less immediate but no less important. By identifying mutated forms of a gene, researchers are better able to understand what a gene does when it functions normally and they are better able to target specific gene pathways that are implicated in specific forms of cancer. By understanding the biochemical processes by which a cancer grows, scientists get closer to understanding how we might prevent such cancers. Because all cancers are genetic—whether they are caused by an inherited mutation or an acquired one—the more we learn about the genetics involved in the development of cancers, the better prepared we will be to treat all cancers—and to prevent them.

Another thing: Inheriting a cancer gene does not mean that you will get cancer—it means that you have an increased risk of getting that particular type of cancer. People who inherit a form of a gene that causes cancer in 100 percent of the cases rarely survive childhood. When scientists say that they have "found" a cancer gene, they mean that they have found a gene that, when mutated, increases a person's risk. For example, even though scientists refer to the recently discovered BRCA-1 gene as the breast cancer gene, they are not being accurate. No woman really has a breast cancer gene—a gene whose function is to cause cancer. Instead, she may have inherited a copy of a gene that contains a specific mutation affecting the ability of that gene to function properly. The side effect is to increase her predisposition toward breast cancer.

Many of the so-called cancer genes are two-hit genes. Because we inherit chromosomes (DNA) from each parent, in many instances we have two working copies of a particular gene. If one doesn't work, the other covers for it. In many genetically linked cancers, a person inherits a working copy of the gene from one parent and a nonworking copy from the other. The odds of that person getting an acquired mutation in the one working copy in a particular cell of the body are much higher than the odds for people who have two working copies of the gene. People with two working copies would need to get *two* acquired mutations—a mutation in each copy of the gene in the same cell—to develop the same cancer. Other cancers require two mutations in two different genes, or the same copy of a gene. One mutation usually won't cause the cancer, but two will. This is true, for example, with certain eye cancers called retinoblastomas. Because there are millions of cells in the eye, the chances of an acquired mutation occurring in any one cell is relatively high. The chances of two acquired mutations occurring in exactly the right places is relatively low. However, we know that certain people are born with one of the mutations already. Hence, the odds of their developing another mutation over their lifetimes are extremely high, making them genetically predisposed to developing this type of cancer.

Recently, inherited links have been discovered for certain types of breast and colon cancers, allowing us to identify people who are predisposed to developing each of these diseases. Such mutations account for a minority of all such cancers. For example, in breast cancer, genetic predisposition is thought to account for less than 4 percent of all cases. However, genetic predisposition is implicated in nearly a third of all breast cancers that develop in women under age forty, showing just how much having one of these genes can affect one's risk.

Testing positive for a cancer gene can make your RealAge dramatically older, as you would then have the same likelihood of developing cancer as a much older person. For example, a thirty-five-year-old woman who tests positive for the BRCA-1 breast cancer gene and whose mother and sister both developed breast cancer before age forty has a RealAge that is seventeen years older. That is, her RealAge would be fifty-two. By knowing she has the gene, she can make choices that make her RealAge younger. The dilemmas involved in this scenario are extremely complex, and individual counseling is recommended.

Identifying cancer genes is a big step for science. Unfortunately, this research is still in the beginning stages. The more we understand about genetically inherited cancers, the more we will understand about cancers in general. For example, the recent identification of a specific mutation in a gene linked to an increased risk of colon cancer among Ashkenazi Jews has helped researchers identify a gene pathway that is believed to be implicated in as many as 90 percent of all cases of colon cancer. That discovery opens numerous doorways for treatment and prevention. There are numerous other examples. The more we learn, the better prepared we will be to stave off the aging that cancer can cause.

What If You Get Cancer?
How Does It Affect Your RealAge?

No doubt some of you are cancer survivors and most of us know someone who is. How much effect does a positive diagnosis have on a person's RealAge? Well, that depends. Clearly, some cancers are much more harmful than others. They attack the body much more quickly and aggressively. On the other hand, some cancers grow slowly, resulting in little damage. The removal of a tumor, chemotherapy, radiation, and other therapies can often stop the spread of a cancer throughout the body. Some people have a tumor removed in their thirties and live until their eighties. The effect of the disease on your aging depends on the type of cancer you have, how it is treated, and how long you are free from cancer after treatment.

Let's use the breast cancer example again. A fifty-eight-year-old woman who has had a malignant lump removed from her breast without indication of significant spreading in the lymph nodes has a RealAge of sixty-five. If that same woman undergoes chemotherapy and still shows no signs of tumor growth in the next five years, her RealAge will shift from being seven years older to being only two years older. In general, the longer a person goes disease-free after treatment, the less effect a cancer diagnosis has on his or her RealAge.

The best thing, of course, is to avoid cancer altogether, and that means avoiding cancer-causing substances and strengthening the immune system so it can act as it did in your youth and effectively scavenge early cancers. By becoming as young as you can be, your immune system will be in better condition and more able to wipe out any possible cancer cells in your body. Fortunately, there are foods, supplements, and behaviors that can help you keep your immune system young.

Let's consider some of those elements. Diet, vitamins, exercise, and preventing stress are all key ways of slowing aging of the immune system. In fact, these are so important, I have devoted whole chapters to those topics. Here, though, let's consider three examples of immune system aging—prostate cancer, skin cancer, and periodontal disease. As diverse as they are, they have something in common—the failure of the immune system.

Let's start with prostate cancer. Here are two things that may help men prevent it.

JUST FOR MEN: TOMATO PASTE AND GREEN TEA HELP TO KEEP YOU CANCER-FREE

Ask any man what he fears most about aging, and he may tell you heart disease or cancer, but, in his heart of hearts, what he fears most is impotence. Impotence is psychologically and emotionally devastating. Since virility is a sign of youthful manhood, losing the ability to perform is something that makes men feel most acutely that their bodies are failing and that they are getting old. There are four major causes of impotence: arterial disease, stress, psychological upsets, and prostate problems. Of the four, prostate enlargement and cancers are by far the most common—and predictable—reasons for the loss of sexual function.

The prostate is a small gland at the base of the penis. As men age, the prostate tends to become enlarged and often cancerous. In fact, most older men show signs of having microscopic cancers in their prostates. The enlargement, from cancers and other causes (called benign prostate hypertrophy when it is not associated with cancer), can be painful and uncomfortable. A swollen prostate cuts off urine flow, increases the need to urinate, and often makes urination painful. Sexual performance can become limited. And that ages us— physiologically and psychologically. Although drugs can be given to reduce the size of an enlarged prostate, they are not especially effective and have side effects, such as impotence or an increased risk of cancer. Fortunately, there are ways of preventing prostate cancer and the aging it causes.

Prostate cancer is the most common cancer found in men. Some 250,000 new cases are diagnosed each year, and it causes 40,000 deaths annually—second only to lung cancer among cancer fatalities for men. More than 60 percent of men over age eighty will develop cancerous prostate cells. For those of us who plan to live into our eighties—healthily, heartily, vibrantly, and as young as sixty-year-olds—we need to be especially careful to protect ourselves from this kind of cancer. The best weapon against prostate cancer, or any cancer, is to avoid getting it in the first place.

Treatments for prostate cancer—surgery, chemotherapy, and radiation—are just as devastating as all cancer treatments but have an added side effect: Almost all the therapies are associated with a significant loss of sexual function in more than 50 percent of the cases. Despite this grim news, there is something that can give us hope—the tomato.

Tomatoes and Lycopenes

Studies have shown that the risk of developing prostate cancer is as much as one-third lower among men who frequently eat foods containing tomatoes or tomato paste than among men who rarely eat such foods. Men who eat tomato products ten or more times a week have significantly lower levels of prostate cancer—a 34 percent reduction in severe metastatic prostate cancers—than do men who eat tomatoes less than twice a week.

The reason appears to be the antioxidant power of tomatoes. A substance found in tomatoes—lycopene—apparently helps retard or reverse the aging of cells in the prostate that can promote cancer growth. Lycopene is one of several kinds of carotenoids that are known for their antioxidant properties (see Chapter 8). Carotenoids, pigments found primarily in yellow, orange, and red fruits or vegetables, are similar to vitamins in that they help facilitate specific chemical reactions. Unlike vitamins, we do not require them to survive. A key function that carotenoids perform is to attach to free radicals, packaging them so they can be washed out of the body and preventing them from damaging our cells and chromosomes. Since the prostate is especially vulnerable to damage from environmental factors, it is especially vulnerable to damage from free radicals. Hence, the importance of the antioxidant powers of lycopene.

A study investigating a wide range of populations in Hong Kong, Tokyo, Milan, New York, Chicago, and Albuquerque found that the incidence of microscopic prostate cancer was the same for all groups, no matter their geographic location or genetic heritage. The chances that these microscopic cancers would develop into full-blown prostate cancer varied wildly across locations, with the number of fatalities due to prostate cancer differing significantly. The areas of the world with the lowest levels of severe, or metastatic, prostate cancer are Mediterranean countries, especially Greece and Italy—where tomato-based foods are central to the diet. In areas where tomato-based foods are not common, the risk of cancer increased markedly.

A long-running question about prostate cancer has concerned the increased risk of the disease for African American men. It is interesting to note that studies have found that African Americans are less likely to eat tomato-based foods. Although no studies have been undertaken to show with certainty that dietary differences account for the higher incidence of prostate cancer for this population group, the data suggest that such could be the case.

Tomato paste, raw tomatoes, and cooked tomatoes all contain lots of lycopene. Our bodies, however, cannot absorb lycopenes except in the presence of fat. Drinking a glass of tomato juice by itself or eating slices of raw tomato without salad dressing does not provide us with lycopene. Some experts question whether we can absorb lycopene from raw tomatoes even in the presence of fat. Tomatoes cooked lightly in oil—as in tomato paste or pasta sauces—result in a two- to threefold rise in lycopene concentrations in the bloodstream the day after ingestion. In contrast, people who drink lots of tomato juice do not show this rise in lycopene levels because the juice lacks the fats that help the body absorb the nutrients. Although slight cooking appears best, raw tomatoes with a little olive oil, sun-dried tomatoes in oil, and probably even tomato juice eaten with a bit of cheese or other fat may also increase lycopene levels.

Studies have found that most men get their lycopene from tomato sauce on pizza. Although that is certainly one way of getting lycopene, pizza with cheese, not to mention pepperoni and sausage, tends to be extremely high in saturated fats. Ways of getting tomato products without so much fat include eating tomato sauces on pasta, eating a roasted tomato with a drizzle of olive oil as a salad, eating tomato-based soups, putting salsa on meats or salads, and even eating ketchup (see Table 5.1).

TABLE 5.1

The RealAge Effect of Tomatoes

FOR MEN

	Servings of Tomato-Rich Foods Eaten Per Week*				
	Less than 1	1 to 3	4 to 7	8 to 10	More than 10
Calendar Age			RealAge		
35	35.3	35.1	35	34.9	34.8
55	55.7	55.2	55	54.8	54.3
70	70.8	70.3	70	69.6	69.2

*A serving is the amount of tomato paste on one slice of pizza.

FOR WOMEN

A diet rich in carotenoids—the antioxidants found in tomatoes and other red, yellow, and orange vegetables—has many beneficial effects for everyone. Therefore, even though women cannot receive the lycopene benefit for prostate cancer, they should still eat a diet heavy in carotenoid-rich fruits and vegetables (see Chapter 8).

Lycopene appears to have other benefits as well. A 1997 reanalysis of the data gathered in the historic EURAMIC study found that men and women with the highest levels of lycopene in their bodies had the lowest risk of arterial aging. Although there has only been one study to date, the reduction in mortality from atherosclerosis was 65 percent. Translated into RealAge terms, that would make ten helpings a week of tomato paste produce more than a five-year younger benefit for the average fifty-five-year-old man.

If you are trying to build up lycopene levels in your blood, do not eat potato chips or other foods containing the new fat substitute olestra (brand name, Olean). This fat "fake" leaches fat-soluble vitamins, such as D and E, from your system and dramatically reduces the amount of lycopene in the body. One study found that eating just six olestra chips every day for a month reduced the amount of lycopene in the body by 40 percent, and eating sixteen chips a day reduced lycopene by as much as 60 percent.

Green Tea: A Cure for Prostate Cancer?

Another substance that appears promising in the prevention of prostate cancer is green tea. Several East Asian studies found that men who consume large amounts of green tea appear to have lower rates of prostate cancer. Studies at the University of Chicago have isolated the hydroxy "8" molecule in green tea that retards prostate cancer in laboratory animals. This molecule is reputed to be one of the most powerful antioxidants yet discovered, even more powerful than vitamins E and C. However, the green-tea molecule is notoriously fragile. The freezing and dehydration processes that imported green tea must undergo destroy the chemical compound that is linked to the reduction of the growth of prostate cancer cells. Unfortunately, to get any benefit from green tea, a person must drink as much as fifty cups a day. So far, there are no commercially available pills containing the green-tea extract in its proper form. While doubt remains, green-tea extract may well be an aid in preventing prostate cancer. Keep your eyes open for any new information on the subject. An extract supplement may be available soon if the studies continue to show promising results. Other preliminary research indicates that green tea—and black tea, too—may have other cancer-fighting abilities.

In both examples of the prevention of prostate cancer, a nutrient in our diet can affect our risk of getting cancer. Eating is one way we interact with our environment and one way we can lessen the impact of environmental factors on our risk of developing cancer. Another environmental cause is, as most of us know, sunshine. How exactly does the sun age you?

SUNNY SKIN:
HOW MUCH SUN IS TOO MUCH?

There is no temptation like the sun. Although that tan may look great now, we all know that in the long run, it can cause wrinkling and, worse, skin cancers. Wrinkles not only make you look and feel older than you want to be, but are actually signs of skin damage and aging. Wrinkles show that your skin, one of your most important organs, is losing the elastin that keeps it young and healthy. Some forms of skin cancer make your RealAge significantly older very fast.

Everyone needs some sun each day. Sun allows our bodies to turn specific kinds of food-derived cholesterols into vitamin D, an important nutrient that helps decrease aging of the cardiovascular and immune systems. In turn, the liver and kidneys convert vitamin D into vitamin D_3, the active form of the vitamin. In fact, ten to twenty minutes of sunlight a day appears to be the optimal amount of exposure to the sun that each of us needs and can make your RealAge 0.7 years younger. If you do not get some sun every day, substitute vitamin D daily (see Chapter 7). Studies on mood elevation show that sunlight and exposure to broad-spectrum light help improve our mood. Seasonal affective disorder (SAD) and other types of depression can be improved by exposure to sunlight. So, some sun is good, but how much sun is too much?

In general, your risk of skin cancer is determined by how much sun exposure you received in your youth. People who had severe sunburns as children are at much higher risk of skin cancers than those who never burned. Since most skin cancers are slow to develop, the sun exposure you get later in life is less damaging than the exposure you get in childhood. That doesn't mean you shouldn't be careful. If you plan to be in the sun for more than ten or twenty minutes a day, you should take precautions.

Exposure to ultraviolet light not only ages your skin by destroying elastin and promoting wrinkles, but also damages the chromosomes in your skin cells. Chromosomes are the strands of DNA contained in each cell in your body. If you look through a microscope at sun-damaged skin cells, you can see actual breaks in the chromosomes where they have been damaged by solar radiation. This chromosomal damage can lead to cancers. Amazingly, the sun can even damage the chromosomes in cells not directly exposed to sunlight.

There are essentially three major kinds of skin cancers: basal cell cancers, squamous cell cancers, and malignant melanomas. Ninety percent of the roughly 400,000 reported cases of skin cancers each year are either basal or squamous cell cancers. Although these forms are rarely fatal and can usually be removed surgically without major repercussions, they are often disfiguring. In contrast, malignant melanomas are very serious and can be fatal. Approximately 34,000 cases of malignant melanomas are reported each year. Although Caucasians suffer skin cancers at somewhat higher rates than Asians, Hispanics, or African Americans, anyone can get skin cancers. More important, skin cancer rates are increasing annually among all population groups.

People who are at a particular risk are those with a family history of skin cancers and those who were excessively exposed to the sun, especially those who had severe burns, during childhood. If you have moles or a family history of moles, you need to be especially attentive to skin cancers. Look for changes in the color, size, or shape of moles. If you note any changes, see your doctor immediately. A mole that looks irregular, has variable colors, or is larger than a quarter of an inch in diameter should be examined by your doctor. Do self-examinations regularly. And have a family member, spouse, or friend check the places that are hard for you to see for any suspicious moles or changes in moles.

Use sunscreen. If you plan to be in the sun for more than twenty minutes, you should use a sunscreen of at least SPF-15. SPF stands for "sun protection factor," and the number fifteen means that you get fifteen times the level of protection that you would get if you wore no sunscreen at all. Everyone under the age of thirty should use at least that level of protection, no matter how long he or she is in the sun. Likewise, SPF-30 means you get thirty times the protection. But SPF is only the beginning. More important, you need broad-spectrum protection.

There are three kinds of ultraviolet (UV) rays. Ultraviolet A (UVA) rays, the rays with the longest wavelength, are the rays that cause you to tan. They are the safest of the ultraviolet rays but can cause cancers and definitely promote wrinkles. Ultraviolet B (UVB) rays are somewhat more dangerous and are the most common cause of sunburn and skin cancers. Ultraviolet C (UVC) rays—those with the shortest wavelength—are the most dangerous, causing high rates of cancers. Luckily, the ozone layer blocks out most of these UVC rays, although in such Southern Hemisphere countries as Australia and New Zealand, where the ozone layer is damaged, you need to be particularly careful and use sunscreen that protects against exposure to UVC.

Different sunscreens use different chemicals to block out rays. Some use PABA; others use benophenones or parisol 1789. Each composition is better than the others at blocking a particular type of UV ray. Studies on albino rats show that mixing all three—thus getting protection from all the kinds of UV rays—provides the best overall protection. Consider using two or three different sunscreens at once, a PABA-based one, a benophenone-based one, and a parsol 1789–based one. If you are going to be out a long time, you should also use zinc oxide on areas particularly vulnerable to skin cancers, like the lips and nose. If you are planning on exercising or being in the water, make sure to apply water-resistant products or, better yet, waterproof products. Finally, apply products liberally and often. The consistent use of sunscreen helps preserve your skin, preventing skin cancers and wrinkling.

Don't think that you need to cover only your face. Skin cancers can appear anywhere on the body, even on areas that have not had excessive exposure to the sun. Although cancers are more likely to occur in areas that the sun has reached, it has recently been shown that too much sun can cause cancers anywhere on the body. For example, construction workers who get tan only on their necks and arms can develop skin cancers on parts of their bodies that have never been exposed to the sun.

Finally, avoid tanning beds, which emit a lot of UVA rays. Remember that

TABLE 5.2

The RealAge Effect of Sun and Vitamin D

FOR MEN

	Daily Sun Exposure and Vitamin D			
	No sunburn blisters; 10 minutes of sun per day or 400 IU of vitamin D per day	No sunburn blisters, no regular sun, and no vitamin D	Blisters, but only after age 30	Blisters prior to age 30
Calendar Age	RealAge			
35	34.9	35.2	35.4	35.9
55	54.7	55.3	55.6	56.4
70	69.6	70.3	70.7	71.5

FOR WOMEN

	Daily Sun Exposure and Vitamin D			
	No sunburn blisters; 10 minutes of sun per day or 400 IU of vitamin D per day	No sunburn blisters, no regular sun, and no vitamin D	Blisters, but only after age 30	Blisters prior to age 30
Calendar Age	RealAge			
35	34.9	35.2	35.4	35.8
55	54.9	55.3	55.5	56.1
70	69.8	70.3	70.7	71.3

UVA rays cause wrinkling. If you decide to use a tanning bed, do not expose yourself for more than ten minutes a day and wear a physical block sunscreen like titanium dioxide or zinc oxide on such vulnerable areas as the lips, nose, ears, and shoulders. If you insist on having a tan, consider using the no-sun tanning cream dihydroxyacetone. It poses no known risks, and most experts believe that it is safer than baking in the sun.

So, remember, some sun is good (see Table 5.2). It helps to promote the production of vitamin D and to prevent certain kinds of depression. Just be careful about getting too much sun. Overexposure can make your RealAge 0.9 years older. Also, don't neglect to take vitamin D supplements and to eat a diet rich in vitamin D (see Chapter 7) because the sun probably won't give you enough.

Now that we've talked about cancers and environmental risk, let's consider other kinds of immune system aging. Did you know that flossing your teeth is one of the best and easiest ways to keep your immune system young?

KEEP SMILING:
KEEPING YOUR TEETH—
AND HEART—YOUNG

If I asked you to list things that mark the transition to old age, I bet that the word *dentures* would be near the top of the list. In all the cartoons and stereotypes, the typical "old" person wears dentures. Tooth loss, through cavities and disease, makes us feel and look old like almost nothing else. But it's not just our vanity that's at stake. Dental disease and tooth loss don't just make us *look* older, they *make* us older. Indeed, periodontal disease can make our RealAge more than 3.4 years older.

Two major studies and another smaller study confirm that the presence or absence of cavities doesn't seem to make a difference in your overall health or longevity, although cavities do lead to dentures faster. The presence of gum disease, called gingivitis, or diseases that destroy the underlying jawbone, called periodontal diseases, do affect the rate of aging. These studies show that the presence of periodontal diseases, diseases most common in people with tooth loss, actually affects longevity. The best of these studies, done at Emory University in conjunction with the Centers for Disease Control, indicated that people with gingivitis and periodontitis have a mortality rate that is 23 percent to 46 percent higher than those who don't. When translated into RealAge terms, these dental diseases make you more than 3.4 years older. Why? They are linked to increased rates of cardiovascular disease and strokes, as well as to an increase in mortality from other causes, such as infections. Conversely, the absence of periodontal diseases makes you 6.4 years younger than the median person. Table 5.3 shows the effect of dental disease.

TABLE 5.3
The RealAge Effect of Dental Disease

FOR MEN

	Gum Disease and Tooth Loss			
	No Disease	Gingivitis	Periodontitis	Periodontitis and Tooth Loss
Calendar Age	RealAge			
35	33	34.6	36.1	37
55	52.4	54.4	56.6	56.6
70	63.6	69.5	73.4	73.6

FOR WOMEN

	Gum Disease and Tooth Loss			
	No Disease	Gingivitis	Periodontitis	Periodontitis and Tooth Loss
Calendar Age	RealAge			
35	33.7	34.6	36	36.9
55	52.7	54.7	56.3	56.3
70	65.4	69.5	73	73.2

When I first read these studies, I couldn't believe the findings. Why would dental health affect arterial health? I've never been one to savor a visit to the dentist, and I had always regarded dental health as primarily a cosmetic issue. We want healthy teeth because a nice white smile looks good. I assumed that the correlation between dental disease and higher death rates was due to confounding factors: I assumed that people with other bad health habits—smoking, overeating, too much alcohol consumption—would also be more likely to develop dental disease. But I was wrong, very wrong. Flossing your teeth daily can make your arteries younger. The probable reason: Flossing helps keep your immune system young. For example, men under age fifty who have advanced periodontal disease are 2.6 times more likely to die prematurely and three times more likely to die from heart disease than are those who have healthy teeth and gums. Why would this be so?

Although the data remain sketchy, a plausible hypothesis is that the same bacteria that cause periodontal disease also trigger an immune response, inflammation, that causes the arteries to swell. The swelling of the arterial walls results in a constriction of blood flow that can lead to a higher incidence of cardiovascular disease. Inflammation and constriction cause a buildup of lipid deposits along the arterial walls. Furthermore, this inflammation destabilizes already existing plaques. Indeed, a bacterial strain commonly found in tooth plaque has also been found in the fatty deposits that can clog your arteries. Other studies have shown that periodontal disease leads to a higher white blood cell count, which is an indicator that the immune system is under increased stress.

Hence, it appears that the same plaque that causes tooth decay—the sticky coating of bacteria, salvia, and food deposits—also needlessly ages both your immune system and your arteries. Whether the arterial-swelling theory is true, my "confounding-factors" theory was disproved. All the major studies done on dental disease and longevity had adjusted for the very confounding factors I was worried about, such as smoking, alcohol, and cholesterol levels, and still found a distinct relationship between the incidence of periodontal disease and a shortened life span. Poor oral hygiene and particularly increased tooth loss are important indicators of your risk. (The fewer teeth you have, the greater your risk of gum infections.)

What should you do to prevent this unnecessary aging? Do the things you already know you should do. Brush your teeth with a fluoride toothpaste several times a day, especially after eating. (Some studies suggest that it may be more effective to brush with no toothpaste, but these findings are still preliminary.) If you cannot brush after a meal, chew sugarless gum instead. When you brush, make sure to brush your tongue, to get rid of bacteria that can cause gum disease and bad breath. Also, floss every day. Flossing is perhaps the most important thing you can do to prevent periodontal disease and the element of our daily routine that we are most likely to skip.

Other factors that appear to increase the incidence of periodontal disease are smoking and stress. So there's yet another incentive to quit smoking and to learn to manage stress (see Chapter 6 for smoking and Chapter 11 for stress). Finally, go to the dentist at least once, but preferably twice, a year to have your teeth cleaned and examined. And keep smiling, because each time you floss, you are making yourself younger.

THE IMMUNE SYSTEM: THE FINAL WORD— OR JUST THE BEGINNING

This chapter has been an introduction to the immune system. The rest of the book tells you even more about the aging of the immune system and, more important, what you can do to prevent it. More and more, we are learning that our choices and behaviors change this rate of aging. *All of us can do things to keep our immune systems strong and young, and there's no better way to prevent cancer and the myriad other autoimmune diseases that age us.*

6

Environmental Hazards

JUST BECAUSE IT'S A TOUGH WORLD OUT THERE DOESN'T MEAN IT HAS TO MAKE YOU OLD

Living young means living smart. And that means planning ahead to avoid situations that can cause aging. Simple decisions like choosing the nonsmoking section of a restaurant or having safe sex help you to stay young. Accidents and unintentional poisonings are the third leading killer in the United States. Even though we don't equate traffic, domestic, or work-related accidents with aging, they can temporarily or permanently disable you and cause a decline in your quality of life. In RealAge terms, accidents will age you. Environmental toxins—whether from cigarettes, pesticides, or air pollution—are major contributors to cancers and other diseases. Learn to be proactive in spotting potential dangers before they make you older. Whether it's quitting smoking, avoiding drugs, or having safe sex—lots of it!—you can help keep yourself young. Learning how to live safely in the world around you will make your RealAge as much as twelve years younger.

- No surprises: Smoking makes you get old fast. Indeed, smoking can add eight years to your RealAge. Secondhand smoke causes aging, too. Just one hour in a smoke-filled room is the equivalent of smoking four cigarettes. Whatever the source, smoke increases your risk of heart and lung disease, weakens your immune system, and is a proven carcinogen. If you're a smoker, learn tricks that can help motivate you to quit once and for all. Celebrating "year-younger" parties, taking walks at lunchtime, and making bets with other "quitters" can help you resist the urge. Learn how to manage the roller coaster of stopping and starting while on your way to becoming smoke-free. The RealAge benefit of quitting smoking: You get back seven of the eight years that smoking has taken from you. Heavy exposure to secondhand smoke can age you almost seven years, too.

Difficulty rating: Most difficult

- Eighty percent of all accidents are avoidable. Taking proper safety precautions in everything you do, whether at home or on the job, can help make your RealAge one to six years younger.

Difficulty rating: Moderately easy

- What, you ask, do seat belts and helmets have to do with staying younger? By taking routine safety precautions, like wearing a seat belt when driving, or wearing a helmet when biking, you can make your RealAge 0.6 to 3.4 years younger. Although avoiding accidents has nothing to do with biologic aging per se, it has a lot to do with the length and quality of our lives.

Difficulty rating: Quick fix

- Air pollution, exposure to toxic chemicals, and living in houses with high levels of radon or asbestos can increase your cancer risk to the level of someone five to ten years older. Learn how to recognize potential environmental hazards and how to avoid exposure to toxins that can make your RealAge 2.8 years older.

Difficulty rating: Moderately difficult

- Sex and drugs, the symbols of wild youth, can keep us young or make us old. Fast. By enjoying sex within the confines of a mutually monogamous relationship or practicing safe sex during casual sexual encounters— avoiding high-risk partners and knowing their sexual histories, and always using a condom, and using it correctly—you can make your RealAge as much as 0.9 years younger. Better still, having lots of sex may prevent aging even more. Having sex more than once a week, the national average, can reduce your RealAge, too. Although these data are preliminary, several studies indicated that having sex frequently is associated with a RealAge that is two to eight years younger. By not using drugs and seeking counseling if drug use is a problem, you can make your RealAge more than eight years younger.

Difficulty rating: Moderately easy to difficult

Anything that keeps you healthy keeps you young. You don't exist outside the world but in it, and everything with which you come in contact affects the rate at which you age. The three leading causes of death and disability are arterial aging; immune system aging; and environmental hazards, such as accidents and unintentional injuries. It is easy to understand how damaging your arteries or weakening your immune system may make you older. But how do preventing accidents, avoiding environmental hazards, and reducing the risk of injuries keep you young?

Environmental factors affect your health and the length of your life much more than inherited genetics do. Your environment consists of everything that is not the body itself: the air you breathe, the city or town you live in, the food you eat, and the people you know. Learning to navigate through the world around you so it doesn't harm you is one of the keys to staying young. And that means using some common sense.

Although we don't tend to think about things like wearing seat belts or bicycle helmets as factors related to aging, I think they should be regarded as such. The aging caused by accidents isn't cumulative but sudden. Many accidents, particularly auto accidents, are fatal—and these fatalities can often be avoided. This is the kind of "instant aging" all of us hope to avoid. An injury from an accident can trigger a chain reaction in which you give up other Age Reduction strategies as well. For instance, you get into a car accident. Because you don't wear your seat belt, you injure your back. That prevents you from staying active and exercising. When you quit exercising, you gain weight, so your cholesterol and stress levels increase and your arteries begin to show signs of age. The injury prevents you from keeping active and involved. All of a sudden, you are living the life of someone much older. Just because you forgot to buckle that seat belt.

The same is true for toxins in the environment around us. Whether it's cigarette smoke in the office or radon in your home, these toxins can lead to increased aging. Avoiding exposure to known carcinogens, whether they are pesticides or asbestos, can help keep you young longer. Not smoking, abusing drugs, or having unprotected sex are all behaviors you can adopt to keep yourself from aging too fast. By choosing to protect yourself against the risks you face in the world around you, you are building your own youth-protection plan.

TOBACCO:
WHERE THERE'S SMOKE, THERE'S FIRE

Not even the tobacco companies deny it: Smoking kills. There is not a soul who doesn't know smoking is bad for health, not a soul who doesn't know that it causes cancer and lung disease. Smoking can be blamed for nearly half the premature deaths each year, more than four hundred thousand. Smoking remains the greatest public health hazard we face.

Even if it doesn't kill you, smoking will make you older. A lot older. The effects are not something that show up thirty years down the line. Smoking makes you older right now. Today. You see it as new wrinkles in your face; tobacco smoke ages the skin prematurely. You notice it as shortness of breath; smoking decreases the amount of oxygen that gets to your cells, causing them to age faster than they should, causing emphysema and a high incidence of respiratory illnesses. You also feel it as a loss of stamina and energy. Smoking damages your cardiovascular system, causing high blood pressure and clogging of the arteries.

If you look at the American population as a whole, smoking makes us more than 250 million years older than we need to be. At 350 billion dollars in settlements, the tobacco industry is getting off cheap. If we valued each year of life lost to cigarettes at fifty thousand dollars, the tobacco companies would owe us fifty times that amount. If you're a smoker and have a pack-a-day habit, stop right here and add eight years to your RealAge. Think you're fifty? How does fifty-eight sound? Think you're forty? Try forty-eight on for size. Even if you smoke just four cigarettes a day, barely any at all, your RealAge is 2.6 years older. Even if you don't smoke, but live with a smoker or work in a smoke-filled environment just four hours a day, your RealAge is almost seven years older.

To start smoking is easy, to quit is hard. Cigarettes are both physiologically and psychologically addictive, and the habit is very hard to kick. That's why nearly one out of three Americans smoke—some 33 percent of men and 28 percent of women—continue to smoke despite the warnings and despite repeated attempts to quit.

If everyone stopped smoking tomorrow, 30 percent of all cancer-related deaths, 30 percent of all cardiovascular disease-related deaths, and 24 percent of all pneumonia- and influenza-related deaths would be eliminated. Unfortunately, it's not easy. Of the 50 million Americans who smoke, 70 percent want to quit, and more than a third of them try each year. Only about 3 percent actually succeed.

Why? In large part, because of the highly addictive nature of cigarettes. But that is only part of it. We often see the risk of cigarettes as something far off in the future. "It may hurt me some day, but what's one more cigarette today?" smokers often say. That's the wrong way to think about it. Thinking about the diseases or risks associated with smoking makes the job of quitting too onerous.

Instead, start thinking about smoking as a choice—a choice you make about how fast you will age. Every cigarette you smoke is a choice you make to get older faster. Every cigarette you don't smoke—every time you fight that urge and win—is a choice you make to get younger.

As I mentioned in Chapter 1, I first developed the RealAge concept to help a friend quit smoking. Those eight extra years caused by smoking were enough to make him sit up and take notice, and he kicked the habit. In the past thirteen years, Simon has gone from a RealAge that was fourteen years older than his calendar age (when all factors, including smoking, were considered) to one that is five years younger than his calendar age. Back then, he was forty-nine with a RealAge of sixty-three; now he's sixty-two with a RealAge of fifty-seven. And the effect: He lives younger now than he did thirteen years ago, with much more vigor and energy than he ever could have imagined. If you are a smoker and give up the habit, you will get younger, too. (See Table 6.1.)

Miraculously, the effects of smoking are largely reversible. Although smoking a pack a day makes a person eight years older in RealAge, the cessation of smoking can win back seven of those years. The net effect of being a *former* smoker is that a person is only about one year older in RealAge. And the benefits of not smoking start almost immediately. Within just twelve hours of quitting, the body begins to get younger. Carbon monoxide levels decrease, and the blood can carry more oxygen to the cells in the body. In only a few weeks, damaged nerve endings in the mouth and throat begin to regenerate, and the bronchial tubes begin to open.

Go just two months without a puff and you can celebrate your first year-younger party. After five months, you pass the point where you feel worse because you quit, since the nicotine cravings subside, and you start feeling better overall. The immune system will show signs of being stronger. You will be at a lower risk of getting colds and other kinds of respiratory tract infections. The gain: two years younger. Within eight months, your lungs will be clearer and your stamina will increase. After one year of not smoking, you will be three years younger. How's that for a New Year's resolution? Three years younger in just one year. In two years, your risk of having a heart attack and stroke will decrease considerably, and after five smoke-free years, your level of arterial aging will return almost to that of people who have never smoked. The risk of developing cancer and other forms of immune system aging will equal the average risk of nonsmokers. Another way of saying it is this: If you give up a pack-a-day habit, you will become a year younger (and can celebrate year-younger parties) at two, five, eight, thirteen, twenty-two, thirty-two, and sixty months from the time you quit.

When Mary Jane came to run the library in my department, she had been a smoker for thirty-five years. Her smoking habit was causing her enormous harm. She was asthmatic, diabetic, and sixty pounds overweight. Her once-

TABLE 6.1

The RealAge Effect of Smoking

FOR MEN

| Calendar Age | History of Smoking* | | | | |
	Never Smoked	Ex-Smoker	1–19 Pack-Years	20–39 Pack-Years	40 or more Pack-Years
			RealAge		
35	34.2	34.9	38.8	39.5	40
55	53.7	54.6	58.6	61.3	61.7
70	68.3	69.4	77.0	77.6	79.8

FOR WOMEN

| Calendar Age | History of Smoking* | | | | |
	Never Smoked	Ex-Smoker	1–19 Pack-Years	20–39 Pack-Years	40 or more Pack-Years
			RealAge		
35	34.1	35.2	38.8	39.8	40.3
55	53.9	54.9	59.7	61.2	61.5
70	68.5	69.8	75.7	79.8	80.4

*The "pack-year" quantifies a person's history of smoking in terms of the number of cigarettes smoked per day and the number of years smoking occurred at that rate. For example, if you smoked, on average, one pack of cigarettes a day for five years and then two packs a day for eight years, your history of smoking would be $(1 \times 5) + (2 \times 8)$, or 21 pack-years.

an-hour run for a smoke outside had slowed to a walk, with lots of pauses to catch her breath. She also routinely missed more than her allotted number of sick days, suffering recurrent bouts of upper respiratory tract infections.

As often as she considered the idea of quitting, she couldn't actually quit. Many mornings she'd say, "I'm never going to smoke again." Usually by the next day, she'd be puffing away again. Then she found she needed to have a major operation. Her diabetes and asthma were both out of control, and her health was in a crisis state. Finally, she decided she had to quit. "In life you have to make choices. I had to make the choice: Was I going to live or die? When you realize that the alternative is dying, quitting's not that hard."

Mary Jane had her doctor prescribe nicotine patches and pills that helped ease her cravings. She walked a lot. She avoided situations in which she knew she might encounter smokers.

Giving up smoking was one of the hardest things Mary Jane ever had to do. Those first few months were especially difficult. Today, she hasn't even had a puff in more than three years. No longer smoking made her RealAge six years younger. And this is not even the best part. She's also managed to get her diabetes and asthma under control, and she lost sixty-five pounds. "I feel one hundred percent better," she told me proudly. "I can't imagine going back to smoking again."

We celebrated Mary Jane's first year-younger party just two months after she smoked her last cigarette. A year later, at her third year-younger party, the department gave Mary Jane some of those days she used to take as sick days as vacation days—her reward for all the new energy she was putting into her job and for sticking to her commitment to kick the habit once and for all.

Beyond the Smoke Screen: How Smoking Ages You

If you're a smoker, you don't want to hear preaching. You know it's bad for you. Maybe you've even tried to quit. Most of all, you're tired of the self-righteous attitude that nonsmokers can have. I don't blame you. My intent isn't to preach, but to give you the facts and let you decide. That's how I've helped seventeen of the last eighteen smokers I've worked with kick the habit. I'll simply present the studies and explain scientifically how smoking ages you. The choice to quit is yours, and all the credit for quitting will be yours, too. The whole point of RealAge is that the age you are—how young you are and can be—is in large part controlled by you.

So, what are the facts? How, exactly, does smoking cause the body to age? Smoking affects the whole body, aging all of its major systems and organs. It causes arterial and heart disease and is responsible for more than 80 percent of all deaths from heart disease in those under fifty. And, of course, as we all know, it causes cancer, lung disease, and emphysema. In addition, smokers have more colds, cases of pneumonia, and other infections than do nonsmokers.

Smoking and Cardiovascular Disease

To understand the physiologic effects of tobacco smoke, let's consider one example—cardiovascular disease. For decades, doctors have known that smokers suffer considerably more heart attacks than nonsmokers. Heavy smokers are at ten times the risk of a heart attack as nonsmokers. Studies have reported that as many as 40 percent of all stroke victims are smokers. How exactly does smoking cause cardiovascular aging?

Cigarettes contain more than four thousand identifiable contaminants besides nicotine, which is generally considered to be the addictive component in tobacco. Since cigarette smoke increases carbon monoxide levels in the blood, the delivery of oxygen to the heart and other tissues decreases. Cigarette smoke also inhibits the ability of the breathing tubes to clear secretions properly, increasing the number of infections.

As I discussed in the chapter on arterial aging, the elasticity of the arteries (their ability to dilate) is directly tied to their youthfulness. The more elastic your arteries, the younger you are. Components of tobacco smoke inhibit the ability of the arteries to dilate. When exposed to the contaminants in cigarette smoke, the arteries are unable to expand properly and remain unnecessarily narrow, a condition that increases the likelihood that they will become clogged. Why does this happen? Scientists speculate that the toxins in cigarette smoke damage the lining of the arteries (the endothelium) and may inhibit the body's production of the chemical component that allows the arteries to expand when the flow of blood increases—for example, when you're exercising. Even in "passive smokers"—people who don't smoke but are often exposed to secondhand smoke—the ability of the arteries to dilate is less than 50 percent of that in people who are never exposed to tobacco smoke. But this is just the beginning.

To make matters worse, smoking also increases the amount of atherosclerotic plaque, the fatty buildup that clogs arteries. Exposure to the toxins in cigarette smoke makes the platelets in the blood more prone to clotting. As if all that were not enough, studies have found that plaques are more likely to rupture suddenly in smokers than in nonsmokers. If a plaque ruptures, it can create a rough surface on which a clot can form or flow through the bloodstream, potentially causing a heart attack or stroke. In addition, the nicotine in cigarette smoke, when present in the bloodstream, raises blood pressure, significantly affecting the rate at which the arteries age. For reasons that are unclear, smoking reduces the level of HDL ("healthy") cholesterol in your bloodstream.

One study found that women who smoked a pack and a half a day had five to seven times the risk of heart attack as women who had never smoked. But don't kid yourself: No level of smoking is safe. Even women who smoked only one to four cigarettes a day had a risk of heart attack that was 2 1/2 times higher than that of nonsmokers. Keep in mind that the impact of cigarette smoking is not gender specific: Both men and women suffer from the arterial aging smoking causes.

Smoking and Cancer

Then, of course, there's cancer. Lung cancer is the most common cause of deaths from cancers, accounting for 34 percent of the fatal cancers in men and 18 percent of the fatal cancers in women. Smoking can be blamed for nearly 90 percent of all lung cancers in the United States and more than 130,000 deaths from lung cancer deaths annually. Among the four thousand chemical compounds that are commonly found in cigarettes, more than 40 percent are known to interact directly with DNA to cause genetic changes that lead to cancer.

Many of the components of tobacco smoke are oxidants, which increase the number of free radicals in the body. Free radicals, you will remember, are the waste products of "oxidant" metabolism that have extra or unbalanced electrons that damage our organs and DNA. These free radicals accelerate aging by causing premature cellular aging and by promoting cancers. Exposure even to low amounts of cigarette smoke can measurably increase the amount of free-radical damage to the DNA within your cells. For example, in animal studies, dogs that were exposed to the smoke of just one cigarette—not enough to increase their heart rates, blood pressure, or other physiologic measures—had twice the amounts of free-radical damage as dogs not exposed to cigarette smoke. Hamsters exposed to the secondhand smoke equivalent of just six cigarettes a day had twice the number of antioxidant enzymes in their lungs—an indication that their bodies were gearing up to repair significant free-radical damage.

Tobacco ages the immune system in two ways. First, it contains toxins that damage DNA, causing cancers. And, as I mentioned in Chapter 5, two protective systems fight aging of the immune system and cancer in particular. Smoking knocks both of those systems out of kilter, making the immune system less vigilant about catching cancers. And it is not just lung cancer. Smoking increases the risk of mouth, throat, kidney, and bladder cancers, as well. A Danish study found that women who had smoked for more than thirty years were 60 percent more likely to develop breast cancer than nonsmokers.

Some people seem to be more susceptible than others to the carcinogenic effect of smoke because they have higher levels of specific enzymes that activate the carcinogens contained in smoke. Nitrosamines, by-products of cigarette smoking, interact with the body's own enzymes to create a new chemical that is highly carcinogenic, or damaging to DNA. Some people have much more or much less of the human acetylator enzyme that helps the body remove certain carcinogens from the body. The people who produce less of this enzyme than others, called "slow acetylators," are predisposed to breast cancer, as well as other kinds of cancer. Don't bank on the fact that you may have better genes for fighting cancer. The ingestion of any tobacco products, whether through smoking, chewing, or inhaling secondhand smoke, increases immune system aging.

Smoking and Emphysema

To add to the list of dangers associated with smoking, it is also the primary cause of emphysema, the premature aging of the lungs. More than 2 million people in the United States (and possibly many more than that) suffer from emphysema, the fourth leading cause of death in the United States. Emphysema occurs when the air sacs in the lungs die. Scientists have long suspected that emphysema is caused by an autoimmune response, a chemical reaction in the smoker's body that causes the body to kill its own lung cells and air sacs. Normally, the immune response is well gauged to react to the low-level assaults of everyday living. The immune system habitually kills off single cells that show signs of distress. When the lungs are exposed to the constant irritation of cigarette smoke, this normally protective system overreacts. When many, many cells show signs of distress, the body begins to kill off its air sacs en masse. And when many of the cells needed for taking in oxygen and expelling carbon dioxide are gone, the smoker is barely able to breathe.

Smoking and Other Aging Effects

As if cardiovascular disease, cancer, and emphysema were not enough, smoking has been tied to other kinds of aging effects as well. For example, since smokers have a decreased immunity to disease, they suffer many more respiratory infections. Smokers were more than twice as likely as nonsmokers to become impotent or unable to experience orgasm, and report reduced sexual pleasure. Heavy smoking also leads to an increase in macular degeneration, an eye disease commonly associated with old age, at a rate more than 2 1/2 times that of nonsmokers. Smokers are twice as likely to get diabetes, and diabetics age at twice the normal rate if the disease is not properly managed (see Chapter 12). For people with mild thyroid disorders (more than 10 percent of Americans), heavy smoking can trigger failure of the thyroid gland, seriously raising cholesterol levels and further accelerating arterial aging.

Unfortunately, smoking amplifies other risk factors disproportionately. For example, in families with a history of heart and arterial disease, smokers have fifteen times the risk of heart attack as nonsmokers from the same families. When people with high cholesterol levels are compared, the smokers have thirty-five times the rate of heart attacks as the nonsmokers. Alcohol and cigarettes are another deadly combination: People who drink alcohol and smoke are at a much higher risk of mouth, throat, and liver cancers than people who do either one or the other. Alcohol causes the body to make enzymes that metabolize tobacco smoke into highly carcinogenic substances.

Not a very pleasant picture, is it? By triggering all these responses in the body, cigarette smoking is triggering an aging response. Most of what I have just described is probably a restatement of facts you already know, but there is still the big sticking point that keeps most smokers smoking: How do you beat the addiction?

No More Cigarette "Buts": Kicking the Habit

If you are really serious about quitting, this book is probably just the beginning. Or, better said, one more beginning. For most smokers, quitting is an on-again, off-again routine. You stop. You struggle with it for a few days, weeks, or months. Then the craving gets you, and you decide, "What's one cigarette?" You light up, and you're back to square one, a smoker once again. Since this book is about the effects of aging, rather than the techniques for beating an addiction, I am not going to go into all the details here. There are many, many services and information sources that help smokers quit—everything from high-priced inpatient clinics to free support groups at community centers. If you are serious about quitting, talk to your physician, search for smoking-cessation programs and support groups in your area, buy a few books about kicking the habit, and consider nicotine patches or chewing gum and pills to help ease your cravings. Different methods work better for different people. Thinking about quitting in terms of aging may be just the ticket for you: Eight years is a lot of time to give up to just one habit.

There is no question that cigarettes are psychologically and physiologically addictive. For example, laboratory mice used in smoking studies learn what times of day they will be exposed to smoke and race expectantly to the side of the cage where the smoke comes out at the appointed hour. They need their smoke! To be fair, it's hard for me even to imagine what it's like to quit since

I've never been a smoker. But having watched friends and my patients struggle through it, I know that it's a major battle. People who successfully quit and stay away from cigarettes deserve a lot of credit.

Years of research on cigarette smoking have brought us closer to understanding the biochemical processes by which the body becomes addicted to nicotine. Brain-scan studies have shown that smoking triggers a release of dopamine in the brain. Dopamine, a chemical that dulls the body's response to pain and makes you feel pleasure, is involved in everything from muscle control to emotional state. Many addictive drugs, including cocaine and even caffeine, trigger a dopamine reaction, too. The more you smoke, the more your body adjusts to a higher level of dopamine release. These elevated levels become your body's normal state. When you quit, the body goes into withdrawal. The question is, How can you beat the cravings long enough for your body to readjust to its smoke-free state?

If you are a typical smoker, you will quit smoking. Again. And again. And *again*. You will kick the habit, start up anew, and then have to kick it all over. Almost no one can quit in one try. But don't become disheartened—just keep trying. One of the problems with quitting is that at first you feel worse. For the first several weeks, you feel intense cravings and, since nicotine is a stimulant, rather sluggish. After a few weeks, those feelings will subside. Just stick to your guns.

Only 2 percent of smokers can successfully quit the first time. Using nicotine patches doubles the success rate to 4 percent. One study found that combining the patch with anticraving pills boosted the effectiveness to almost 60 percent. In my own practice, the success rate has been much higher—seventeen of the last eighteen patients who tried to quit did so. Many had been pack-a-day smokers for a decade or more. By combining the patch and the pills with RealAge planning, they stopped smoking and started getting younger. (For my patients, I prescribe bupropion—100 mg of the slow-release formula of Wellbutrin, twice daily, the dosage adjusted to body weight. Three days later, I advise them to apply a nicotine patch, throw away all cigarettes and cigarette items, and begin additional exercise. Talk to your doctor about the best regimen for you.)

If you are a smoker, don't try to quit "cold turkey." See your doctor and develop a plan. Ease the physiologic cravings by getting patches and pills and ease the psychologic urge to smoke by developing a support system that will keep you away from cigarettes. And don't forget to include "year-younger" parties in your plan: You need to celebrate your successes.

Changing little day-to-day habits can make quitting easier. For example, increasing the amount of exercise you get helps reduce the craving for cigarettes. Avoid environments where smokers congregate and, instead, frequent places where smoking is prohibited—museums, libraries, or theaters. Regimented programs provided by smoking-cessation clinics and community support groups give some people the willpower and supportive environment they need to stop smoking.

Smoking and the Weight Gain Blues

One of the biggest fears that people have about quitting smoking is the weight gain that often follows. On average, men gain about ten pounds within six months of quitting, and women, about eight pounds. Weight gain should be the least of your worries. The risk of smoking is far greater than the risk of being overweight. And the weight gain is often temporary. For example, women commonly lose six of the eight pounds that they gained in the first six months within the next eighteen months. With careful planning you can prevent the weight gain altogether.

Here are some tips:

- Chew sugarless gum. It can help ease the oral cravings.

- Have lots of chopped vegetables and low-fat snacks on hand. Popcorn without butter is good to munch on. Fruits, especially small ones like grapes or berries, are another great snack.

- Integrate regular exercise and walking into your daily routine. It will help fight the cigarette urge, as well as help keep off the weight.

- Don't quit smoking during the holidays. All that rich food will only increase the temptation to overeat.

- Find something to do with your hands. Many smokers find comfort in having something to hold. Buy yourself a bunch of desk gadgets or other objects to fiddle with and divert all that nervous energy.

- When you feel the temptation to smoke, close your eyes and take a deep breath. Remember all the reasons you quit smoking in the first place. Keep a list of those reasons and add the new benefits of being a reformed smoker to the list as you discover them: more energy, fewer colds, years younger.

- Don't downplay your accomplishment. Reward yourself for quitting. You deserve those year-younger parties. Buy yourself a present or give yourself a special treat. Being smoke-free is something to celebrate.

Other tips: Stay busy. It will help keep your mind off cigarettes. Also, throw away all cigarettes and smoking paraphernalia. Avoid coffee, alcohol, and other drinks or food you associate with smoking. Instead, drink lots of water, fruit juices, and herbal teas. Eating small meals instead of one big one keeps blood sugar levels constant, which helps quell the nicotine craving. Avoid behaviors and situations you associate with smoking. If you used to smoke after meals, try to do something else at that time— take a walk, do the dishes. Do positive things that boost your self-image. Go to the dentist and have your teeth cleaned. Have your smoky-smelling clothes cleaned at the dry cleaners. *Reward yourself.*

If you start smoking again, don't become disheartened. It's not a catastrophe, just a temporary setback. Remember that each time you quit, the easier it will be to quit the next time. And each time you'll get closer to your goal.

One final note: It's never too late to quit. In fact, the older you get, the more important it becomes to quit. Smoking causes relatively more aging among smokers aged forty to seventy-five than younger ones. Smoking is to aging what putting the gas pedal to the floor is to driving. Smokers in their fifties have more than seventeen times the risk of having a major health event than smokers in their thirties because the rate of smoking-induced aging has accelerated. That acceleration is measurable at least through age seventy-five. (Beyond that age, there may not be enough smokers still living to say with any accuracy what happens to aging.) Even if you've smoked for ten, fifteen, or twenty years—or especially if you have—you should quit. Do not think, "Well, I've smoked this long, why quit now?" Quit now, precisely because you've smoked this long.

Cigar Smoking

Cigars have become the new chic. In the past several years, cigar smoking has tripled in the United States; more than 3 billion cigars were sold in 1996 alone. Cigar bars are opening all over the country as baby boomers take up a habit that was once reserved for the "old fogy" set.

Since cigar smokers smoke less frequently and do not inhale to the same degree, they believe they are at a lower risk than cigarette smokers. But they are wrong. Cigars are a particularly dangerous form of tobacco. They produce more carbon monoxide and more particulate matter than cigarettes do. Just like cigarettes, they produce benzoapyrene, hydrogen cyanide, and ammonia. Cigars produce more particulate matter, making them more dangerous, not just for the smoker, but for those around him or her as well. Cigars produce a more toxic form of secondhand smoke than cigarettes, so don't think that sitting in that cigar bar without smoking is not doing you harm. Although cigar smokers claim not to inhale, this claim is often untrue. Most former cigarette smokers continue to inhale when they take up the cigar habit.

Cigar smokers are at greater risk of cancers of the lip, mouth, pharynx, and esophagus than cigarette smokers and at about six times the risk of nonsmokers. Such cancers are often fatal and, even when nonfatal, can age and disfigure you. No comments, please, about long-lived cigar smokers like Winston Churchill or George Burns. Although we don't know why these people lived so long (good genes or good habits), we do know that other cigar smokers, such as Babe Ruth and Ulysses S. Grant, died young from throat cancers caused by cigar smoking. Smoking one cigar a day makes your RealAge 2.6 years older. Smoking five cigars a day makes your RealAge eight years older.

Passive Smoking

You should not tolerate an environment in which you are exposed to passive smoke. If you live with a smoker, ask that person to go outside to smoke. You'll be giving the message that it's time to quit. Although it may feel like you're being intolerant or uncaring, what you're really saying is that you care enough to make it a whole lot of hassle to smoke. Remember, you're not doing you or your partner any good when you become the passive recipient of that person's smoking habit.

If people smoke around you at work, talk to them to see if there is a way for them to smoke somewhere far away from you. Generally, a solution can be worked out. If your office doesn't have a provision to ensure that you are not exposed to secondhand smoke, talk to your boss or office manager about implementing some kind of policy to ensure a smoke-free environment. If there appears to be no solution to the workplace smoking problem, talk to your local board of public health or Better Business Bureau to find out if there is a city or state no-smoking ordinance. The federal Americans with Disabilities Act requires employers to provide a work environment that will accommodate employees having a variety of disabilities. That means employers must provide a smoke-free environment if they have employees who have either asthma or allergies to smoke.

If you work in certain environments—restaurants or bars, for example—it may be hard to avoid secondhand smoke. See about installation of air filters that recycle the air and decrease particulate matter. This will be good not only for you, but for all the customers, even the smokers.

To minimize your exposure to secondhand smoke, avoid smoke-filled bars, and at restaurants ask to sit in the no-smoking section. Many hotel chains now offer no-smoking rooms, and car rental companies offer no-smoking cars. If you spend more than four hours a day in a smoke-filled environment, your RealAge may be as much as 6.9 years older.

Smokeless Tobacco

Dip, chew, spit? More than 5 million Americans use smokeless tobacco, and its use is on the rise. Over the past twenty-five years, its use has increased ten-fold, making it the fastest-growing segment of the tobacco market.

Many tobacco users think they are avoiding the risk of tobacco by using it in its smokeless form, as snuff or chewing tobacco. They are wrong. Although the risk of lung cancer is lower among people who use chew or snuff, the risk of other cancers is considerably higher.

Smokeless tobacco causes mouth and throat cancers, dental problems, cardiovascular disease, and nicotine addiction, just like smoking does. And just like smoking, it's hard to kick the habit. In fact, the amount of nicotine and other chemicals found in the blood of people who chew is even higher than that found in the blood of smokers.

ACCIDENT PREVENTION: PROTECT YOUR YOUTH

In 1994, approximately 150,000 Americans died from injuries; 61 percent of these deaths were considered accidental, and 80 percent of those accidental deaths were preventable. For American adults age thirty-five to forty-five, accidental poisoning (primarily drug overdoses), motor vehicle accidents, and firearm accidents are the first, second, and third major causes of death, according to a report by the National Center for Health Statistics. Motor vehicle accidents are the third leading cause of death among Americans under age sixty-five, resulting in over 45,750 deaths and 500,000 serious injuries each year.

Although we tend not to think of avoiding accidents as something we can do to stay young, it is a quick and easy way to do just that. Not only do we risk death in traffic accidents and such accidents as falls (the second leading cause of accidental death), the injuries we sustain are likely to cause aging because they can make us less mobile, less likely to be active, and more prone to chronic pain. And accidents not only directly cause physical disability and impairment from the injury, they also cause aging from stress.

As a doctor, what I find maddening about the accident statistics in the

United States is that so many accidents are preventable. For example, drunk driving is a leading cause of car accidents, accounting for about 40 percent of all traffic deaths and 9 percent of all injuries (see Chapter 10 on alcohol use and abuse). Although we all know better than to drink and drive, too many of us still do so. The cost of a cab is nothing compared with the cost of your life. But we persist. The question is, Why tempt fate?

I ask that question every time I see a patient who gets hurt because a loaded gun was stored in the house. Or because he thought it would be a good idea to climb out on the roof to clean the gutter but slipped and fell. Or when I see someone in a cast from a ski injury received when playing the daredevil. Although so many accidents are one of a kind in their particulars, they often have something in common: no common sense. If that little voice in your head says, "Don't do it," don't do it. If something "feels" risky, don't risk it. Promptly fix potentially hazardous situations. Don't let the accident-waiting-to-happen become the accident that happened. It's one of the best ways to keep yourself young.

Remember, it's not just at home but at work, too, that you need to pay attention to safety. Most Americans between twenty-two and sixty-five (more than 120 million of us) spend 40 percent of their waking hours at work. Most jobs carry a certain amount of risk from accidental injury. Whether it's the risk of developing carpal tunnel syndrome from typing at a computer or lung cancer from breathing toxic fumes in a factory, your job can be dangerous. Each year, 6,500 Americans die from work-related injuries, and 13.2 million suffer non-fatal injuries. Think about the risks you face on the job and what steps you can take to avoid them. Make choices that help protect your youth. No job is worth getting older for.

These are the general statistics, but what about the particulars? What safety advice should you follow? Let's consider the biggest cause of accidents: transportation. Whether it's a car, bike, or motorcycle, you can get younger while getting from here to there.

Seat Belts: Buckle Up, Youngster!

As an anesthesiologist, I think about car safety all the time. Every month, I see the victims of auto accidents as they are rushed into the operating room for emergency surgery, clinging to the last thread of life. Perhaps nothing brings it into focus like seeing one of your own there. This past summer, a colleague of mine almost died. Her child did die. A summer vacation in the mountains that should have been perfect but wasn't. It was raining, and the road was slick. Their rented van was winding up a curvy mountain road when a flash flood hit. The van hydroplaned and plummeted over a precipice. Everyone in the van was wearing a seat belt, except my colleague and her child, who were thrown from the van. The child was killed, and my colleague suffered serious internal injuries and broken bones. The fact that she survived at all was a miracle. No one wearing a seat belt was hurt at all.

This is a shocking story that has a very real point. The moral is to buckle your seat belt. It can save your life. And it will make you younger. A recent study estimated that seat belts and air bags reduce a person's risk of severe injury by 61 percent. Simply using a three-point seat belt—one that crosses over both the lap and shoulder—reduces your risk by as much as 45 percent.

Because seat belts have a proven safety record, most states now require that you wear one whenever you are riding in a car. Strap on a seat belt every time you get in a moving vehicle, whether it's your car or a cab or anything else with wheels. Wear a seat belt even if you are sitting in the backseat and make sure that every seat belt has both a lap and a shoulder harness. Keep all seat belts in good working condition. If you have an older car, make sure that the seat belts are up to standard, even if you have to replace the old ones. If you are under 5 feet 2 inches tall, have a small frame, or have children who regularly ride in the car, check to make sure the shoulder harnesses fit properly. If they don't, go to a service dealer and have them adjusted. Don't deliberately slip out of the shoulder strap, either. The shoulder strap significantly reduces the amount of damage to internal organs that would occur if you get into an auto accident.

Also, have your car inspected annually or every five thousand miles. Have the oil, tires, and engine checked. If you are about to go on a long trip, have a mechanic look the car over to make sure it's in good working order. Finally, by making safety a priority when you shop for a car, you are choosing to get younger. Look for cars with a strong safety record. It's worth a little more money for the added youth protection such a record provides.

New cars are required to have air bags. If your car doesn't have them, consider trading it in for a car that does. Air bags reduce the risk of death by 9–16 percent among drivers who use seat belts and by as much as 20 percent among drivers who do not wear seat belts. Experts estimate that air bags have prevented some 1,600 fatalities from head-on collisions over the past six years.

Despite the recent furor over air bags, they still, car per car, accident per accident, save lives. The concern has been that, in rare instances, air bags have deployed rapidly, hurting and even killing the passengers they were supposed to protect. Air bags have been shown to pose risks for only two groups: young children and adults (almost exclusively women) who are shorter than 5 feet 2 inches. Almost all of the adults who died in accidents involving deployed airbags were not wearing seat belts.

Another auto safety youth rule: Drive within five miles an hour of the speed limit; it can keep you three years younger in RealAge. Although it sounds easy, this one is far easier said than done. In developing the RealAge concept, I have run hundreds of people through the computer program that calculates their RealAge. At the end of the run, the computer gives a RealAge reading and makes suggestions for reducing that age even further. A vast majority of people who have taken the test admit to speeding on a regular basis. When the computer asks them if they would be willing to modify their behavior, most of them say, "No way!" Indeed, more people say that they would rather give up smoking than speeding! It is amazing that so many people refuse to budge on this one: Slowing down and staying close to the speed limit is a reliable way to keep your RealAge younger. Indeed, for drivers under age thirty-five, the most frequent cause of auto accidents is speeding (see Table 6.2). For drivers over age seventy-five, the most frequent cause is unsafe or ill-timed left turns against traffic. Finally, if you can do so, use a cell phone only when you are not driving. Using a cell phone while driving focuses your attention on the conversation; this diversion of attention increases the accident rate.

Motorcycles: Don't Forget the Helmet

We associate motorcycles with wild youth. The truth is, few things can age you so quickly. Five seconds is all it takes to go from "young" to "dead." A motorcyclist is thirty-five times more likely to be killed on the road than the typical car owner. And it is not surprising that most motorcycle deaths and serious trauma come from head injuries. Emergency room doctors have been known to refer crudely to motorcyclists as "organ donors" because so many victims arrive at the emergency room brain dead, the rest of the body's vital organs intact. Although it sounds harsh, the point is well taken. The risk of death aside, motorcyclists who do survive accidents often endure injuries that are disabling or crippling, including paralysis from spinal cord injury, loss of limbs, and severe and multiple fractures.

Although that youthful urge to hit the road may grab you, choosing to ride a motorcycle is choosing to get older. If you do decide to ride one, try to avoid roads with lots of traffic, go at moderate speeds, wear protective clothing, and make the most important choice for youth—wear a helmet. Comparisons of helmeted and nonhelmeted riders have found that the use of helmets decreased the number of fatalities by as much as 27 percent and that nonhelmeted drivers had two to four times the number of head injuries. Helmets

TABLE 6.2

The RealAge Effect of Speeding

FOR MEN

| Calendar Age | Driving the Following Miles Over the Speed Limit | | | |
	Less than 5 mph	5 to 9 mph	9 to 14 mph	15 mph or more
	RealAge			
35	34.8	35.7	36.6	43.1
55	54.9	55.2	55.3	59.2
70	69.8	70.1	70.2	72.7

FOR WOMEN

| Calendar Age | Driving the Following Miles Over the Speed Limit | | | |
	Less than 5 mph	5 to 9 mph	9 to 14 mph	15 mph or more
	RealAge			
35	34.8	35.3	35.5	42.1
55	54.9	55.1	55.1	56.9
70	69.8	70	70.1	71.2

don't make motorcycle riding safe, just safer. After California passed a mandatory helmet law, serious head injuries from motorcycle accidents decreased by 34 percent. In the year after passage of a helmet law in Texas, the number of motorcycle fatalities due to head injuries decreased by 57 percent, and the number of severe injuries to the head in motorcycle accidents declined by 54 percent.

Other safety tips: Keep your headlights on at all times. The risk of fatal day-time crashes decreases by 13 percent simply by keeping the lights on. You should also wear heavy leather boots and such thick clothing as heavy jeans and a leather jacket when riding, to keep your arms and legs covered. This habit helps prevent injury to the feet, legs, and arms. I was shocked to learn from a television sports producer who had covered motorcycle races that professional motorcycle racers rarely finish their careers without losing at least part of a foot. That's not something to look forward to as you age.

Of course, never ride a motorcycle when under the influence of drugs or alcohol. True to the rebel image we associate with motorcycle riders, the rates of driving under the influence are much higher for motorcyclists than for those who drive cars and other types of motor vehicles. More than half of those injured in motorcycle accidents have elevated blood alcohol levels, and more than 40 percent test positive for marijuana use.

Bicycling: A Hardhead for Youth

So you think that taking your bike out for a ride will help lower your RealAge? Indeed it will. You burn more than 450 calories an hour just riding at a moderate pace. Incorporating this type of stamina-building exercise into your life can reduce your RealAge by as much as six years (see Chapter 9). On that same bike ride, you can do something else that will help make you even younger. Wear a helmet. Wearing a helmet can help make your RealAge 0.4 years younger than that of nonhelmeted riders (when calculated at a rate of fifty days per year of bike riding).

Each year more than half a million Americans end up in emergency rooms because of bicycle accidents. Head injuries account for one-third of these emergency room visits, two-thirds of the hospitalizations, and three-fourths of the deaths. And cyclists who suffer head injury are twenty times more likely to die than are those who are injured elsewhere. A recent study found that the use of helmets by bicyclists reduced the risk of head injuries by as much as 85 percent and reduced the risk of brain injury by more than 88 percent. The "take-home message"? Choose youth. Wearing your helmet will help reduce your risk of injury and will keep your RealAge young.

Does wearing a helmet mean that you won't get a head injury? No. But it does make it less likely. Communities that have promoted extensive bike-safety education and encouraged the use of helmets have seen a 50 percent increase in the use of helmets and a corresponding decrease in head injuries requiring emergency or hospital care. In the event you do bump your head, with or without a helmet, see a doctor. Many cyclists who fall and hit their heads but don't have any other injury requiring medical care, often do not go to the doctor. Remember, head injuries can be very serious and often don't produce symptoms right away, sometimes not for months or even years. If you receive a hard knock on the head, it is always best to have a physician look you over.

Also, if you have an accident while wearing a helmet, replace the helmet. Even though it may not look damaged, it might be. Many manufacturers have a crash-protection guarantee, agreeing to replace a helmet for free if you are in a crash. Once you buy a helmet, treat it carefully. The helmet can be damaged by extremes of hot and cold. Consider replacing your helmet every five years because helmets can begin to deteriorate internally with time and use. The quality of helmets has improved so much in the past five years that we can assume that the helmets manufactured five years from now will provide even better protection.

Finally, take these extra safety steps for youth: Make sure your bike is in good working order. Have it tuned up regularly and make sure that you have good tires; that the brakes work; and, of course, that the bike fits you properly. Try to ride on bike paths and avoid roads with heavy traffic. Wear reflective clothing when you ride on roads where there is automobile traffic, especially at night, and have reflectors or lights on the bike itself. You might even consider getting a light for the back of your bike. If you're biking to reduce your RealAge, you might as well take a few steps to make your RealAge younger still.

Other Precautions: Making Safety an Issue

Driving, motorcycling, and biking are obvious activities in which we might get injured. Other activities have risks, too. If you participate in an adventure sport—whether downhill skiing or scuba diving—make sure you have the proper equipment and proper training. No matter what the activity, if there is a reasonable chance of a head injury, wear a helmet. If you play a racket sport or basketball, wear eye protection. All you have to do is look at professional basketball players with their wraparound glasses or professional bikers with their helmets on to know that the people at the top take safety seriously. Even sports like in-line skating require safety precautions. Enter an emergency room on any nice spring Saturday afternoon, and you will see it packed with skaters who forgot to put on their knee pads, wrist guards, and helmets. Boating accidents are another common source of injury, often because people forget that drinking-and-driving rules apply to the waterways, too.

THE AIR YOU BREATHE: AGE POLLUTANTS

According to a report published in 1991 by the Environmental Protection Agency (EPA), 164 million Americans, fully two-thirds of the population, live in areas where the air quality does not meet federal air-quality standards. That means that the majority of us are affected by aging that is due to pollution. Just how much? That depends on where you live.

The effects of pollution are difficult to quantify because air quality varies so much from area to area, even block to block, and day to day. If one were to generalize about the effect by determining the difference in deaths from all causes in areas with heavy pollution versus areas with little pollution, the

TABLE 6.3

The RealAge Effect of Air Pollution

FOR MEN

	Of Exposure to the Following Concentration of Air Pollution Particles per Cubic Meter of Air (µg/m³)*				
	Less than 9	9 to 15.5	15.6 to 20.7	20.8 to 28.4	More than 28.4
Calendar Age	RealAge				
35	34.2	34.7	35	35.2	35.4
55	52.8	54.4	55	55.2	55.6
70	68.8	69.2	70	70.2	70.7

FOR WOMEN

	Of Exposure to the Following Concentration of Air Pollution Particles per Cubic Meter of Air (µg/m³)*				
	Less than 9	9 to 15.5	15.6 to 20.7	20.8 to 28.4	More than 28.4
Calendar Age	RealAge				
35	34.5	34.7	35	35.1	35.3
55	53.0	54.6	55	55.1	55.5
70	68.9	69.3	70	70.2	70.7

*In these tables, the concentration of air pollution has been expressed as the amount (in micrograms) of particles that are smaller than 2.5 microns in diameter, per cubic meter of air (µg/m³). You can obtain the numbers for your specific area by consulting the PM-10 pollution numbers at the Web site of the Environmental Protection Agency (www.epa.gov/oar/oaqps/greenbk/pr/state.html) or the 1996 publication of the National Resources Defense Council: *Breathtaking: Premature Mortality Due to Particulate Air Pollution in 239 American Cities* (see Web site www.nrdc.org/nrdcpro/bt).

TABLE 6.4

The Ten Worst Metropolitan Areas in the United States (1990–94)

Highest Concentration of Air Pollution (PM-10s or smaller)

	Average Annual PM-10 Concentration ($\mu g/m^3$)
Visalia-Tulare-Porterville, California	60.4
Bakersfield, California	54.8
Fresno, California	51.7
Riverside–San Bernardino, California	48.1
Stockton, California	44.8
Los Angeles–Long Beach, California	43.8
Phoenix, Arizona	39.5
Spokane, Washington	38.7
Reno, Nevada	38.5
Las Vegas, Nevada	38.3

Highest Annual Per Capita Death Rates Attributable to Air Pollution

	Deaths Per 100,000
Visalia-Tulare-Porterville, California	123
Bakersfield, California	122
Fresno, California	115
Riverside–San Bernardino, CA	95
Stockton, California	93
Los Angeles–Long Beach, California	79
Steubenville, Ohio/Weirton, West Virginia	78
Las Vegas, Nevada	76
St. Joseph, Missouri	76
Phoenix, Arizona	74

Other cities and areas among the top fifty for premature deaths attributable to particulate-matter air pollution include: Spokane, Washington (ranking, 14); Cleveland, Ohio (20); Reno, Nevada (20); Tampa–St. Petersburg (22); Philadelphia (25); Pittsburgh (28); San Diego, California (28); Providence, Rhode Island (32); Omaha, Nebraska (34); St. Louis, Missouri (34); Chicago (37); Detroit (37); Nashville, Tennessee (37); Atlanta, Georgia (44); and Mobile, Alabama (46).

Data pertain to 1990–94 and were taken from the 1996 publication of the National Resources Defense Council, *Breathtaking: Premature Mortality Due to Particulate Air Pollution in 239 American Cities* (see Web site www.nrdc.org/nrdcpro/bt for a more comprehensive listing).

RealAge difference would be 2.8 years. That statistic, though, can be misleading, as different health effects are brought about by different pollutants. (In addition, heavily polluted areas may have other kinds of factors that affect mortality as well, like higher population density or increased crime.) Nevertheless, pollution appears to have a measurable aging effect. The different kinds of pollutants include sulfates, ozone, large particulate matter, small particulate matter, lead, asbestos, and aerosols.

Air pollution can aggravate arterial and respiratory problems. A study published in the *British Medical Journal* found that changes in the level of air pollutants, specifically ozone and black smoke, led to an increase in mortality from all causes, primarily because of an increase of as much as 5 percent in cardiovascular and respiratory aging. Air quality may also significantly influence the development of asthma, a disease affecting as 15 million Americans. Researchers suspect that some people have a genetic predisposition to asthma, which manifests when the body is confronted by the wrong stressors. Asthma rates are increasing in intensely urban areas, such as in the inner cities of New York and Chicago, suggesting that poor air quality may trigger the onset of the disease. Air quality also affects the number of sinus infections and respiratory illnesses people suffer.

Air quality is measured in particulate matter (PM). The higher the concentration of particulate matter of a certain size, the more likely you are to suffer from premature aging from heart and lung disease. The smaller the particle, the more potentially injurious. Particles that are 10 microns (PM–10s) or less in diameter are the most easily (and therefore the most commonly) measured particles for analysis of air pollution. (See Tables 6.3 and 6.4.)

Air pollution does not occur only outdoors. Generally, it has been shown that indoor air pollution parallels that of the air outside. Sophisticated air-filtration systems don't seem to make much difference. Sometimes the indoor air quality is actually worse. "Building sickness," essentially a malady caused by poor indoor air quality, is a real illness. Those who work in poorly ventilated buildings have more respiratory infections and complain of fatigue, headache, and nausea more often. If you work or live in a building you think could be causing you health problems, have the building checked.

A particularly notorious indoor pollutant is radon, a naturally occurring gas that is a known carcinogen. Radon, the product of decaying radium and uranium in the soil, seeps into houses from the ground below. A 1995 report in the *Journal of the National Cancer Institute* estimated that exposure to radon contributed to as many as 10 percent of the deaths from lung cancer. A more recent report by the National Research Council (NRC) boosted that figure to 12 percent. The report also said that smokers are at a particular risk because smoke and radon interact. The NRC report estimated that 6 percent of American homes had excessively high levels of radon. How do you know if your home is one of them? You can buy a radon-testing kit at your local hardware store for about fifty dollars. Choose one that is certified by either the EPA or the state. The best variety are the "alpha-trak" or "electret" versions, which are used for ninety days. These versions give a better reading than short-term monitors that do not track changes in gas levels, which can vary over the year. If your house has high levels of radon (over 4 picocuries per liter of air), call the local public health board or the EPA hot line (800-426-4791) to find out how to fix the problem. The usual remedies include having the basement foundation properly sealed and having appropriate ventilation systems installed.

Asbestos is another indoor pollutant, and one that has been associated with higher incidences of lung cancer and other cancers. Asbestos is found in many houses and apartment buildings, especially those built in the 1940s through the 1970s, when asbestos was a major component of many building materials. It is found in insulation, such as that used to wrap water pipes; in certain kinds of flooring; textured paints; old roofing materials; and other sources. Asbestos is not a risk as long as it is contained in a properly sealed wrapping. However, those protective wrappings can crack with age, causing asbestos fibers to leak into the air. As airborne fibers, asbestos particles are extremely carcinogenic. Since it is so expensive to have asbestos removed from your home, most experts recommend leaving it alone unless it is exposed. There are ways of sealing asbestos-containing materials so they present no health risk. For more information, call your local health board or the EPA at the number provided earlier.

Other air pollutants that can cause aging are smoke and carbon monoxide. These are a particular risk at home. Some toxic fumes are specific to your choices at home: household cleaning fluids, laundry detergents, exterminator pesticides, garden sprays, and dry-cleaning and rug-cleaning fluids. Others are more generalizable. About 15 percent of all deaths of adults from poisoning are due to the inhalation of such vapors as carbon monoxide and gas. Buy a smoke detector and keep it in good working order, with fresh batteries. Smoke detectors have been shown to reduce the risk of death and injury from smoke inhalation by as much as 70 percent in home and apartment fires. Having a carbon monoxide monitor in the home is another quick and easy way to protect your youth. A recent study by the Centers for Disease Control found that having a functioning and well-maintained carbon monoxide monitor could cut the risk of inadvertent carbon monoxide poisoning in half. Since deaths from carbon monoxide poisoning and smoke inhalation are relatively rare, the RealAge benefit is just six to ten days. Nevertheless, why risk that kind of aging when having two silent monitors can protect you?

We've considered what you can do to minimize aging from toxins, pollution, and accidents, but that's no fun! Let's look now at the RealAge risks and benefits of sex and drug use. Although drug use makes you age, sex (safe sex) makes you younger. The more, the better!

SEX AND DRUGS

A Prescription for Youth?

In 1996, the first baby boomers turned fifty. Those who grew up during or after the age of "sex, drugs, and rock and roll" now outnumber those who came before. Which means that sex, drugs, and rock and roll aren't just for kids anymore. Nearly 50 percent of Americans age fifteen to fifty-four admit to having tried an illegal drug at least once in their lifetimes. And the person who spends a lifetime with just one sex partner is increasingly rare. Just how does our sexual history or our encounters with illicit drugs affect our RealAge?

By enjoying sex within the confines of a mutually monogamous relationship, by practicing safe sex during casual sexual encounters, by avoiding high-risk partners, by knowing your partner's sexual history, and by always using and correctly using a condom, you can lower your RealAge by as much as 0.9 years. And having lots of safe sex can make you even younger. Having sex at least twice a week can make your RealAge 1.6 years younger than if you had sex only once a week. And having sex frequently might make your RealAge younger still. By avoiding drug use and by seeking counseling if drug use is a problem, you can reduce your RealAge by more than eight years.

Sex: The Most Fun You Can Have Getting Young

This book is about getting younger. But what are we getting younger for? To enjoy life more. One of those enjoyments is sex. Sex keeps us young and makes us want to stay young. It's one of life's greatest pleasures, and not one that we want to give up because we're too old. Emotionally, physically, and mentally, remaining sexually active will help make your RealAge younger no matter what your calendar age. Why? It decreases stress, relaxes us, enhances intimacy, and helps form the foundation of strong and supportive personal relationships. No matter what your calendar age, nineteen or ninety, sex is a first-rate age reducer. Nevertheless, there are risks associated with sexual behavior. With divorce, the relaxation of social roles, an increase in sexual freedom, and changes in gender expectations, more and more of us have chosen and will choose to have sex with more than one person over our lifetime. However, having multiple partners or not practicing safe sex puts us at an increased risk of sexually transmitted diseases (STDs). Some STDs are life threatening—AIDS, for example. Others are more subtle; they do not cause immediately identifiable symptoms but have long-term health consequences. Exposure to human papillomavirus, for example, which results in no problems in the short run, increases a woman's odds of cervical cancer later in life. Learning how to have fun while being safe is the key to getting the most out of your sex life.

Sexually Active: The Benefits of Sex

Surveys show that the average sexually active American has sex about once a week (fifty-eight times a year, to be precise), although there is clearly a variation. Married people tend to have more sex than single people. Frequency also varies over age, economic, and social and ethnic boundaries. One of the first studies to track aging longitudinally, done at Duke University beginning in the 1950s, found that the frequency of sexual intercourse (for men) and the enjoyment of sex (for women) correlated with longevity. In other words, people who had more sex more often lived longer. Other studies found that sexual satisfaction became a predictor of the onset of cardiovascular disease: Both men and women who were less satisfied with their sex lives were more likely to have premature aging of the arteries. Although the early studies provided thought-provoking insights, they unfortunately failed to provide accurate data; they did not control for confounding factors and failed to consider underlying physiologic factors. Some new studies are beginning to fill in the gaps, although the data are still not conclusive.

The recently published Caerphilly study from Great Britain suggests that men who have sex considerably more than the once-a-week average—over two orgasms a week—have lower rates of mortality (from all causes combined). In RealAge terms, they stay younger longer. The results suggested that there might be a dose-response relationship: The more sex a person has, the less aging he or she will undergo. Again, this study was preliminary, identifying only a correlation between sex and longevity and not a cause-and-effect relationship, and unfortunately took only men and not women into consideration. This study is the strongest proof we have that sex can actually help us get younger and stay younger. If the numbers from this study prove true, we can say that having sex twice a week (twice the national average) can make a person's RealAge 1.6 years younger. And if we extrapolate linearly, something the early evidence suggests that we can do, the person who has sex almost every day (350 times a year) and is happy with his or her sex life could have a RealAge as much as eight years younger. Indeed, I believe so much in the therapeutic value of sex that I have even prescribed sex for several of my patients, going so far as to write it out on a prescription pad! What these patients needed wasn't another pill but a bit more fun to keep them young.

Sex-ercise

One of the questions I'm frequently asked is: How much energy do you expend during sex? Men and women get various workouts depending on position, vigor, and duration, but the calories spent per orgasm are about the same. During their sex studies in the 1950s, Masters and Johnson found that both men and women burn seven to twenty-five calories per orgasm.

Unfortunately, few studies have been done since then, so more recent data are lacking. Some recent studies have shown, however, that sex is good for cardiovascular health. But there is little information on sexual interactions that do not include orgasms or that detail the differences between women and men. Although sex can provide a lot of exercise, most of us probably don't think of it as a supplement to a workout. If the Masters and Johnson data are correct, to get your full RealAge workout from sex—and to hit the recommended 3,500 calories per week physical exercise quotient—you would have to have at least 140 orgasms a week!

SEXUALLY TRANSMITTED DISEASES: THE DOWNSIDE OF SEX

Because of the AIDS crisis, we hear a lot in the media about safe sex. When it comes right down to it, most information isn't as explicit as it needs to be. We still have a Puritan streak, which often keeps us from talking about the actual mechanics of sex. But that doesn't help anyone because there are important issues that need to be explained, such as which diseases we are really at risk of contracting or how to use a condom properly.

The safest sex is with a disease-free partner in a mutually monogamous relationship. For some people, however, this is not a realistic option. The next best thing is to use condoms. Using a condom every time you have intercourse—and using it correctly—drastically reduces your risk of contracting an STD.

Beyond correct condom usage, the choice of partners is another key element in practicing safe sex. High-risk groups include men who have sex with men, intravenous drug users, and former prisoners and their sex partners—no matter what their sex. Know the person you're sleeping with before you sleep with him or her. Talk to your partners about their sexual histories and about

TABLE 6.5

The RealAge Effect of Sex Practices

FOR MEN

	Casual Sex Practices			
	Mutual Monogamy	Low-Risk Partner Safe Practices Condom Use	Low-Risk Partner Safe Practices No Condom Use	High-Risk Partner No Condom Use
Calendar Age	RealAge			
35	34.1	35.1	35.9	40
55	54	55.1	56.1	62
70	69.6	70	70.5	72.9

FOR WOMEN

	Casual Sex Practices			
	Mutual Monogamy	Low-Risk Partner Safe Practices Condom Use	Low-Risk Partner Safe Practices No Condom Use	High-Risk Partner No Condom Use
Calendar Age	RealAge			
35	34.1	35.3	36.2	42
55	53.9	55.2	56.1	62.2
70	69.6	70.1	70.6	73

yours. Remember, too, that younger partners aren't necessarily less risky. Quite the opposite. Two-thirds of STDs are diagnosed in people under age thirty-five.

Although AIDS is clearly the biggest worry, we shouldn't forget about other diseases as well. The Centers for Disease Control estimates that 20 million Americans will contract some form of STD each year. Others estimate a more conservative 12 million. A study by the Allan Guttmacher Institute in the early 1990s estimated that one in five, or over 50 million Americans, have had some kind of STD.

How much does having an STD age you? Statistically, only 0.9 years. But this statistic is misleading. Contracting HIV is a way of becoming old overnight. A thirty-five-year-old man who contracts HIV experiences twelve years of aging from the disease in a short period and more aging as the disease progresses. His risk profile changes to that of a much older man as soon as HIV is diagnosed. In light of the current improvement in treatment for HIV, the aging effect correlates directly with the quality of care. Other diseases are more uncomfortable than life threatening, but they can lead to long-term aging of the immune or cardiovascular system.

Unfortunately, data on the relationship between safe sex and aging is hard to correlate, partly because STDs are so different. One of the biggest problems with getting statistics on STDs is that it is virtually impossible to do controlled studies on sexual behavior. Researchers can't create the kind of double-blind study populations that we can create for studies like drug tests. We can't tell a group of people that half of them should have lots of casual sex and the other half should be monogamous. We can't even divide the monogamous group into two subgroups and tell one to have sex only once a week, and the other to have sex every day.

More important, statistics are only general trends. For example, although the group having the highest incidence of STD infection consists of unmarried people under age thirty-five, STDs can affect anyone. Either through divorce or widowhood, a lot of people find themselves back on the "dating scene" when they hit their forties and fifties. If this is you, play it "safe." Don't risk an STD.

AIDS-HIV infection is clearly the biggest risk, as it is a fatal disease for which we have not found a cure. Although the new, better drugs have made it possible for many HIV-positive patients to live symptom-free for years after infection, it appears that these drugs only delay the onset of full-blown AIDS; they do not prevent it. Moreover, this delay is achieved only when HIV-positive patients rigorously maintain a complicated and expensive medication schedule. If you believe that you may have been exposed to the disease or are changing sex partners, it's a good idea to get an HIV test. If you think you've been exposed, early treatment can prevent permanent infection (by early, I mean within one to four hours).

Although HIV is a fairly difficult disease to contract, exposure to other STDs reduces the immune system's defenses and increases the likelihood that HIV will actually infect a person who has been exposed. Estimates are that a person with genital lesions (for example, from syphilis or herpes) is one hundred times more likely to contract HIV during a single sex act than someone who has never had an STD.

When it comes to safe sex, remember three rules.

1. Look out for number one. *Always* take care of yourself. Don't depend on your partner for protection. No matter who your partner is or what your partner says, make sure you use a condom. No matter how it feels at the moment, don't take needless risks.

2. Talk before you act. Talk honestly and forthrightly with your partner about your respective sexual histories and safe sex before you ever get to the bedroom. Trust is an important part of sexual intimacy.

3. Don't believe your partner. As I said, trust is an important part of sexual intimacy. Honest talks and full disclosure of past behaviors are essential for practicing safe sex. But they aren't enough. Your partner may tell you in good faith that he or she has no STDs but may be wrong. Since many STDs are "silent," a person may be unaware of the infection for years but still be capable of transmitting the disease. Also, many people have problems talking about STDs, a potentially embarrassing topic. Surveys show that a large percentage of people say that they would lie if asked about past sexual behavior. And a recent study of sexually active HIV-positive patients showed that four of ten had not told their partners about their disease status.

One of the most difficult issues concerning safe sex is deciding when it is okay to stop playing it safe. When do we just get a RealAge benefit from sex, with none of the risk of disease that can cause us to age? All the information about safe sex suggests that you either use condoms or maintain a mutually monogamous relationship. Yet, many people have to make the transition. When does the "new" partner becomes the "one-and-only" partner? When can we give up on the condoms?

If you are in a monogamous relationship and making the decision to switch from condoms, first talk about it. Then, both you and your partner should go to a doctor for a full workup of tests. That way each of you will know the facts. If one of you tests positive for an STD, then you can make an informed decision about the best way to proceed.

Women who are pregnant or considering getting pregnant should get checked for the presence of any STDs, since these diseases can sometimes be harmful to the developing fetus or newborn. Usually, an STD doesn't interfere with pregnancy; rather, extra precautions are taken to prevent mother-to-child infection.

Wear It, Wear It Right

Studies of condom use consistently show that people just don't get it right. There are six essential steps to using a condom properly, but most people perform only three or four of the six steps correctly. Don't assume you know. I admit I felt a little silly when I used a banana to show my son how to use a condom, but, silly or not, I am reassured that he now knows exactly what to do.*

1. Buy only latex condoms and use a new condom for each episode of intercourse—even if you don't ejaculate each time. Make sure you use condoms that say they protect against STDs. Joke or novelty condoms may not provide protection. Make sure that the condoms have not passed their expiration date, that the foil pack is intact, and that the condoms have not been left too long in some place where they could get damaged (for example, in the sun—or in a wallet!).

2. Open the package carefully and be sure to avoid damaging the condom with either your fingernails or any other sharp object.

3. Place the condom on the erect penis prior to any intimate contact (some STDs, such as gonorrhea, can be transmitted even without penetration). Roll the condom down to the base of the penis, where the penis connects with the body. Make sure the fit is snug.

4. Leave a space at the tip of the condom and remove any air pockets from that space.

*This group of six steps needed to correctly wear a condom is modified from the report of U.S. Preventive Services Task Force, *Guide to Clinical Preventive Services, 2nd Edition.* U.S. Department of Health and Human Ser133vices Office of Public Health and Science, Office of Disease Prevention and Health Promotion, 1996, p. 732.

5. Use only water-based lubricants, such as KY jelly or spermicidal foam or gel. Never use oil-based lubricants, such as petroleum jelly (for example, Vaseline), lotions, or mineral oil, because they destroy the latex. Also, many condoms are treated with nonoxynol–9, a spermicide and lubricant that seems to provide some added protection against HIV and other types of STD infection. It is probably a good idea to use this type of condom, since it will give you some added protection just in case.

6. Withdraw immediately after ejaculation, while the penis is still erect, holding the condom firmly against the base of the penis.

The following are the most common sexually transmitted diseases:

AIDS-HIV

Human immunodeficiency virus infection—the infection that causes or is presumed to cause AIDS—has traditionally been associated with gay men and intravenous drug users. However, its incidence is growing in other sectors of the population. Between half a million and a million people in the United States are infected with HIV, with six times as many men being infected as women. Infection rates are higher in the African American and Latino communities, presumably because of other associated risk factors, such as higher rates of poverty and drug use. In nine major American cities, AIDS is the number one cause of death for women aged twenty-five to forty-four. Since women are more susceptible to contracting the disease than are men, experts expect AIDS to increase among women.

The reason that AIDS spread so quickly among gay men in the 1980s was that many had sex with multiple partners without using condoms, and many engaged in practices that are now known to increase the likelihood of disease transmission, notably anal sex. Studies consistently show that people who have sex with HIV-infected partners but use condoms are at minimal risk of contracting the disease. No matter who you are, straight or gay, choose your partners carefully and always wear a condom.

HIV-AIDS is a two-stage disease. A person who is infected with HIV can remain virtually symptom-free for years, but nevertheless is infectious. AIDS is the disease stage of HIV infection. By rendering the immune system basically useless, the disease destroys the body's primary line of defense. Infections, cancers, and other immune diseases then can attack the body, causing horrible and painful illnesses. A person goes from a young healthy adult to a disease-ridden old person in a matter of months or years.

Because of recent advances in HIV treatment, people who are infected with HIV who get a proper regimen of medications can stay virtually symptom-free for years. If you discover that you are HIV-positive, seek medical care immediately. Proper management of the disease can add years to your life. Each year, more effective treatments for the disease emerge, so the longer an infected person survives, the better the odds of living until a cure is discovered.

Chlamydia

Chlamydia is the most common bacterial STD in the United States. The greatest problem with chlamydia is that its symptoms are largely "silent." Seventy-five percent of those who are infected show no symptoms. Primarily affecting women, chlamydia can cause internal scarring of the fallopian tubes, ectopic pregnancy, and infertility. Symptoms, when they do occur, include painful urination, vaginal discharge, and abdominal pain. Although men are usually not affected by the disease, they should seek treatment if they are exposed because they can transmit the disease to their partners. Ask your gynecologist or general physician to include a chlamydia screen in your routine battery of tests, particularly if you have recently changed sex partners. Fortunately, chlamydia can easily be treated with antibiotics.

Gonorrhea

"The clap" can affect anyone. Although as many as two-thirds of women and 40 percent of men who are infected with gonorrhea are asymptomatic, painful urination, unusual vaginal discharge, and menstrual spotting can be signs of infection. Gonorrhea is highly contagious and can be transmitted simply through genital contact, even without penetration. It can cause ectopic pregnancy or infertility in women and seems to increase a person's susceptibility to HIV. Nonoxynol-9, the spermicide most often used on condoms, helps block the transmission of gonorrhea. Untreated, the disease can cause cardiovascular aging. Gonorrhea can usually be treated with antibiotics, although some antibiotic-resistant strains are appearing. Infections from these strains can be cured with a more vigorous and difficult series of treatments.

Hepatitis B

Hepatitis B is not officially classified as an STD, but its most common mode of infection is through intercourse. Hepatitis B can cause severe damage to the liver. There is no effective treatment, although many people recover on their own. A hepatitis B vaccine is available (see Chapter 12), and getting vaccinated is a quick, easy way to help yourself stay young, particularly if you are sexually active and plan to have more than one sex partner in your lifetime.

Herpes

Estimates are that one in five sexually active Americans has genital herpes, an increase of 15–20 percent since the mid-80s. This increase has occurred despite "safe sex" education and programs that encouraged the use of condoms. Many people who have been infected remain asymptomatic and unaware of the disease, yet they are still infectious and spread the disease to their partners. Within the first week or two after infection, symptoms can include fatigue, muscle aches, and itching. Ten days or so after infection, a small blister usually emerges in the genital region. The blister can burst and remain for several weeks, causing pain and discomfort. Once the initial outbreak heals, victims remain infected for the rest of their lives and may suffer recurrent outbreaks. Although herpes can be both painful and embarrassing, it is not life threatening and has no particular long-term health consequences. Creams and antiviral medications can treat the symptoms and reduce the number of outbreaks but cannot cure the underlying infection, which remains within a person for life. Although transmission is most common during outbreaks, transmission can occur between outbreaks as well, in a process known as "viral shedding." Women are more likely than men to contract the disease from an infected partner, and herpes can cause more serious consequences if they become pregnant.

Human Papillomavirus

Human papillomavirus is the most commonly transmitted STD. Some experts have estimated that as many as 80 percent of the sexually active population is infected with the virus. However, little is ever said about this disease. In general, the virus is benign. Since it increases a woman's risk of developing cervical cancer considerably, we can say it accelerates aging of the immune system. Some strains cause small genital growths or warts that can be uncomfortable, but these growths can be easily removed. If you have had more than two sex partners in your lifetime or your partner has had more than two sex partners, chances are you have been exposed to the virus. In general, human papillomavirus infection doesn't do much, and there are no treatments. Once you have it, you have it.

Women who have been exposed to the virus are more likely to develop cervical cancers. In fact almost all women with positive results on a Pap smear show evidence of having been exposed to the virus. For men, exposure seems to have little effect, and penile cancers are rare. Men can transmit the virus to their partners and can develop growths or warts, sometimes inside the urethra, which can cause discomfort. Recent studies have found that the virus may be implicated in some anal and rectal cancers, as well as in some oral cancers. Women should remember to get annual Pap smears, which can detect precancerous cells. Treatments can then be given to prevent the development of full-blown cervical cancer. Positive Pap smear results do not mean you have cancer. Most positive results merely identify an increased risk of developing cancer. If you do get a positive result, you will want to be especially careful about having the condition monitored. Your gynecologist may recommend biannual or quarterly Pap smears or treatments to remove precancerous cells.

Syphilis

If gonorrhea is the "sailor's disease," syphilis is the disease of kings. Famous in the eighteenth and nineteenth centuries because of its ravages on the European aristocracy, syphilis is once again on the rise. The incidence of syphilis has doubled since the early 1980s. Symptoms include genital lesions, aches, fevers, rashes, hair loss, and skin and mouth sores. If untreated, syphilis can infect the eyes, heart, brain, and other organs, causing irreparable structural damage. In addition, it accelerates the rate of arterial aging. Syphilis is easily treated with antibiotics and, if detected early, leaves no lasting damage.

Sex is a great thing. The more, the better. There's no way to get younger that's more fun! Just remember: *Be safe. Use a condom, get tested, and pick your partner carefully.*

Illegal Drugs: Staying Young Without Them

Illicit drugs may be illegal, but that doesn't mean that people aren't taking them. About 40 to 50 percent of Americans aged fifteen to fifty-four admit to having tried an illegal drug at some point in their lives, and over 15 percent say they have done so in the past year. Estimates suggest that 5 to 10 percent of the population use illegal drugs regularly, and many admit being addicted. The more than $3 billion spent each year on drug rehabilitation programs is just a small part of the major impact that drug use has on our society. Although we tend to associate drug use with teenagers, rock stars, or inner-city poverty, it's not an accurate picture. People from all segments of society use and abuse drugs. And drug use, it is not surprising, accelerates aging.

Drug addiction is a serious problem that has physiologic and mental effects. The problems associated with drug use are complicated and warrant more discussion than I can provide here. For the purposes of this book, there is only one question: How does illicit drug use contribute to aging?

Most hard drugs are illegal for a reason: They're dangerous and addictive. Cocaine, crack, heroin, and a whole array of hallucinogenic (mind-altering) drugs can cause serious health problems. Unnecessary aging associated with drug use can be as much as eight years. Drugs like heroin and cocaine top the list. They can kill a person almost instantaneously. An overdose, if not fatal, is always serious and puts a person's life at risk. Although trying a drug once probably won't do much damage by itself, it may cause addiction. Many people crave more and then are on the path to drug addiction. Addiction affects a person's physiology, making him or her more likely to suffer real physical aging that is manifested in many ways. The mental effects of drug use tend to disrupt social ties, often causing users to lose their friends, families, and jobs.

People who use drugs are more likely to make bad decisions. They are more likely to get into accidents and have unsafe sex. For example, cocaine and crack use are associated with higher rates of HIV transmission, not because using the drugs increases susceptibility to the HIV virus, but because users take risks (unsafe sex, needle sharing) that make them more likely to be exposed to the virus.

Marijuana, by far the most popular illegal drug, is less immediately dangerous or addictive than other drugs. Smoking "pot," even if you "didn't inhale," makes your RealAge older. Marijuana contains 50 percent more carcinogens and four times as much tar as cigarettes. Studies show that the heavy use of marijuana can cause residual neurologic effects that decrease cognitive functioning. Heavy users actually experience aging less from the drug itself than from the behaviors it tends to induce, most notably a lack of motivation. For example, users are less likely to exercise or eat a healthy diet or to maintain the kinds of social networks that can help protect against stress. They are also more likely to engage in risky behaviors, such as unsafe sex or driving under the influence of either drugs or alcohol.

When it comes to illicit drugs, the best advice is not to start. If you do use drugs, consider quitting. If you find you can't stop "cold turkey," you have an addiction problem and need to seek help. Although overcoming a drug addiction is difficult, addiction is one of the most pernicious agers of the body, and ending a habit of drug abuse will make you younger and, consequently, feel better. It could even save your life.

7

Take Your Vitamins

TURNING VITAMINS
AND SUPPLEMENTS INTO
AGE REDUCERS

Can vitamins make you younger? Yes. The right nutrients in the proper amounts help protect your body from needless aging. Although we often hear about the recommended daily allowance (RDA), the minimum needed to prevent disease from deficiency, we should start thinking instead about the "RealAge Optimum" (RAO), the dose you really need to stay as young as you could be.

- Hundreds of vitamins, minerals, herbs, and supplements are available for sale. Learn some general guidelines for taking those that can keep you young and avoiding those that will make you older. Taking the wrong combination of vitamins or needless vitamins can make you 1.7 years older.

  Difficulty rating: Quick fix

- Antioxidants are all the rage because of their supposed antiaging effect. This section investigates those claims. What is oxidation? How does this bodily equivalent of "rusting" age your body? Vitamin C and vitamin E, when taken together, work as an antioxidant team, keeping your arteries, immune system, organs, and bones young. When taken consistently, these vitamins can reduce your RealAge by as much as six years.

  Difficulty rating: Quick fix

- Frail bones and arthritis are hallmarks of aging. The danger of these conditions can be reduced by getting the proper levels of calcium and vitamin D. Getting 1,200 mg of calcium and 400 IU (International Units) of vitamin D a day can help make you 1.1 years younger.

  Difficulty rating: Quick fix

- Despite the hype over cholesterol, you may have to worry about something else even more: homocysteine. Homocysteine is an amino acid that is a by-product of various metabolic processes. High homocysteine levels correlate with the early onset of heart and vascular disease more than almost any other factor. But not to fear—by getting adequate amounts of folate (folic acid) daily, you can make your RealAge more than 1.2 years younger.

  Difficulty rating: Quick fix

- We would all like to eat a balanced diet, but not all of us can or do. The hectic pace of real life interferes. If you do not eat a regularly balanced diet, including six to eight servings of fruits and vegetables each day, you can get all the vitamin and mineral nutrition you need by taking a multivitamin daily in addition to the other supplements recommended in this chapter.

  Difficulty rating: Quick fix

- Besides vitamins E, C, and D; calcium; and folate, what should you be getting in your diet? Here we consider some of the latest nutrient fads. What are the possible benefits or side effects of such highly touted micronutrients as chromium picolinate and selenium, and such herbal remedies as echinacea? Avoiding inappropriate supplements and fads will make you one to four years younger.

  Difficulty rating: Quick fix

Vitamins, vitamins, vitamins. How many times have you been told to take your vitamins? Your mother told you to eat your vegetables to get your vitamins. Now, more than likely, you take vitamins out of a bottle. But do you really know what and how much you should be taking?

Walk into a health-food store or down the vitamin aisle at your local drugstore, and you will see shelves overflowing with vitamins of all sorts, not to mention minerals and a whole panoply of supplements. There are multivitamins, individual vitamins, vitamin cocktails, stress vitamins, energy vitamins, herbs, minerals, pills, capsules, and drops; the same vitamins in different dosages and different formulations; and no clear instructions about what you should take, how much, or how often.

In the 1960s, Nobel Prize–winning chemist Linus Pauling asserted that by taking high doses of vitamin C, you could prevent the common cold. His assertions became a kind of folk remedy, and people readily began to take vitamin pills. Now 25 percent of all adults in the United States gulp down vitamin supplements regularly, and half take them occasionally.

I didn't realize exactly how consuming and confusing all this could be until Frank T. walked into my office one day, opened up a bag, and began pulling out bottles. Brown bottles, blue bottles, small bottles, big bottles. When he was done, he had thirty-five containers of vitamins, minerals, and supplements lined up on my desk.

Incredulous, I asked, "You take all of these every day?"

"Absolutely," he replied. "Some of them I take twice a day." In all, he took some fifty tablets daily. Clearly, here was one organized man. This was a full-time job. At fifty-four, Frank was in good shape. He exercised vigorously and often, was trim, enjoyed a happy marriage, and was at the peak of his career. Recently he'd had a prostate scare, and that made him worry. He began reading up on his health and asking people at the health-food store. The results of his research—all thirty-five bottles' worth—were now spread out in front of me like a Thanksgiving feast. Now he wanted to know what I thought.

"Fifty pills a day is too much," I told him. "Some of them are good for you, but some of them could be bad for you." Then I gave Frank some basic guidelines for taking vitamins and outlined a specific plan that could do exactly what he wanted—keep him young.

General Rules About Vitamins

Before getting into the details of what vitamins you should take and which ones you shouldn't, I think it's worth pointing out some *general* considerations that apply to vitamin usage. To say that there is a difference between the practices advised by medical doctors and those advised by practitioners of alternative medicine would be an understatement. There has been a long history of debate between the two sides. Since this is clearly a controversial issue, let me make some points that can help you understand and untangle the debate. It's not so much that medical practice has dismissed alternative medicine outright—not at all—but, rather, that medical doctors, for the most part, like to have strong and convincing evidence that treatments help their patients before they advocate those treatments.

For doctors, one of the most frustrating aspects regarding the vast array of vitamins and supplements available is not that they don't work, but that we have no idea if they actually *do* work. With the exception of a few basic vitamins (C, D, E, B, and A) and a few minerals (calcium and iron), we have limited scientific information about the role and optimum dosages of most of the supplements on the market. Although for many minerals and vitamins, we have basic information about the minimum amounts of essential nutrients that we need to survive or prevent deficiency diseases (the recommended daily allowance, or RDA), we know much less about the optimum doses we need for health and youth. Most of what you learn in health-food stores has not yet been proven. It may prove right, it may prove wrong—we just don't know.

There have been few or no scientific studies on the vast majority of vitamins and supplements on sale in any local health-food store. Most of these supplements are sold without any description of what they are, why they are good for us, or how we should take them. Many of them are unnecessary—and some can even be harmful. Comfrey, for example, long given as a cough suppressant, can actually cause severe and irreversible liver damage—a big price to pay for easing a cough. For most herbs, as well as most minerals and other food supplements, the research has just not been done.

Nutritional supplements—because they are classified as food products and not medicines—aren't regulated by the strict standards governing the sale of prescription and over-the-counter drugs, so manufacturers can sell them in any quantity or combination they want. Nor does the law require that they do any scientific studies to back up their claims, as they would have to do for any new medicinal drugs. There are no industry standards or federal requirements. Different brands of the same supplement might contain very different elements. It is not uncommon to find bottles containing ingredients and even contaminants not listed on the ingredient list. When you do buy vitamins or supplements, make sure you buy them from a large and reputable manufacturer. In addition, do not take any supplement without getting a recommendation from a reputable source.

Another caveat: I advise against taking any supplement "cocktail" sold at a health-food store, from a vitamin aisle at a store, or from a catalog (many are sent from Canada where the laws are even more lax). These supplement cocktails are *mixtures* of herbs, vitamins, and minerals. I do not object to "cocktails" in principle, just in practice. For one thing, they claim to provide everything from "prostate cancer prevention" to "menopause ease" to "muscle building" but often don't even list what they contain—or how much of any one ingredient is included—since the companies that sell them aren't required by law to do so. You—the consumer—could be taking all kinds of things that you don't want. Most of these wonder pills are probably harmless, but we cannot say for sure. I can guarantee that they are not "wonder" pills. If you are trying to be smart about Age Reduction, don't start taking a pill or cocktail just because a store clerk or infomercial tells you to do so. If you don't know what it is, don't take it.

That said, what *do* we actually know about vitamins, minerals, and supplements? Which ones should we take? And which ones should we definitely not take? In general, if you eat a balanced and healthy diet, with four servings of fruits and five servings of vegetables a day and plenty of grains, you should get all the nutrients you need. However, that's not always realistic. Most of us have busy lives and hectic schedules, which means that it's not always easy to eat a balanced and nutrient-rich diet.

To make up for such inconsistencies, I recommend taking a multivitamin every day, in case you have missed out on a little bit of one mineral or the other. Choose a multivitamin without added iron, and one that has less than 8,000 IU of vitamin A. If you are worried about whether you are eating a balanced diet rich in vitamins and nutrients, talk to your doctor or schedule a session with a clinical nutritionist to review your eating habits and to develop basic dietary guidelines. (You can take the nutrient profile from your RealAge Age Reduction planning session, available at *www.RealAge.com*, with you to facilitate the process.) Vegetarians and others on special or restricted diets should be vigilant to ensure that they are getting the basics.

What other nutrients and vitamins should we be getting? What do they do for us? What shouldn't we take?

OXIDANTS AND ANTIOXIDANTS: RUSTPROOFING YOUR BODY

One of the biggest trends in vitamins these days is the use of antioxidants, because they purportedly can help prevent the oxidation damage that has been linked to cancers and other types of aging. It's true: Taking the right amounts of antioxidants can make your RealAge as much as six years younger. Many people, however, wrongly believe that if a little bit of antioxidant is good, a lot is better. Too many antioxidants—especially of the wrong type—can actually cause oxidation damage. My recommendation: antioxidation in moderation. Eat a balanced diet, with four servings of fruits and five to six servings of vegetables a day. Then, each day, take 600 milligrams (mg) or more (up to 2,000 mg) of vitamin C in divided doses separated by at least six hours, plus 400 IU of vitamin E. That should give you all the antioxidation, antiaging protection you need. Here's why.

To understand antioxidants, let's first think about the oxidant, oxygen. We all know that oxygen is necessary for our bodies to function at all. Breathing is fundamental to living. When we breathe, oxygen enters our bloodstream and is transported to our cells. Once it enters our cells, oxygen forms the basis of many of our cells' most fundamental processes. You probably learned these facts in elementary school, but what you probably didn't learn was that this same oxygen, in the form of oxygen radicals, can oxidize our tissues. In a sense, it can cause those tissues to rust. Oxygen waste products, called lipofuscins, build up in organs like the heart and brain, leaving brown discoloration on the tissues. These spots are signs of aging. The older you get, the more prevalent they become.

Why? Imagine apples. If you slice an apple and leave it out in the air, it will soon turn brown. Exposed to air, the surface of the apple oxidizes. The process is similar to what happens when oxygen radicals build up in your body. If you were to take that same apple and sprinkle lemon juice on the slices, they would stay white. The apple does not turn brown because lemon juice is full of vitamin C, which works as an antioxidant. Lemon juice stops the oxidation process and keeps the apple from "rusting." In your body, antioxidants like vitamin C and vitamin E do the same thing.

Think of your body as an exclusive club. Free radicals are the visitors who crash the scene without an invitation. They are so pesky, the body can't get rid of them without some help. Antioxidants function as a kind of security system, the bouncers. They seek out the roving oxygen radicals and bind to them—a kind of chemical handcuff. Bound together, the free radicals and the antioxidants form an entity that the body can then flush out. As long as you have enough bouncers, free radicals and lipofuscins won't build up in the body.

How does this "rusting" affect us? Mainly, oxidation ages your arteries. As you get older, your arteries are more likely to become clogged with fat deposits. These clogs contain high levels of oxidized lipids—that is, fats that have been chemically altered through interaction with high levels of free radicals. Therefore, oxidation plays a significant role in the aging of our arteries. Oxidation affects us in other ways, too.

Oxygen free radicals are an unstable form of oxygen that cause genetic damage. Each cell in your body contains DNA (deoxyribonucleic acid) that instructs the cell what to do and when to do it. Every time your cells divide, DNA is copied into the new cell. Oxidation interferes with this process, causing DNA damage. This can lead to cancer and the premature aging of solid tissues. It can also damage the immune system, your body's backup security system to ensure that cancer cells don't spread (see Chapter 5 on immune system aging). Finally, oxidation ages our eyes. It can damage the lenses (promoting cataracts) and the retina. The gradual loss of sight is one of the very first things that can make us feel old.

There are still many gaps in what we know about oxidation, and a lot of what we do know is based on circumstantial evidence. We do know that people with lots of buildup of oxidized fats in their bodies have much higher rates of heart disease and that their bodies appear to age more quickly in other ways, too. The hypothesis is that there is a connection between aging and oxidation—although we still can't verify it completely. Regardless of the exact reasons why oxidation seems to age us, we know that people who consume the antioxidants vitamin C and vitamin E at the levels I recommend have substantially lower rates of coronary disease, cancer, and other forms of aging. Let's consider why I recommend that you take vitamin C and vitamin E supplements, but not vitamin A, for antioxidation.

THE DAILY BASICS: VITAMINS C AND E

The two most important Age Reducing vitamins are C and E. These vitamins exert powerful antioxidant activity. Taken together, they help keep your cardiovascular system healthy by reducing the amount of harmful buildup on the walls of your arteries. In addition, vitamin C strengthens the immune system, improves both eye and lung function, and helps the body heal. Vitamins E and C, taken in combination, help keep the arteries relaxed and elastic. Taking 600 mg or more (up to 2,000 mg) of vitamin C a day as supplements (in divided doses of no more than 500 mg in any six hours) and 400 IU of vitamin E a day, in addition to eating a balanced diet with lots of fresh fruits and vegetables, can reduce your RealAge by more than six years! What could be easier?

Vitamin C and vitamin E are powerful antioxidants that complement one another. Vitamin C is water soluble, whereas vitamin E is fat soluble. What does that mean? Your cells are made up of two components: the cell membrane and the cell interior. The cell membrane, the outer casing of the cell, consists of lipids, or fats. Since vitamin E dissolves in fat, it works to prevent oxidant-induced aging in the membrane. It is in the cell membrane that you see the buildup of lipofuscins, those brown spots. In contrast, the inside of the cell is made up mostly of water. Since vitamin C dissolves in water, it can enter the center of the cell and collect the free-radical oxidants lurking there. Together, these two vitamins keep oxidants from damaging your cells, both inside and out (see Table 7.1).

TABLE 7.1

The RealAge Benefit of Vitamins C & E

FOR MEN

Of getting the RAO* dose of vitamin C:
>At age 55: 2.8 years younger
>At age 70: 3.2 years younger

Of getting the RAO dose of vitamin E:
>Age 55: 2.5 years younger
>Age 70: 2.8 years younger

FOR WOMEN

Of getting the RAO dose of vitamin C:
>Age 55: 2.2 years younger
>Age 70: 2.6 years younger

Of getting the RAO dose of vitamin E:
>Age 55: 1.5 years younger
>Age 70: 2.2 years younger

THE DAILY DOSE, AT THE RAO LEVEL

Vitamin C:

600 mg or more as a supplement, plus five servings of fruits and vegetables, to total 1,200 mg/day, in divided doses, separated by at least 6 hours (not to exceed 2,000 mg a day)

Vitamin E:

400 IU (international units)

*The RealAge optimum, the dose recommended for the greatest Age Reduction.

Vitamin E

As mentioned, vitamin E is fat soluble. That makes it an especially vigorous antioxidant. Vitamin E goes right to work on oxidized lipids that clog the arteries, shrinking their size and preventing the initial buildup in the first place. It hampers the attachment of dangerous LDL cholesterol along the arterial walls.

Vitamin E can lower the risk of heart attack in women by as much as 40 percent and in men, by about 35 percent. If a person already has arterial disease, but not fibrotic or permanently hardened arteries, vitamin E can decrease the risk of heart attack by as much as 75 percent. That's an astounding impact! Something as simple as taking 400 IU of vitamin E a day will give you a younger, healthier cardiovascular system and all the vigor and energy that goes along with it. Moreover, like aspirin, vitamin E thins your blood, making clots less likely to form. The quinone in vitamin E has powerful anticlotting powers. Studies have found even lower levels of platelet aggregation when vitamin E is taken in conjunction with aspirin, something you should be doing anyway (see Chapter 4).

Recent claims have also been made for vitamin E as a preventive against lung and prostate cancer and other cancers as well. The antioxidant properties of vitamin E are believed to help stop the immune system from aging. Further studies still need to be done on the exact details of the cancer–vitamin E connection, but the evidence appears promising. Vitamin E may also help the body build muscle strength. Finally, as I mentioned, vitamin E has been shown to help prevent cataracts, and preliminary studies suggest it might help prevent macular degeneration, the leading cause of visual impairment associated with aging.

There are several caveats you should be aware of before taking vitamin E. This vitamin therapy works only to reduce the size of fatty buildup *before* the arteries have become fibrotic, or permanently hardened (that is, when there is fat buildup but no irreversible changes). Vitamin E seems to help reduce the size of small or medium-sized lesions in your arteries but not severe ones. That is why you want to start taking these vitamins as soon as possible—to foil aging before it begins.

How much vitamin E should you take, and where is it found? Vitamin E is found in fatty vegetables, such as avocados, and in some vegetable oils. It is also found in nuts, leafy green vegetables, and some grains. It is virtually impossible to get the necessary antiaging dose of vitamin E from foods. The RDA is only 12 to 15 IU a day; that is, 12 to 15 IU are all you need to survive without showing signs of deficiency disease. But the RAO—the

RealAge optimum—is 400 IU. To prevent aging, you need 400 IU daily. Since most multivitamins tend to follow RDA recommendations and contain only 15 to 30 IU, do not rely on multivitamins to get your vitamin E; the level of vitamin E in most multivitamins is usually 370 IU short of the anti-aging optimum.

How often do you need to take vitamin E? Since vitamin E is fat soluble, it resides in your body for quite a while. One tablet a day is just the right dose. There is little risk of a vitamin E overdose unless you ingest more than 1,200 IU a day, and vitamin E is probably safe up to 3,000 IU a day. If you have high blood pressure, get the high blood pressure treated, and start slowly with 200 IU of vitamin E a day. After a week or so, increase the dose to the 400 IU level. One additional note: Several studies have noticed an increase in bleeding when vitamin E and aspirin are used in combination, a condition implicated in both ulcers and strokes. It is rare, but discuss this risk with your physician, especially if you have a history of ulcers or other blood-clotting problems.

Vitamin C

Have you ever noticed that the minute you get a cold, everyone from the checkout man at the grocery store to your mother starts telling you to take vitamin C? That is the legacy of Nobel Laureate Linus Pauling. All of us know that vitamin C is good for us, but most of us probably couldn't say why.

What exactly does vitamin C do? Like vitamin E, vitamin C helps to keep the arteries clear by inhibiting the oxidation of fat in the walls of your blood vessels. It converts cholesterol to bioacids, so they can be washed out of the body easily and not add to the problem of lipid buildup. Since vitamin C is water soluble, it enters the cells that make up the wall of the vessels themselves, binding to free radicals lurking inside the cell, precisely in the place where those free radicals are likely to cause DNA damage. Because of its healing capabilities, vitamin C helps maintain a healthy matrix in the blood vessels, repairing the vessel walls when they become damaged. When it comes to keeping the cardiovascular system healthy, vitamin C seems to help men more than women, and vitamin E helps women more than men. Regardless of your gender, you should take both vitamins (see Table 7.1).

In addition, vitamin C helps reduce high blood pressure, prevents cataracts, and promotes healing. It improves lung function, preventing aging of the respiratory system. And it really does keep your immune system young. Pauling thought vitamin C helped cure colds. We now know it decreases our risk of the one ager we all want to avoid—cancer!

Since vitamin C is water soluble, it washes out of your body when you urinate. It is important to get several doses of vitamin C a day. I recommend at
least two, usually three, doses daily. I do this by combining food and supplements. In the morning, I drink a big glass of orange juice, I take a multivitamin
with 200 mg of vitamin C in it, have an orange or a grapefruit at lunch, and then
take a 500-mg supplement at night, just to make sure I'm getting enough. I also
get vitamin C from other things I eat, just in smaller amounts, such as tomatoes
or salads. The RAO for vitamin C is about 1,200 mg a day from food and supplements, taken in smaller amounts spread throughout the day. The RDA is just
60 mg, way short of the antiaging optimum. Vitamin C tends to leach out of
packaged or cut vegetables. Moreover, cooking reduces vitamin C levels even
more. It is important to make sure you eat plenty of fresh fruits and vegetables
every day. Eat some fruit or take some of your vitamin C one to two hours
before you exercise. Exercise causes the buildup of oxidants.

It doesn't matter what kind of vitamin C you take, either natural or synthetic. Your body can't tell the difference. Personally, I stay away from chew-
ables because they are hard on the teeth. Although it costs a little more, I prefer taking vitamin C that contains calcium ascorbate, which helps prevent the
stomachaches that straight ascorbic acid (vitamin C) can cause. If you have a
sensitive stomach, take the calcium ascorbate form of vitamin C. Besides, it's
another source of calcium, and, as you will see in the next section, you want
to get as much calcium as you can!

Two more comments on vitamin C. A recent headline said that vitamin C
caused cancer by causing breaks in DNA. What the headline didn't say was
that at the 500-mg dose, vitamin C appeared to prevent, or be associated with
repair of, far more DNA damage than it caused. If you take 500-mg pills, take
them no more frequently than one every six hours to get the optimum balance.

Finally, I have to respond to the question, Does vitamin C prevent colds?
The answer is no. But it does lessen their effect. To get this effect, when you
begin to show signs of a cold, increase your dosage of vitamin C to as much
as 4 grams (4,000 mg) a day, taken with plenty of water (eight glasses for 4
grams). Although this amount won't cure your cold—Pauling wasn't exactly
right—it will lessen the severity of the symptoms. For example, when I have
a cold and take my C, I find I can keep exercising.

Now, let's consider the last big antioxidant vitamin, vitamin A. What is it
about A that makes it an aging vitamin, not an antiaging one?

VITAMIN A

In 1988 Americans spent less than $8 million a year on vitamin A supplements. Now they spend $80 million on vitamin A, often sold in the form of beta carotene. They may be doing themselves more harm than good.

This is an example of too much of a good thing. In the late 1980s, a study came out showing that people who ate foods with lots of vitamin A in them tended to have lower rates of cancer. People interpreted this result to mean not that they should be eating more fruits and vegetables, but that they should be taking vitamin A supplements. The market boomed. Sales of vitamin A and beta carotene, a substance the body breaks down into vitamin A, went through the roof.

More recent studies have found that we jumped the gun. First, the correlation between vitamin A and the prevention of cancer is not as strong as was once thought. Second, too much vitamin A can actually be harmful. Although it is important to get sufficient vitamin A, you should do this by eating well, not by taking supplements. Especially avoid megadosing. Do not take more than 8,000 IU a day, which is a standard dosage in many vitamin supplements. In choosing a supplement, try to find one that has the vitamin A in the form of beta carotene because the body will not convert beta carotene into vitamin A if it has no need for it.

Vitamin A is a necessary and important nutrient, but taking large doses of it can be dangerous. Why? Because vitamin A is a nutrient that is "level sensitive." When levels of vitamin A are moderate, it works as an antioxidant and is important to the functioning of your body. However, when you megadose, the surplus vitamin A does the opposite. Rather than functioning as an antioxidant, high doses of vitamin A work to oxidize tissues. So taking too much vitamin A makes you age faster.

A 1993 study in Finland showed that people who took vitamin A had an increased risk of lung cancer; atherosclerosis; and, for smokers, stroke. Several other studies have confirmed these findings. Excessive amounts of vitamin A may cause liver damage. Smokers need to be especially careful about taking any kind of vitamin A, even the beta carotene form; when combined with smoke, vitamin A can be toxic.

Although health-food stores still push vitamin A and beta carotene, remember that you probably get enough in a multivitamin and in your daily diet. For basic antioxidation, rely on vitamin C and vitamin E. Carotenoids (such as lycopene found in tomatoes) and flavonoids (found in onions, garlic, and grape products such as wine) also seem to have antioxidant power. Likewise, they help decrease aging of the arterial and immune systems. We discuss them in Chapter 8. As good as vitamins E and C are, remember this: When it comes to vitamins, antioxidants are just the opening act. Another great duo is calcium and vitamin D.

CALCIUM

Bone weakening, or osteoporosis, affects more than 25 million Americans. It is the major underlying cause of hip fractures and bone breaks in the elderly— about 1.25 million bone fractures, including 300,000 hip fractures, are caused annually by osteoporosis. Although osteoporosis affects women dispropor- tionately, especially small-boned women of northern European or Asian descent, we are all at risk. Twenty million women suffer from the disease, but so do 5 million men. As more men live longer, they, too, will be at increased risk of osteoporosis.

We often forget that our bones are living tissues that need proper care. After we have completed our growth cycles, it is easy to forget about them. Just as we can make our arterial and immune systems younger, we can make our bones younger as well. Doing so protects us for the long term, reducing our overall RealAge. How do we make our bones younger? By making them stronger. We can do that by taking 1,000 to 1,200 mg of calcium a day.

Osteoporosis is a condition involving the loss of bone density. As you age, your bones lose calcium, becoming progressively weaker. Why? Your body stores excess calcium until you reach your early thirties, at which time you reach your peak level of bone density. After that, your body stops storing extra calcium. You must then get all the calcium you need from your daily diet, or you will begin to deplete the calcium stores in your bones. Just imagine your skeleton as the structure of a house. Your bones are the beams that buttress your body. In a house, you have to worry about termites: they hollow out the beams from within until the beams become so weak they collapse. As your body depletes the calcium stored in your bones, they become weaker and weaker, until, finally, like termite-eaten beams, they are almost hollow. Then, *snap*. They break. And a broken bone, especially a broken hip, is one of the things that can age you the fastest. Just six months of immobility can reverse all your RealAge progress by a third or more. Each day you go without activ- ity, you get older.

Why is breaking a hip so bad? It's not the fracture itself that ages a person but, rather, the complications that stem from such an injury. A hip fracture may be the beginning of a downward spiral, triggering a chain of aging events. When a person is bedridden, the body weakens, becoming susceptible to pneumonia and other infections that can often be fatal. With less exercise and movement, arteries start showing signs of aging, becoming less elastic and more prone to disease or failure. Also, the immune system becomes more vulnerable. For older people, the mortality rate from hip fractures is as high as 20 percent (12–20 percent of older women who have had hip fractures die within six months). Furthermore, 40 percent of those who survive that initial six months require long-term nursing care. More than half never regain their former quality of life.

Hip fractures are astoundingly common. Thirty to forty percent of women over calendar age sixty-five have fractured their spine or vertebrae, and twenty-five percent of such women will suffer a fractured hip. Doing what you can to prevent a fracture is one of your best protections against aging. Remember, it's not just women, either.

Men traditionally have been much less susceptible to bone fractures than women. Just 5–10 percent of men over age sixty-five have these kinds of debilitating fractures. Since historically men have not lived as long as women, however, we know less about the strength of men's bones as they age. It appears that men also suffer bone loss as they get older, although they start out with higher bone density than women. I predict that as more men live longer, bone loss and severe fractures will become an increasing problem for them, too.

If you are working to make all the rest of you younger, you should make sure that your bones also stay young. For the best RealAge advantage, men and women should make sure to get enough calcium—that is, 1,000 to 1,200 mg a day for men and 1,200 mg for most women over thirty (pregnancy and other conditions may change the requirements slightly). Take 500 or 600 mg twice a day. (This refers to the amount of actual calcium, not calcium in combination with citrate or carbonate. If the label reads 1,000 mg of calcium citrate, read on to find the amount of calcium by itself.) Any kind of calcium supplement, even over-the-counter antacid tablets, should fit the bill, just as long as you are getting the right milligram amount. I advise against taking calcium supplements that contain bone meal, dolomite, and/or oyster shells, as these can contain lead or other heavy metals that may be toxic. Calcium carbonate is best absorbed when taken with food. Calcium citrate may be taken at any time (either by itself or with food). Both forms can cause constipation. If you notice this side effect, eat more fruits and vegetables or rely on that old standby, a prune a day. Some recommend taking about 300 mg of magnesium in conjunction with the calcium (see the section on magnesium later in this chapter).

Although calcium is plentiful in dairy foods (milk, cheese, and yogurt), most people do not eat enough dairy products to get adequate amounts of calcium from diet alone. Eat dairy foods for extra calcium, but do not rely on them as your only source of calcium unless you eat and drink a lot of dairy products (and, of course, remember to eat *low-fat* versions). If you consistently drink three or four glasses of milk a day (most adults do not drink anywhere near that amount), then you can modify the amount you take in supplemental form accordingly. But be very careful to make the 1,000- or 1,200-mg marker daily. And a reminder to anyone under thirty, or even thirty-five, who's reading this: You should get lots of calcium to build bone strength for the future because the calcium the body stores in bone then becomes the surplus stores for the rest of your life.

Not only does calcium help your bones, it may also help lower your blood pressure. A recent study showed that men who took 1,000 mg of calcium a day had a 12 percent reduction in blood pressure. This evidence remains controversial, as other studies have reported no such lowering of blood pressure. Although there is as yet no consensus on this finding, lower blood pressure may be just one added benefit of taking calcium, which is something you should be doing anyway. Another side note for people with high blood pressure: A common treatment for high blood pressure is the administration of calcium channel-blocking drugs. These drugs have nothing to do with calcium supplements, so don't be concerned. Go ahead and take calcium supplements.

VITAMIN D: THE STRONG-BONE, ANTICANCER VITAMIN

There are some pairings where you can't imagine one without the other: Bonnie and Clyde, Abbott and Costello, Charlie Brown and Snoopy. The same is true for calcium and its vital partner, vitamin D.

Vitamin D is essential for proper absorption of calcium. Vitamin D helps strengthen bones and prevents the joint deterioration that accompanies arthritis. Vitamin D and its metabolites appear beneficial in reducing certain kinds of breast, colon, prostate, and lung cancers. No one is exactly sure why it works as an anticarcinogen, but both animal studies and one major epidemiologic study on humans showed this to be true. One of the most important vitamins in your Age Reduction Plan might be vitamin D.

Vitamin D may also help protect the body from the onset and aging effects of arthritis itself, but this finding is still somewhat speculative. Osteoarthritis is a disease that afflicts more than 10 percent of the population sixty-five or older. It is painful, disabling, and aging. Recent studies from Framingham, Massachusetts, and elsewhere have shown that taking calcium, vitamin C, and particularly vitamin D can retard the progression of arthritis and perhaps even prevent it. These studies found that those who had high levels of vitamin D in their bodies had less joint deterioration and fewer of the painful bone spurs and growths that can accompany arthritis as it worsens. Arthritis patients with low levels of vitamin D and calcium were reported to be three times more likely to suffer the rapid progression of the disease than those who had high levels of these nutrients in their bodies. Arthritis caused them to age faster.

Importantly, vitamin D seems to help prevent cancers. Although no one knows exactly why, and confirming studies are yet to be done, three primary theories try to explain how vitamin D works as a deterrent to cancer. All three have some validity, as evidenced by both animal and test-tube studies, but we still lack confirmation from studies on humans.

The first theory speculates that the D_3 form of the vitamin kills cells which contain DNA mutations. Somehow, vitamin D_3 is directly lethal to mutated, possibly cancerous, cells. The second theory suggests that vitamin D_3 promotes the death of cancerous cells. The body has an internal mechanism by which it is able to recognize mutated cells, and vitamin D_3 is an essential component used in the body's attempt to rid itself of these cells. The final theory proposes that vitamin D_3 promotes protein transcription; that is, it helps make proteins from the P53 gene, a gene that is one of the body's cancer watchdogs. Vitamin D appears to be vital for the proper functioning of the P53 gene. This gene helps prevent cancer by regulating the protein production of specific oncogenes—genes that, when mutated, can cause cancers. Indeed, vitamin D not only helps in the proper functioning of the gene but also appears actually to help safeguard the P53 gene from genetic damage.

Although studies still need to be done to confirm the link between vitamin D and cancer prevention, it is very possible that vitamin D does double duty by helping to prevent aging of not only the skeletal system but also the immune system. When I think of vitamin D, I think of "defense." Vitamin D helps you defend yourself.

Most American adults do not get enough vitamin D. Estimates are that 30 to 40 percent of adults are vitamin D-deficient. You get vitamin D from two and only two sources: first, the sun; and second, food and supplements. Let me explain how our bodies produce vitamin D from sunlight.

Vitamin D production is a three-stage process. In the first stage, the body takes in food that contains a kind of cholesterol that is the precursor to vitamin D. Our bodies can't use this cholesterol form of the vitamin without first converting it. Only a few foods, such as cod liver oil and certain fatty fishes (tuna; salmon; sardines; oysters; mackerel; herring; and, to a lesser extent, cod itself) naturally contain vitamin D in the form that can be used by our bodies. For conversion, the second stage, we need sun. Solar radiation is necessary to create the right chemical reaction in our bodies to turn these cholesterols into vitamin D. In the final stage of the process, the liver and kidneys convert that vitamin D into yet another form of the vitamin, vitamin D_3, the active form that our bodies can use. As mentioned in the section on sun exposure (see Chapter 5), you need just ten to twenty minutes of sunlight a day to ensure that your body is producing enough vitamin D. Most of us do not get enough sun, particularly in northern climates. In Boston or Seattle, for example, it is almost impossible to produce the necessary levels of vitamin D from sunlight alone from November through February. After we reach our seventies, the precursor to vitamin D generally found in our skin diminishes three- or fourfold, making it increasingly difficult for us to produce vitamin D naturally.

The second and less risky way of getting enough vitamin D is through food and supplements. Some foods, mainly fish and shellfish, contain vitamin D naturally. Such foods as milk (the major source of vitamin D in food) and most breakfast cereals contain vitamin D as an additive. These additions, which help prevent rickets (a vitamin D-deficiency disease) in children, are synthetic. When it comes to getting vitamin D, it is no better for us to drink milk than to take a pill. When you drink milk—and please drink *skim* milk!—you get the added benefits of calcium and protein. As I mentioned earlier, most adults do not drink milk in sufficient quantities to get their vitamin D from diet alone.

So how much vitamin D do you need to get the maximum antiaging protection? The RDA of 55 IU only ensures a level of vitamin D that prevents a deficiency disease, such as rickets. I recommend that you consume at least 400 IU of vitamin D a day in a vitamin supplement if you are under seventy years old, and 600 IU if you are older than seventy, unless you are absolutely sure that you are getting enough from your diet. This amount is what I consider the RAO. That means four glasses of no-fat milk a day (for 400 IU). Vitamin D overdoses are exceedingly rare among adults. To develop toxic levels of vitamin D in your blood, you would have to consume more than 2,000 IU a day for more than six months.

In addition to the supplement, I recommend getting some sunlight. Ten to twenty minutes a day outside without sunscreen should provide sufficient vitamin D protection, although the farther north you live, the less likely it is that you can produce all the D you need this way. If you are going to be in the sun for more than twenty minutes, put on sunscreen. Note that an SPF 8 sunscreen reduces your vitamin D production by 95 percent, and SPF 30 cuts it to zero. The risk of skin cancer from a little bit of sunlight is probably less than the benefits you gain from having healthy vitamin D levels, especially the older your calendar age. Finally, if you are worried about vitamin D deficiency, you can ask your doctor to test your blood levels. The test will quickly determine whether you are getting enough vitamin D.

Vitamins E and C work as a team. Calcium and vitamin D work as a team. Now let's look at a vitamin that works all on its own—folate, a member of the vitamin B family.

THE RISK OF HOMOCYSTEINE, AND THE FOLATE COUNTERATTACK

Every time I visit my lawyer, he asks me for a health tip. The last time I went to see him, he asked me, "So, Mike, what's the latest thing I should be doing to get younger?"

Without hesitation, I said, "Taking 400 micrograms of folate a day as a supplement."

"Folate? What for?" he replied.

"To reduce your homocysteine," I said.

"My what?"

"Homocysteine. It's worse for your arteries than a sixty-four-ounce steak."

"I thought cholesterol was the worst thing."

"If cholesterol is petty crime, homocysteine is grand larceny." Then I gave him some free medical advice in exchange for some paid legal advice. Lawyers!

Homocysteine is an amino acid that is a by-product of various metabolic processes that may build up in the blood. As you age, your homocysteine levels increase. No one is exactly sure what homocysteine does to the arteries, but it is well established that people with high levels of homocysteine have considerably more arterial disease and much higher rates of atherosclerosis than those who don't.

People with high levels of homocysteine in their blood are at a significantly higher risk of the early onset of arterial disease and suffer markedly greater rates of arterial aging. Elevated homocysteine levels triple the risk of heart attacks and stroke. More than 42 percent of people with cerebrovascular disease, 30 percent of those with cardiovascular disease, and 28 percent of those with peripheral vascular disease have homocysteine levels that are too high. Getting 400 micrograms (mcg) of folate a day can reduce homocysteine levels dramatically, essentially removing any excess from your bloodstream and stopping its aging effect. It's a quick, easy, and painless way to make your arteries younger. By religiously taking 400 mcg of folate a day, you can reduce your RealAge by 0.6 years in just three months. If you already have elevated levels of homocysteine, you can reduce your RealAge by three years in just three months.

As I discussed in the chapter on arterial aging, one of the main causes of arterial aging is atherosclerosis. For some reason—no one knows for sure—high levels of homocysteine seem to disturb the endothelium, the inner lining of the artery. Some scientists believe that homocysteine causes small openings in the cell layer, leading to deterioration of the arterial wall and the buildup of plaque. There are other hypotheses as well. Homocysteine may decrease the production of relaxing factors that let our blood vessels dilate. It may stimulate blood clots by changing the shape or form of the cells that form the endothelium. Homocysteine might also oxidize low-density lipoproteins (LDL—remember "L" for lousy—cholesterol), promoting the buildup of plaque along the walls of the arteries.

Although we don't know all the reasons, there is a clearly established link between high homocysteine levels and arterial aging and a clearly established link between high folate levels and arterial health. One study estimated that if everyone had proper levels of folate, the number of heart attacks in the United States could be reduced by as much as 40,000 to 150,000 cases a year, and this number may be too conservative! The risk-factor statistics predict that a more realistic estimate would be a reduction of one-third in the rate of heart attacks in the United States a year. In other words, perhaps as many as 450,000 heart attacks occur a year because we don't get enough folate.

As folate levels drop, homocysteine levels increase, and vice versa. The two compounds are part of a complex chemical reaction involving many steps, but the end result is that more of one means less of the other. The more folate you take, the lower your homocysteine levels.

Folate (in its natural form)—or folic acid (in supplements)—is part of the B-complex family of vitamins. Folic acid is often prescribed for pregnant women because it is essential for the normal development of the brain and spinal cord of the fetus. Although we tend to think of folate as being essential during infancy, we need it as adults, too. As you age, folate concentrations drop. The most common vitamin deficiency found in older people is a deficiency of folate. More that 50 percent of all Americans do not get enough folate daily. On average, American men consume 281 mcg of folate a day and

American women, just 271 mcg. Older people ingest even less. All are far below the ideal intake of 1,100 mcg of folate in food or 675 mcg of folic acid in supplements a day.

Lots of foods contain folate. A glass of orange juice has 43 mcg of folate, and many breakfast cereals average 100 mcg a serving. Still, to get enough folate, you would have to drink about twenty-five glasses of orange juice a day! A slice of white bread has only 6 mcg of folate and a green salad, just 2 mcg.

Since the average intake of folate is approximately 275 mcg from diet, a 400-mcg supplement is what you should take to get the 675-mcg-a-day RAO, the RealAge optimum. If you are trying to get all your folate from your diet, you will have to consume even more—as much as 1,100 mcg—since the body will absorb only about half the folate found in food. For example, 700 mcg of folate found in food is equivalent to about 400 mcg of the folic acid found in supplements. Don't worry about an overdose of folate. Toxicity occurs only when more than 1,500 mcg is ingested a day on a regular basis.

You will need to take folate consistently for the rest of your life. Studies show no known side effects of folate consumption. If your kidneys are not working properly, you should probably not only take folic acid supplements, but also eat a low-protein diet. This will help control homocysteine levels, which normally increase with a high protein diet. Vitamin B_6 also lowers homocysteine levels, so you may want to consider that option. Consult your physician.

Should you have your homocysteine level checked? Probably not. The test is expensive and difficult to perform. It is far easier to try to get adequate folate every day. If homocysteine is high, folate will bring it down. If it is low, folate will help keep it low.

As a medical student, I was taught that high homocysteine levels were associated only with a rare disease. In those days, we "hotshot" medical students and residents used to laugh at the "old, out-of-date clinicians" who gave their elderly patients shots of B_{12} and folate as placebos, often to make them feel better. Perhaps those "old fogies" knew something we young hotshots didn't. Getting enough folate makes your RealAge at least 1.2 years younger.

By the way, make sure you get adequate B_{12} (25 mcg) and B_6 (4 mg) each day, as well. The highest quantities of B_6 are found in almost all beef, parsley, many fish (cod, catfish, crab, halibut, herring, mackerel, salmon, sardines, and tuna), bananas, avocados, some fortified cereals, whole grains, eggs, chestnuts, peanuts and sunflower seeds, beans (garbanzo beans, lima beans, green beans, pin beans, and lentils), soybeans, spinach, potatoes, and green peppers. Most of us get this much B_6 and B_{12} from our diets or multivitamin, but vegetarians may need to take supplements of these two vitamins (see Chapter 8).

TABLE 7.2

The RealAge Effect of Vitamin B$_6$

FOR MEN

	Daily Intake of Vitamin B$_6$ (mg)				
	Less than 1.2	1.2–1.5	1.51–2.2	2.21–3.7	More than 3.7
Calendar Age			RealAge		
35	35.9	35.1	35	34.3	34.2
55	56	55.2	55	54.2	54.1
70	71.1	70.2	70	69.1	69

FOR WOMEN

	Daily Intake of Vitamin B$_6$ (mg)				
	Less than 1.2	1.2–1.5	1.51–2.2	2.21–3.7	More than 3.7
Calendar Age			RealAge		
35	35.7	35	35	34.6	34.5
55	55.8	55.1	55	54.5	54.3
70	71.2	70.2	70	69	68.9

MINERALS, HERBS, AND MISCELLANEOUS SUPPLEMENTS

We have reviewed the four basic vitamins—E, C, D, and folate—and one mineral—calcium—that I recommend you get each day to retard aging. What about the panoply of others? What else do you need? First let us review the seven other minerals (besides calcium) your body needs to function. Then we'll consider a few of the more popular herbal remedies.

Minerals

Besides calcium, a number of other minerals are found in either large or trace amounts in our bodies, all of which are necessary for basic metabolic function. Magnesium, potassium, sodium, chloride, sulfur, and phosphorus are, like calcium, needed in relatively large quantities. Most people's diets provide sufficient quantities of all these minerals, and, in the case of sodium, we may get far more than we require. People with salt-sensitive high blood pressure, arterial disease, and excess weight gain often need to reduce their sodium intake. Trace minerals that we need include chromium, copper, cobalt, iodine, iron, fluoride, manganese, molybdenum, selenium, and zinc. Our bodies demand these minerals in much smaller amounts, and we generally get them from our diet. Silicon, vanadium, nickel, lithium, cadmium, and boron are other trace minerals we seem to need, but scientists know much less about them. If you are eating a well-balanced diet, you can make sure you're getting enough of all these minerals by taking a multivitamin at least once a week. Do not take extra mineral supplements.

Why? Minerals are insoluble elements that come from the earth's crust. Many of them are heavy metals, which can be toxic in excess amounts. With minerals, you want to make sure to get enough without overloading. Extra minerals can build up in the body. Iron is a perfect example.

Iron

Unless you have been diagnosed with an iron deficiency—a condition seen almost exclusively in premenopausal women, growing children, and occasionally vegetarians—it is more likely that you have to worry more about getting too much iron than not enough. Men and postmenopausal women are at the lowest risk of iron deficiency, and most of us—no matter who we are—get plenty of iron from meats, fortified breakfast cereals, breads, and pastas. In fact, the United States has been criticized for adding too much iron to such foods as breakfast cereals. The critics aren't all wrong; the consequences of taking too much iron can be grave. Iron overload can be life threatening and may make your RealAge older.

Perhaps this news sounds surprising. After all, most of us were raised with cartoon images of Popeye gulping down spinach to revitalize his strength. We all thought we needed iron. Don't get me wrong—spinach is good. It's needless iron in supplements that ages us. Avoid iron unless it is prescribed for you by a physician.

When Jason—a body builder, just twenty-four years old—came to see me, he should have been at the peak of health. Instead he was near death. He suffered from congestive heart failure, unusual for someone so young. A few more months of decline, and he would have needed a heart transplant. Whereas he once had been able to bench-press three hundred fifty pounds, by the time I saw him he could barely get out of a chair. His condition seemed a mystery: A young man to an old one in just three years. Luckily for him, other patients' histories had convinced me of the need to ask everyone about the use of vitamins and supplements, and I learned that Jason was taking 10 grams of iron a day. He thought that it would help him build muscle, but he was wrong. It was killing him. Fortunately, the treatment to remove the excess iron that had built up in his body worked. He recovered completely, his heart intact.

Although iron overload as extreme as Jason's is relatively rare, his story proves a point. Iron stays in the body for a long time and, when present in large amounts, can be toxic. The body rids itself of iron primarily through bleeding, which is why menstruating women are sometimes anemic or deficient in iron. Early symptoms of iron overload include abdominal pain, fatigue, and loss of sex drive. Later symptoms include enlargement of the liver, diabetes, arthritis, and shrinking of the testicles. In severe cases, such as Jason's, iron overload can cause an abnormal heartbeat and even heart failure.

Hemochromatosis—chronic iron overload—is a fairly common affliction, and as many as one of every two hundred fifty people has a genetic predisposition to developing the condition, making hemochromatosis one of the most frequently occurring genetic disorders. Even people who don't carry the gene can develop the disorder, which damages such key organs as the liver and heart and causes needless aging.

Even slightly excessive levels of iron in the body can be damaging. Too much iron may interfere with our levels of zinc. Studies have linked elevated iron levels with increased rates of cardiovascular disease and cancers. Although in both cases the evidence is somewhat preliminary and more studies are needed to prove the links, taking extra iron is not worth the risk. In RealAge terms, it can increase your aging.

There are two possible ways that even low levels of iron toxicity can age us. First, iron appears to contribute to arterial aging. No one knows exactly how, but the theory is that because iron is an oxidant, it increases the oxidation of LDL cholesterol. When LDL cholesterol is oxidized, it becomes especially dangerous, causing atherosclerosis. Some scientists have speculated that one of the reasons menstruating women have lower rates of cardiovascular disease is that they have lower levels of iron in their blood. One Finnish study showed that the rate of heart attacks doubled when the concentration of iron in the blood exceeded 220 mg/dl (milligrams per deciliter of blood). This risk was four times higher for patients who had both high iron levels and an LDL cholesterol reading of 190 or higher. Other studies have been unable to confirm this link, and the claims about the connection have been strongly contested. But, why risk it?

Elevated iron levels have also been linked to cancers. The data remain preliminary, and we still don't completely understand the relationship, but two major theories suggest why this may be the case. First, iron is an oxidant. In contrast to antioxidants, such as vitamins C and E, that remove free radicals from the body, iron enhances the production of free radicals, which, in turn, is linked to an increased incidence of cancer. Second, cancer cells appear to demand more iron than other cells. When cancers do develop, the increased iron in the body may fuel them to grow at a faster rate. Although neither theory has been proven, studies in the United States and Finland have shown an increased risk of cancers for people with elevated levels of iron.

If you are not iron deficient, make sure that your multivitamin does not contain iron. Eat normally. Take iron only if anemia is a chronic problem and you are specifically directed to do so by a doctor. If you are a vegetarian, be sure to have your red blood cell count checked annually just to ensure that you are not developing an iron deficiency. If you are a vegetarian and are eating a balanced diet, you are probably getting enough iron from other sources. If you are a woman and still menstruating, have your iron levels checked before you decide to take iron. Most menstruating women do not require iron supplements.

Chromium

Chromium, a mineral involved in glucose metabolism, is important for the synthesis of cholesterol, fats, and protein. Health-food gurus advocate chromium—usually in the form of chromium picolinate—for everything from weight loss to cholesterol reduction to the alleviation of depression to treatment for hypoglycemia and diabetes. Chromium has also been said to prevent osteoporosis, to build muscle, and to promote longevity. In light of these claims, should you take chromium as a supplement? Chromium is certainly a necessary mineral, but we generally get enough from our diets to provide for our needs. Chromium is found in many whole grains, meats, and dairy products—even in beer! Clearly, having proper levels of chromium in your body is necessary to metabolize blood sugar, and most of the benefits associated with chromium are tied to the process of proper glucose metabolism. Doctors sometimes advise that people with Type II diabetes take chromium to boost the effect of insulin. Regardless, if you have diabetes, you should not take chromium or any drug without first consulting your doctor.

Most of the longevity claims made for this mineral stem from animal studies and seem to be tied to the already well-known fact that a low body mass index increases life span. Several studies in the 1980s glorified chromium as a wonder nutrient, but the results have largely been disproved. It is still unclear whether taking chromium as a supplement promotes safe weight loss, and some studies have indicated that chromium may even cause weight gain. Indeed, one study linked the intake of chromium picolinate with weight gain among already overweight women. As for other claims, studies have shown little evidence that chromium adds muscle mass. Since we know little about chromium toxicity, we don't have much sense of how much a person can take without causing a negative effect. Too much chromium can cause heart palpitations, high blood pressure, and even psychosis. Animal studies have shown that chromium can cause chromosomal damage and so may pose a risk of cancer as well. I recommend eating a balanced diet and taking a multivitamin as a backup. That should provide all the chromium you need.

Selenium

Recently, there has been a big stir over selenium, which has been heralded for its antioxidant properties. Selenium is one of the trace minerals that our bodies need. We get selenium largely from such plant foods as garlic, which absorb the mineral from the soil they grow in. The soil in different regions of the country varies considerably in selenium content.

A recent study in the *Journal of the American Medical Association* reported a 50 percent reduction in cancer deaths among diagnosed patients who took 100 mcg of selenium twice a day. Yet other research has suggested that selenium may have an immune effect as well, boosting resistance to certain viruses. These findings are still preliminary and have been much criticized by some cancer researchers. Unfortunately, all we have are tantalizing tidbits. The National Cancer Institute is funding at least five studies on the potential benefits of selenium, and we should know considerably more about the role of selenium within the next four years. Of the five primary medical advisers on the RealAge team, one thought the data convincing enough that he began taking selenium. The other four chose to wait for more information.

Although we may find that selenium has important antiaging properties, it is a trace mineral that is not easily excreted by the body and can build up to toxic levels, causing needless aging. The current recommended daily allowances for selenium are 70 mcg a day for men and 55 mcg a day for women. I recommend that you get this mineral from your diet, rather than from a supplement. That way, you probably won't overdo it. Most Americans who eat a balanced diet should not worry about a deficiency, since selenium is plentiful in many foods: garlic, whole grains, cereals, meats, and some seafood. Since garlic in particular has been thought to provide numerous health benefits, I recommend getting selenium by loading your meals with lots of garlic.

Potassium

Strokes are the major cause of cognitive aging, or aging of the brain. Thankfully, strokes can largely be prevented. One easy thing you can do to minimize the risk of stroke and the aging it can cause is to increase your intake of potassium. If you already eat a normal diet rich in fruits and vegetables, supplementing that diet with three bananas (or their potassium equivalent) a day can make your RealAge as much as 0.6 years younger in just three years.

What makes potassium so important? Potassium is what is known as an electrolyte, an electrically charged particle, an element the body needs for proper cellular functioning. Every time a nerve impulse is conducted or a muscle is contracted, potassium—because it carries an electrical charge—makes that reflex possible. Potassium, in conjunction with other minerals, regulates blood pressure and allows the heart and kidneys to function properly. Four major studies have shown that increased potassium intake is linked to a decrease in the incidence of strokes and may prevent other kinds of arterial aging, too. How does potassium prevent aging?

We still don't know, but studies on rats have shown that potassium acts as a counterbalance to sodium intake. Whereas rats fed a high-sodium diet normally had shortened life spans, that effect was mitigated when they were fed a high-potassium diet. In human clinical trials, the Rancho Bernardo study found that people who ate comparatively little potassium had 2.6 to 4.8 times the risk of stroke as those who ate considerably more potassium. Of the 287 people who had high potassium intake, no one had a stroke during the study. Among the 572 people with lower potassium intake, 24 had strokes. Possible explanations? Three studies found that increased dietary potassium intake decreased blood pressure, thus decreasing the rate of arterial aging, which can cause both heart attacks and strokes. That could not have been the whole story because the decrease in blood pressure does not account for the entire RealAge benefit. Other biological mechanisms that may account for the RealAge effect include stabilization of arterial plaques, decreased oxidation of lipids, and stabilization of nerve cells when they get inadequate oxygen.

There is no RDA standard for potassium, but nutritionists recommend that you consume about 3,000 mg a day. If you eat a balanced diet, you will probably get a little more than half that amount in normal consumption. Bananas and avocados are, ounce for ounce, the richest sources of potassium. One banana contains about 467 mg of potassium, and both Florida and California avocados contain over 1,000 mg of potassium per fruit. Although avocados are highly caloric because they are high in fat, they are rich in monounsaturated fats—the kind of fats that are good for you (see Chapter 8). Potatoes, citrus fruits, tomatoes, spinach, celery, cantaloupes, and honeydew melons are also excellent sources of potassium, having 400 to 500 mg a serving. Even though they are relatively high in calories, dried apricots and peaches provide over 1,500 mg of potassium per cup, which is all the extra potassium you need in a day. Dairy products, lean meats, and such fish as tuna, mackerel, and halibut contain over 500 mg per serving. Sardines are extremely rich in potassium, with over 1,000 mg per serving. Skim milk and low-fat yogurt are excellent sources of potassium (400 mg per serving). To get the RealAge benefit of potassium, try to eat three bananas (or about 1,400 mg of potassium) a day and get the rest from a well-balanced diet, with plenty of fruits and vegetables rich in potassium. By doing so, your total intake would be about 3,000 mg a day.

Under no circumstances should you take potassium supplements unless advised to do so by your doctor, as overdosing can be a problem. Although most of us do not consume the optimal amount of potassium, actual potassium deficiencies are truly rare, except in people with very specific medical conditions. Since certain medications may deplete potassium supplies, supplements may be advised, but they should be taken only under strict medical supervision. Remember, too, that increasing potassium intake can actually cause aging in people who have kidney disease or are taking certain medications, so talk to your doctor before increasing your potassium intake. For most of us, however, increasing potassium intake through diet is a quick, easy way to make our RealAge 0.6 years younger and to decrease our risk of stroke and the associated cognitive aging it can cause.

Sodium

Although sodium is a vital mineral for proper functioning of your body, you don't need to worry about getting enough of it. Most Americans consume far more sodium than they need. The minimum amount of sodium you need for good health is 116 mg a day, and the average American consumes more than 4,000 mg.

When we hear the word *sodium,* we tend to think of table salt (sodium chloride), but the fact is, sodium comes in many other forms. Approximately 75 percent of the sodium you consume comes not from the salt shaker but as an additive to processed food. Table salt is actually only 40 percent sodium.

High consumption of sodium is associated with higher blood pressure in some, and perhaps all, people. Numerous studies have found this to be true. The most famous study of this kind was the InterSalt study, which evaluated sodium consumption in over 10,000 people in fifty-two study centers. Sodium intake correlated with an increase in blood pressure, and, correspondingly, high blood pressure correlated with an accelerated rate of arterial aging. For years, doctors have been prescribing low-salt diets to those whose blood pressure showed a particular sensitivity to sodium. Indeed, the first correlation between sodium intake and high blood pressure was made by Ambard and Beaujard in 1904. As a result, early in the century, low-sodium diets were frequently prescribed as a way to successfully lower blood pressure. The development of blood pressure medications encouraged many doctors to move away from this approach, except in rare instances in which it could be shown that an individual was "sodium sensitive."

Newer data suggest that perhaps all of us age faster when salt consumption is excessive. The idea of sodium sensitivity is problematic. A chief drawback of the sodium-sensitivity theory is that no one knows who is sodium sensitive until after high blood pressure develops, and by then significant aging has already begun. Many people's sensitivity to sodium changes with age, as their metabolism undergoes other changes as well. The best choice is to cut back on sodium intake. Sodium chloride (salt) restriction, exercise, and weight control form the triad of behavioral changes that can best help you reduce the likelihood of developing high blood pressure and subsequent arterial aging.

Although the average American consumes about 4,000 mg of sodium a day, most reputable medical organizations, including the U.S. Surgeon General's Office, the National Institutes of Health, the National Academy of Science's Research Council, and countless experts in the field, suggest that sodium intake should not exceed 2,400 mg (about a teaspoon of salt) a day. I go further and suggest that for the maximum Age Reduction benefit, try to keep sodium consumption at less than 1,600 mg a day. A fifty-five-year-old man who has consistently consumed only 1,600 mg of sodium a day is as much as 2.8 years younger than his counterpart who has paid no attention to sodium intake.

How can you reduce sodium intake? The easiest way is to decrease your consumption of processed and prepackaged foods, since a lot of sodium is used to preserve these products. Most fast foods are also high in sodium—just one more reason not to frequent Burger Heaven. Alternatively, fresh fruits and vegetables and fresh meats and poultry contain little sodium. If these foods form the basis of your diet, you will significantly reduce your sodium consumption without really trying. When you do buy prepackaged or canned foods, read the labels. Foods that you would never describe as "salty" can have an astounding amount of sodium. Cheese, preserved meats, many condiments, and some shellfish are very high in sodium, so beware. Often similar products have surprisingly different sodium levels; many companies now offer "no-sodium" and "low-sodium" variants of their products. Even though you should cut back on table salt, remember, it is the hidden salts in processed foods that account for most of your sodium consumption.

Although sodium deficiencies are virtually unheard of, strenuous exercise on a hot day can lower salt concentrations in the body, a condition that can trigger other complications that age the body. When exercising, drink plenty of water to keep yourself properly hydrated.

Magnesium

Magnesium is a mineral that is essential for energy metabolism. Muscle contractions, nerve impulses, and even the most basic processes of cellular energy storage require magnesium. Unfortunately, magnesium deficiency is increasingly common. Experts estimate that 40 percent of Americans are getting less than 70 percent of the RDA for magnesium. Life in the modern world seems to be especially hard on our magnesium intake: Stress, sugar, alcohol, and the phosphates commonly found in soft drinks and processed foods all deplete our stores of magnesium. Even exercise, one of the most important factors in preventing aging, can cause magnesium deficiency because we lose magnesium when we sweat. Moreover, magnesium deficiency often provides no symptoms. The first sign that something is wrong can be a heart attack caused by an abnormal heart rhythm.

A ten-year study of four hundred persons who were at a high risk of coronary disease found that those who ate a magnesium-rich diet had fewer than half as many complications from cardiovascular-related problems as did those who ate only about one-third of the recommended amount of magnesium. Overall mortality rates for people who ate a magnesium-rich diet were lower as well. Although this ten-year study was the first in-depth study of magnesium, if its findings are true, it would mean that eating a magnesium-rich diet would lower your RealAge by as much as 0.9 years.

For now, I cannot say with certainty that eating a magnesium-rich diet will lower your RealAge, although both anecdotal and preliminary evidence suggest that it would. It has been known for some time that heart attacks are less common in areas where the water supplies are rich in magnesium. Magnesium is also known to lower blood pressure; dilate the arteries, and, when given after a heart attack, restore normal heart rhythms. Magnesium is especially important in the regulation of calcium. Since we do know that taking calcium helps reduce RealAge, it is also vital to get enough magnesium to allow for the proper absorption of calcium.

The suggested intake of magnesium is about one-third the intake of calcium, which means that women should get at least 400 mg of magnesium a day, and that men should get at least 333 mg a day. Current studies show that the average intake for Americans is less than 300 mg. People who need to be extra careful to get the right amounts of magnesium include pregnant and lactating women, those with kidney disease, diabetics, those on low-calorie diets, and those taking digitalis preparations and diuretics. All these people should consult their physicians before beginning any new regimen.

Magnesium is found largely in whole-grain breads and cereals. Breads made with refined flours unfortunately have little magnesium because most of the mineral is lost during the refining process. Most fortified and whole-grain cereals contain 100 to 200 mg per bowl. Soybeans and lima beans contain 100 mg per serving, and most nuts contain 100 to 300 mg per serving. Such fruits and vegetables as avocados, bananas, beets, raisins, and dates are also good sources of magnesium. When you choose your daily vitamin supplement, check to see that it contains magnesium. If you worry that you are not getting enough magnesium, consider supplementing your diet with 250 to 300 mg daily. As with all Age Reduction behaviors or plans you adopt, check with your doctor first, since those who have kidney problems can accumulate too much magnesium and have serious side effects.

Zinc

Recent claims have linked zinc to antioxidant activity and immune system response. Unless you are a vegetarian or are on a restricted diet, you probably get enough zinc from food. Zinc is most commonly found in animal products but is also found in nuts, legumes, and fortified cereals. Shellfish contain high quantities of zinc. Zinc is vital to the synthesis of DNA and RNA (ribonucleic acid) and is therefore important for cell division.

Zinc deficiencies are rare. As with most trace minerals, I do not recommend that you take extra supplements. Although zinc deficiencies may cause various problems, boosting zinc beyond basic levels appears to do no good and may even cause harm. For example, too much zinc may interfere with the workings of another trace mineral you need, copper. As with most minerals, high intake may prove toxic, and too much zinc can damage the immune system. Take no more than 30 mg daily. The RDA is just 15 mg for men and 12 mg for women. More than that can be harmful. For example, taking just 50 to 75 mg a day can actually reduce your HDL (healthy) cholesterol, something you want to avoid.

Recently, zinc has received a lot of attention for its role in fighting colds. One study found that zinc lozenges may help ease cold symptoms; another showed they did not. We still need more information.

Herbs and Miscellaneous Supplements

I have talked about vitamins and minerals, but what about all those other bottles you see lining the shelves of any health-food store? Again, as little as we know about minerals, we know even less about most herbal remedies and food supplements. Drawn from various folk treatments, as well as from traditional Eastern medicine, herbs no doubt can provide some benefits. More scientific studies are being done on such remedies each year. Most of the herbs are probably harmless, but some cause needless aging. Never, for example, take anything with comfrey in it. This herb is known to cause liver damage. Also, sassafras, chaparral, germander, and pokeroot have been associated with severe and even lethal effects.

If you think you might want to take an herbal remedy or food supplement, find out about it first. Do not simply ask the clerk at the health-food store or rely on a book there. Do research at the local library or on the Internet. With the right search, you can find out about popular claims and the status of that herb in the scientific literature. If you don't have time to do a search yourself or don't have access to the resources, ask your doctor to find more information for you. Sometimes you may decide that you want to try an herb even though its claimed effects remain unproven. As long it is proven harmless, go ahead. It might prevent you from aging, but you want to make sure that it does not cause aging.

Here's my review of some of the more popular herbal remedies and food supplements. The list is almost endless and ever changing.

Coenzyme Q_{10}

Coenzyme Q_{10} has gained popularity recently for alleged benefits in preventing cardiovascular aging. Found naturally in our organs, it helps stimulate energy pathways at a cellular level, notably in the muscle tissue of the heart. Studies have claimed that coenzyme Q_{10} is an antioxidant that can prevent arterial aging. It has gained some popularity for therapy of critically ill patients awaiting heart transplants, and the findings of some clinical studies have supported these claims. Our bodies naturally produce Q_{10} when they are not lacking in vitamin C or any of the B-complex vitamins. There is little information on the effects of the supplemental form of the coenzyme, and there are no guidelines regarding dosage. Currently, the American Heart Association lists it as an experimental drug. Although coenzyme Q_{10} appears safe and beneficial in some studies, no studies have been done on its possible side effects. I cannot recommend taking coenzyme Q_{10} as a supplement, as no scientific data suggest that it has greater antiaging benefits than risks. In any case, the group of patients for whom there is a purported benefit—those with severe and life-threatening heart failure—should take a supplement or medication only under the strict supervision of their physicians.

Echinacea

Come cold and flu season, I always see individuals who are taking echinacea, an herbal powder derived from the leaves and stems of the coneflower. A popular folk remedy, echinacea is purported to boost the body's natural immunity. Unfortunately, the very few studies that have been done on this herb, both in Germany and the United States, have produced mixed results. Some found an immune response, others found no effect. At this stage, we really don't have any proof whether it works. In general, echinacea appears harmless. People with allergies to plants in the sunflower family should steer clear of it, and those with autoimmune diseases will want to talk to their doctors before taking this herb. Do not take echinacea for long periods; even fans of the herb recommend taking it for only a few weeks at a time, when cold or flu symptoms set in.

Ginkgo Biloba

Ginkgo biloba, an herb that comes from the Chinese ginkgo tree, is purported to have antioxidant properties. It is best known for its supposed enhancement of mental clarity. It is also believed to lower blood pressure and have other antiaging properties. Are these claims true? No one knows. Ginkgo biloba does contain flavonoids and other compounds that are known to scavenge free radicals. Several European studies have indicated possible benefits for Alzheimer's disease, but these studies were not performed using proper clinical-trial design, and so amount to hearsay.

Only one scientifically credible clinical trial on ginkgo biloba has been conducted in the United States. It indicated that the herb may help improve cognitive functioning in people who have Alzheimer's disease or other forms of dementia. Published in the *Journal of the American Medical Association*, the study found cognitive improvement in 37 percent of those given the extract, as opposed to 23 percent of those given a placebo. The data offered by the study were preliminary, merely a first-round screening of the supplement. The study relied largely on subjective social indicators—such as whether caregivers of patients suffering from dementia noticed any change in behavior when the patients took the herb—rather than on concrete physiological or psychological tests. More research needs to be done on ginkgo biloba before we know if it really has any effect.

Ginkgo biloba appears to be another of many possible antioxidants found in fruits and vegetables. It is unclear whether it has any unique properties that are not found in other antioxidants. Even if its alleged positive effects were proven, it is not as effective in diminishing the symptoms of Alzheimer's disease as are certain known medications currently prescribed. On the other hand, there are no known side effects associated with gingko biloba.

Ginseng

Ginseng is a root that has long been used in Eastern medicine to boost energy. Recently, medical reports have claimed that it can boost immune response and increase white blood cell count. As with most herbs, there have been very few rigorous studies, so most information we have comes from personal testimonials and word of mouth. One study linked ginseng to a reduced incidence of the common cold and flu, but another showed that the immune systems of mice who were fed ginseng were damaged. Ginseng made the mice suffer more illness and get older faster than they would have normally. There are claims that the American variety of ginseng, not the Asian variety, has more active properties. In general, the evidence for a beneficial effect of ginseng is low. Ginseng is known to increase blood pressure and may negatively affect sugar metabolism. Some reports related to these side effects indicate that ginseng should not be used except for discrete periods of two weeks or so. Since there are no proven benefits and there are known side effects, I cannot recommend the use of ginseng.

Thymus Extract

Because of its alleged antiaging benefits, there has recently been a stir about thymus extract. Should you take it? No. Why not? The thymus is a gland that is active during childhood and adolescence. It helps control and modulate the immune system. By age twenty, the thymus begins to dry up, and by age fifty, it has virtually disappeared. The theory behind taking thymus extract as a supplement is that the extract will help stimulate immune functioning and protect you from cancers, arthritis, and other ailments that age you. Since the thymus is active during our youth, it is assumed (wrongfully) to be something that will keep us young. No studies and no data indicate that thymus extract helps in any way. Furthermore, taking the extract has a potential hazard. Thymus extract that is introduced into the body is different from that produced by your own body. Since supplemental thymus extract is a foreign protein, it may trigger an immune reaction, which, in turn, may cause your body to develop antibodies against itself.

Other Supplements

Many other miscellaneous supplements and herbs could be discussed here. However, except for a few supplements that treat specific conditions—St. John's wort has been shown useful for preventing and treating depression, for example—there are no data on their antiaging effects.

EATING A NUTRIENT-RICH DIET: TAKE YOUR GET-YOUNGER PILLS AND AVOID THE GET-OLDER ILLS

Remember Frank, who came to my office with thirty-five bottles of pills in his knapsack? When he left, he had only three. He kept his bottle of vitamin C, with instructions to take 600 mg or more a day and to get at least two servings of C from his diet, either from drinking orange juice or eating two pieces of citrus fruit. He kept the vitamin E at 400 IU a day and the vitamin D at 400 IU a day. Beyond that, everything hit the trash. Then he had instructions to buy a few things that, incredibly, were not contained in his vast collection. He had instructions to buy calcium and to take 1,000 to 1,200 mg a day and to give his wife 1,200 mg a day. He also had instructions to take an iron-free, low-vitamin-A multivitamin daily and to take a 400 mcg supplement of folate daily. He learned to reduce his sodium intake to 1,600 mg a day and to boost his potassium intake to 3,000 mg a day, all through diet and without pills. Other than that, he had instructions to eat a balanced diet rich in fruits and vegetables, high in nutrients, and low in calories (see Chapter 8).

"Mike," he said, "are you sure I'm getting what I need?"

"Yes, and, more important," I told him as I looked into my wastebasket filled to the brim with bottles, "I'm even more sure you're not getting what could be harmful to you. Those will stay here in the trash, right where they belong."

He laughed as he walked out, carrying a much lighter load.

8

Eat Dessert First

AND OTHER TRICKS OF AN
AGE REDUCTION DIET

Too many of us will only modify our diets to lose weight. We only think of diet when it becomes "I'm on a diet." This attitude hurts us more than it helps us: We get so obsessed about losing pounds that we don't eat right. It is no surprise that food plays an important role in overall health and longevity, but how can you modify your diet so it helps you stay young? Let's consider diet from the unique perspective of aging, especially quantifying the ways in which eating habits can affect your RealAge. Just a few changes in your diet can make your RealAge anywhere from four to twelve years younger.

- Eating a nutrient-rich, calorie-poor diet that includes lots of grains and cereals, as well as fruits and vegetables, can make your RealAge as much as four years younger. Learn the basics of eating right. Simple tricks can help keep you eating young: for instance, my daughter's favorite, eating dessert first!

  Difficulty rating: Moderate

- Most Americans eat far more fat than they need. Staying away from saturated fat and trans fat in particular will help you stay young. Saturated fats and trans fats build up in our arteries and cause our cardiovascular system to age. Eating less fat and eating the right kinds of fats are key to the Age Reduction diet, but that doesn't mean giving up good taste. By eating fewer than 20 grams of saturated fats and trans fats (and fewer than 60 grams of total fat) a day, you can reduce your RealAge by as much as six years.

  Difficulty rating: Moderate

- Just a couple of years ago, cholesterol led the news. Now we see it a bit differently. Learn how to evaluate your own cholesterol levels, what to do if your cholesterol level is over the danger reading of 240 mg/dl, what to do if it's elevated but not in a danger zone, and what to do if your HDL (healthy) cholesterol level is below 40 mg/dl. The RealAge benefit of lowering cholesterol intake from food: 3.7 years younger.

Difficulty rating: Moderately difficult

- Most of us could shed a few pounds, but losing weight and keeping it off is no easy trick. Learn how to calculate your body mass index (your weight-to-height ratio) and how to combine exercise and healthy eating habits to produce sensible, gradual weight loss. Maintaining a steady low weight can reduce your RealAge by more than six years.

Difficulty rating: Difficult

Eating, next to breathing, is perhaps the most intimate way you interact with the world around you. Yet this contact, unlike breathing, is something you consciously control. The decisions you make about when, where, and what you eat make a difference not only in your weight and health but in how fast you age.

Surveys show that the vast majority of Americans know that they should eat more carefully, watching fat and calorie intake, but the overall American diet is getting worse. More Americans are being classified as overweight than ever before. A poor diet—one that is full of saturated fats and trans fats (I explain these terms in detail later) and laden with calories—accelerates aging. In contrast, a diet rich in nutrients, full of fiber, and low in calories can slow the pace at which you age. The difference between being on a good diet and a bad one can be as much as twenty-four RealAge years. A bad diet can make you as much as twelve years older than the average American, and good dietary choices can make you twelve years younger. If you like to eat—and who doesn't?—learn how to eat right. It will buy you added years of good meals.

When I went to medical school in the late 1960s and early 1970s, I received just two lectures on nutrition. First, we learned about diseases associated with vitamin and mineral deficiencies, diseases that are rare except under starvation conditions. Second, we learned—big surprise!—that eating too many calories caused people to gain weight and that eating too few caused them to lose weight. Discussion over. Fortunately, the two-lesson-view of nutrition is a thing of the past. Increasingly, studies show that the food you choose can greatly affect your rate of aging and substantially alter your odds of being stricken with arterial disease, cancer, diabetes, and other disorders.

Why did it take us so long to see the diet-health-youth connection? And what made our attitudes change? I attribute the change to what I call the "industrialized society" paradox. From the 1940s through the 1960s, modern medicine really came to the fore. The discovery of antibiotics and the development of safe vaccines helped us exert control over the infectious diseases that had ravaged earlier generations, and advancements in surgery and internal medicine lowered the rate of other afflictions. Life expectancy increased dramatically. People in the medical community felt a real exuberance, fostering a "we-can-conquer-any-disease" mentality. As the ravages of some diseases decreased, other medical problems became endemic. Cardiovascular disease and cancer emerged as the new killers, becoming the number one and two causes of death in most affluent and industrialized societies. These diseases did not fit the old model of disease. Suddenly, such issues as diet and nutrition that had been ignored began to provide some intriguing clues.

When researchers began investigating cardiovascular disease, they discovered something interesting. People who lived in rural Greece and Italy, and even Albania—in communities less "developed" and less affluent than our own—had significantly lower levels of arterial disease. Certain Asian populations also had slower rates of arterial aging. If we Americans and northern Europeans were so "advanced," why were we so afflicted?

Genetics seemed a clear answer. But studies soon showed that genetic background, though having some impact on the onset of arterial aging and cancer, certainly could not explain the widespread incidence of these diseases. When individuals moved from their rural villages and emigrated to the United States, they developed the same diseases as those around them. The onset of diseases correlated with lifestyle. One of the most important factors seemed to be diet. Researchers learned that eating a diet rich in fruits and vegetables—one that was full of fiber, nutrients, and fish but that had a minimum of meat, calories, and fats (especially saturated fats and trans fats)—caused a major postponement in the onset of arterial aging. In this healthy diet, the primary fat consumed is olive oil, a monounsaturated fat that lowers the LDL-to-HDL ratio (discussed later) while decreasing the amount of harmful LDL cholesterol in the bloodstream. Dairy products that are heavy in saturated fats, such as cheese, are consumed in small amounts. These food choices were found in the diets of the Mediterranean region and throughout Asia, and they seemed to correlate with long and healthy lives.

Within the past two decades, medicine and American society have changed. These nutrition studies have been well publicized, and most of us now know that cutting back on fats and boosting vegetable and whole-grain consumption will help us stay healthy longer.

But knowing we should eat healthier and actually doing so are two different things. What guidelines should you follow?

NUTRITION BASICS

Eat Your Way to Youth?

Many people have a little goblin in their heads that says, "If it's good for you, it will taste bad." This is simply not true. You can eat your way to youth and do so deliciously. All it takes is a commitment, which starts with exorcising all those unhealthy ideas about diets.

Eating should be fun. If your diet is like a prison sentence, you will only end up breaking out. Eat sensibly and reasonably. If once in a while you eat something that's not 100 percent healthy, it's not the end of the world. What's important are general habits, not obsessive compliance. How can you eat for youth without sacrificing good taste?

With eating and weight loss, no quick fixes exist. There are only long-term methods. The best eaters—and the ones most likely to have young RealAges because of their food choices—are those who love to eat and who see healthy, tasty eating as a challenge. Become a food connoisseur, searching out the best and freshest ingredients while expanding your food horizons. Along the way, you might be surprised to find that the best-tasting food is often the healthiest food. Now let's consider twenty things you need to know to eat right, so you can shed pounds and years deliciously.

1. Eat a Nutrient-Rich, Calorie-Poor Diet

Did you know that it takes at least twenty minutes to work off the calories you can eat in about thirty seconds? I'm not talking french fries, but healthy foods like bananas or apples. Whenever you eat, make every calorie count toward getting younger. Make sure the food you eat is full of the vitamins, minerals, nutrients, and fiber you need to stay young. Too many Americans waste their meals on empty calories. We end up devouring foods that contain lots of sugar, fats, empty (few nutrients) carbohydrates, and calories without getting the nutrition we need.

As you get older, your dietary requirements change. As you hit middle age, muscle mass declines, as much as 5 percent per decade, contributing to a slowing of metabolism of as much as 30 percent. This change in your body composition increases the ratio of fat to muscle and decreases bone density. As your calendar age increases, you need to be even more careful to eat less fat and fewer calories. At the same time, you need to be even more vigilant about getting the right nutrients. Medications and certain diseases can affect the rate at which you absorb nutrients and your appetite. Some studies find that as many as 60 percent of older individuals have some kind of dietary deficiency.

2. Eat Less Fat, Eat the Right Fats, and Time Them Right

There is clear evidence that eating a diet that is low in fats, particularly saturated fats and trans fats, can help prevent arterial aging while reducing the risk of plaque buildup, heart attacks, and strokes. Although the evidence is controversial and definitive studies are lacking, such a diet also appears to slow the immune system aging that is linked to cancer. Estimates run the gamut, with experts claiming that 10–70 percent of all cancers stem from eating a diet high in saturated fats and trans fats and low in fruits and vegetables. A report in the *Journal of the American Cancer Institute* said that women who ate more than 10 grams of saturated fats a day had a 20 percent greater risk of ovarian cancer. Consuming red meat more than once a week has also been linked to increased aging from colon cancer, presumably because of the saturated fats contained in red meat.

By limiting your consumption of saturated fats and trans fats, you limit your risk of aging. Stay away from fried foods and don't eat fried fast foods. Be careful about eating too much salad dressing: most contain lots of saturated fats. Try to eat red meat no more than once a week. When eating beef or pork, choose low-fat cuts. For beef, choose "round" or loin cuts. For pork, choose leg or loin cuts and trim the fat from around the meat. Avoid all processed meats, such as frankfurters, salami, and other luncheon meats. Stay away from anything containing palm or coconut oil, as these are saturated fats. Dairy products low in fats include fat-free milk, fat-free yogurt, and cottage cheese.

There are several kinds of fats, and knowing which ones to avoid, which ones to eat, and when to eat them can make a big difference in how they affect your rate of aging. In fact, this topic is *so* important, I have devoted an entire section of the chapter to it (pp.191–195).

3. Keep a Steady Weight

Clearly not all of us are or can be pencil thin. The point is to be the right weight for you. Your aim should be to keep your weight as close to your weight at age eighteen for women or twenty-one for men. Having a low body mass index—or weight-to-height ratio—is one of the things that will help keep you young. Studies of animals have shown that restricting calorie intake can increase longevity. For example, mice that were fed a low-calorie, low-fat diet lived considerably longer than mice fed a more high-calorie, high-fat diet. Low-fat eating, in combination with exercise, is the easiest and quickest way to lose weight and to keep your weight where it should be. The most important point is this: Moderation and balance are the key principles when it comes to eating for youth. Avoid yo-yo weight loss and gain—this is worse for you than simply being overweight. We don't know why, but the data repeatedly confirm this finding. For more information on weight and aging, see the section on Slimming Down later in this chapter (pp. 204–209).

4. Diversify Your Diet

Everyone thinks he or she eats a balanced diet, but it's not so. Forty percent of Americans don't eat fruit daily, even though it is recommended that a person eat four servings every day. And 30 percent of Americans don't consume any dairy products regularly. On average, Americans get less than half the 25 to 30 grams of fiber they need a day.

Why is diversity in your diet so important? Choosing a diverse diet can lower your RealAge. If you eat items from all five food groups daily, you can be as much as five years younger than if you eat from only two food groups. (The five groups are breads and cereals, fruits, vegetables, dairy products, and meats and other proteins; see Table 8.1.) It is also important not just to choose one thing from each food group but to eat diversely within each food group. For example, some vegetables contain lots of one nutrient and virtually none of another. Try to eat four servings of fruit, five servings of vegetables, and six servings of breads, cereals, or grains a day. These amounts will give you the vitamins and fiber you need without excess calories. Eat two or three servings of low-fat dairy foods and no more than two servings of protein—nuts, beans, meats, fish, or poultry—daily.

5. Eat Your Vegetables

One of the tricks to eating a diet that is low in fat, low in calories, and full of nutrients is to eat lots of vegetables. Since they contain lots of fiber, vegetables help you fill up fast. With only twenty to forty calories a serving, they help you feel full and keep your weight down. They also have loads of vitamins, carotenoids, and flavonoids, many of which have antioxidant properties that will help keep you young. Try to eat five or six servings a day.

Just because you hated vegetables as a kid doesn't mean you won't like them now. Try steaming them with a little lemon juice or lightly sautéing

TABLE 8.1

The RealAge Effect of Diet Diversity

FOR MEN

Calendar Age	Number of Food Groups Eaten Each Day		
	1 to 2	3 to 4	5
	RealAge		
35	38.3	34.8	34.7
55	59.4	54.8	54.5
70	75.3	69.8	69.3

FOR WOMEN

Calendar Age	Number of Food Groups* Eaten Each Day		
	1 to 2	3 to 4	5
	RealAge		
35	38.3	34.8	34.7
55	59.4	54.8	54.5
70	75.3	69.8	69.3

* Food groups are bread and cereals; fruit; vegetables; dairy products; and meats and other proteins.

them. Cook green vegetables just until they turn bright green. If they go all the way to gray, you've cooked them way too long. Try to eat some kind of dark green leafy vegetable and one serving of a cruciferous vegetable (broccoli, cauliflower, or cabbage) each day. Remember, too: Yellow, orange, and red vegetables contain essential vitamins and lots of carotenoids, which are natural antioxidants.

Make vegetables your new snack foods. I buy bags of precut baby carrots and other vegetables and keep them in the refrigerator. When I'm looking around for something to munch on, I start there. Cucumbers, celery, peppers, radishes, and even mushrooms all make great snacks. Eaten raw, they keep all the nutrients and fiber that cooking can deplete.

6. Don't Forget the Fruit

The lengthening of the average life span in America has paralleled the availability of fresh fruits. This is a correlation, not a proven cause-and-effect relationship, but the data suggest that increased fruit consumption may contribute to longevity. Fruits are rich in vitamins and dietary fiber and are loaded with carotenoids and other nutrients.

Carotenoids are vitamin-like substances found in many fruits and vegetables. Over six hundred different types of carotenoids are found in foods, the best known being beta carotene, a substance the body turns into vitamin A (see Chapter 7). For a long time, scientists did not know whether most carotenoids had any nutritional benefit, but it is increasingly clear that many of them have antioxidant—and, hence, antiaging—properties. You can spot carotenoids by the red, orange, and yellow color they impart to foods, such as tomatoes, carrots, and apricots—basically any fruit or vegetable with these hues. Also, carotenoids are plentiful in dark, leafy, green vegetables—spinach, broccoli, kale. Lycopene, a carotenoid found mainly in tomatoes, helps prevent prostate cancer (see Chapter 5). Carotenoids are one of the reasons eating a diet rich in fruits and vegetables can help keep you young. Flavonoids are also present in fruits.

Like carotenoids, flavonoids are an antioxidant found in plants and help protect the body against damage from free radicals. One reason red wine has an antiaging effect is because it is rich in flavonoids. The richest sources of flavonoids are onions, green tea, cranberries, broccoli, celery, apples, and grapes. So flavonoids are another reason a diet rich in fruits and vegetables will help you stay young.

Because most fruits have only thirty-five to sixty calories a serving, they are low-cal alternatives to cookies or candy. Dried fruits contain considerably more calories per mouthful, so be careful. If you are tired of common fruits, such as apples, oranges, and bananas, then diversify. Buy exotic or seasonal fruits. I find it easier to have such bite-size fruits to munch on as grapes, cherries, or small plums. I keep a big fruit bowl in my office. That way, I can grab a piece when I feel hungry, and everyone else in my department can grab a piece, too.

When eating fruit, remember to wash it well but keep the peel on. If you peel an apple or pear, you are throwing away all the fiber. Juices don't have the same fiber content as whole fruit. Although drinking fruit juice provides one or two servings a day, don't make these your only servings of fruit. Try to eat two or three pieces of whole fruit a day and make one of them a citrus fruit. It will give you the added vitamin C that you need to prevent immune system aging (see Chapter 5).

7. Fruits + Vegetables = Fiber

A key reason that diets high in fruits, vegetables, and grains are good for you is that these foods contain lots of fiber. People who eat diets high in fiber have significantly lower rates of aging. Eating 25 grams or more of fiber a day can lower a person's RealAge by as much as three years, compared with eating only 12 grams of fiber a day, the national average.

Fiber is found solely in plant foods and is largely indigestible, passing through the digestive tract intact. Since it cannot be digested, fiber contains no calories, but it makes you feel full sooner and helps you control overeating. Fiber seems necessary to keep the digestive tract running smoothly. High-fiber diets speed up digestive processes, adding bulk to stool and helping the body rid itself of waste products more quickly. Thus the exposure time, in the bowel, of potentially carcinogenic substances found in food is significantly reduced. This shorter exposure time appears to help reduce aging from intestinal disorders and from heart disease. High-fiber diets also correlate with a reduction in colon cancer and probably other cancers as well. For example, one study found a connection between low-fat, high-fiber diets and reduced blood estrogen levels in women, possibly helping to explain why women on such diets have a lower incidence of breast cancer. In a study of forty-three thousand participants conducted at Northwestern University, a 10-gram increase in the daily intake of cereal fiber decreased the risk of heart attack by 29 percent (making a fifty-five-year-old's RealAge 1.9 years younger). People who eat less fiber also tend to have worse overall diets and to be more sedentary.

Fiber helps regulate metabolism and digestion, stabilizing blood glucose levels and affecting the rate of absorption of nutrients. Fiber clearly helps reduce the risk of diverticulitis and inflammatory bowel disease, both of which cause inflammation of the gastrointestinal tract. A high-fiber diet also helps reduce the incidence of hemorrhoids, a condition that can be provoked by excess pressure on the bowel walls caused by the forced bowel movements that often accompany a low-fiber diet.

Don't go on a high-fiber diet all at once. Increase your fiber intake gradually. Make sure to drink lots of water, as fiber tends to absorb water. Eat breads and cereals that have whole grains in them. Even healthy-sounding breads made of "wheat flour" have had their fiber removed by the refinement process. Check the labels on processed foods, which are now required to indicate the overall fiber content.

8. Watch Excess Protein Consumption

There is much debate about how much protein we should eat. Recently, some nutritionists have advocated high-protein diets. Unless you consume lots of dairy products as a counterbalance, meat proteins can leach calcium from your bones. A high-protein diet places undue strain on your kidneys, which excrete metabolized proteins. Your body uses only the amount of protein it can consume, and much of the excess must be excreted (some excess is turned into sugars and fat). Studies have shown that excess protein consumption does not promote health, weight loss, or the building of muscles.

Although the average American diet consists of 100 grams of protein a day, the recommended daily allowance (RDA) is only half that amount. I recommend restricting protein intake to 20 percent of your daily total calories. Protein content is highest in meats, poultry, fish, dairy products, soybeans, and nuts, all of which have a protein content of 15–40 percent of their total caloric content. Beans, cereals, lentils, and peas have a protein content under 15 percent. Limit your intake of fish, meat, and poultry to five to seven ounces a day (an ounce is 31.1 grams). Since these foods contain only about 40 percent protein, eating this amount will give you plenty of protein without overloading.

If you are getting your protein entirely from vegetable sources, it is important that you choose from a wide array of foods to ensure you get all the essential amino acids. For example, breads and grain cereals lack certain amino acids, and lentils and nuts may have those amino acids but lack others. If you are a strict vegetarian, you should talk to your doctor or a nutritionist about balancing your protein intake. Generally, protein deficiencies are rare in this country.

9. Remember, Carbohydrates Were Meant to Be Complex

In a well-balanced diet, 50–60 percent of daily caloric intake should come from carbohydrates—preferably complex carbohydrates. Two basic types of carbohydrates exist: simple and complex. Simple carbohydrates are the sugars—both refined sugars and those found in honey and many fruits. Complex carbohydrates—the kind found in cereals, breads, pasta, vegetables, beans, legumes, and some fruits—are starches that the body breaks down into simple sugars. This leads to two obvious questions: If complex carbohydrates break down into simple sugars, why are they any different from the simple carbohydrates found in sugars? Don't they provide the same amount of energy?

Yes and no. They do provide the same amount of calories per sugar mole-

Vegetarianism: Pro or Con?

Only about 5 percent of Americans classify themselves as full-time vegetarians, but increasingly the health conscious are choosing vegetarianesque diets. Many people have eliminated red meat from their diets, and more are choosing to eliminate poultry and fish as well. This choice may be a good thing. Study after study has shown that a diet low in animal protein and rich in fruits and vegetables does the most to keep a person young. Decreasing the consumption of red meat to once a week or less reduces aging of both the cardiovascular and immune systems. However, vegetarians need to be careful. They run the risk of not getting the appropriate variety of foods, thereby missing out on proteins and nutrients that are more plentiful in animal products.

Anyone who adopts such food choices will need to supplement his or her diet with vitamin B_{12}, which is obtained almost exclusively from animal products. If you do not eat any animal products, make sure to take a vitamin containing adequate amounts of folate, B_6, and B_{12} daily. If you decide to go on a vegetarian diet, I suggest meeting with a nutritionist to go over a sensible food choice plan.

cule and the same amount of energy. Most complex carbohydrates are found in foods that are rich in vitamins and nutrients and high in fiber. The body treats complex carbohydrates differently. They break down more slowly, consuming more metabolic energy in digestion and keeping glucose levels more stable. Since they are not concentrated in form as refined sugars usually are, we eat less complex carbohydrates per ounce of food.

Forget those old diet myths that breads and pasta are fattening. Carbohydrates contain far fewer calories per gram than fats: 4 per gram as opposed to 9 per gram. Eating a diet high in complex carbohydrates—fruits, vegetables, and grains—will help you shed excess pounds and gain extra years of youth.

10. Cut Out Excess Sugars

Although the consumption of sugar is not tied to aging itself, it is linked to weight gain. Simple sugars tend to be more concentrated in foods, meaning that you consume more calories per mouthful. Cutting back on overall sugar intake is a quick and easy way to make extra calories disappear from your diet. Some people think that eating too much sugar is associated with the development of diabetes; this is not true. However, foods containing lots of refined sugar are high in calories, and most of these calories are nutritionally empty. Don't

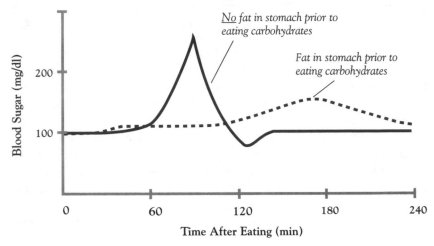

Figure 8.1
If you eat a little fat prior to eating carbohydrates, your stomach doesn't empty its contents into the intestine as quickly. This slowing of stomach emptying has two RealAge Age Reduction effects. First, you feel full faster and stay full longer, so you eat less; and second, since sugars are largely absorbed in the intestine, the amount of sugar in the blood rises slower and peaks at a lower level.

delude yourself: honey and natural sugars are not a healthy substitute for white sugar. In the end, the body breaks them down into the same molecule, and they contain the same number of calories. Finally, though it is not true in all cases, many people find that a diet low in sugar can help provide a more stable blood glucose level. Eating sugar in large doses tends to cause peaks in a person's metabolic level. Eating a little fat first will slow the emptying of the stomach into the intestine, which keeps your stomach fuller and stabilizes your blood sugar levels, so you feel full and eat less. Furthermore, since sugars are largely absorbed in the intestine, delaying the sugar getting to the intestine slows and decreases the rise in the sugar level in the blood (see Figure 8.1). Lots of people find that eating less sugar gives them more energy without after-the-big-meal sleepiness.

11. Eat Fish

Salmon; white fish, such as cod or bass; and other fish contain lots of omega-3 fatty acids, a type of fat that actually reduces triglyceride levels in the blood and appears to lower blood pressure. Eating fish at least once a week may cut the risk of heart attack in half, making the RealAge of a fifty-five-year-old man more than 2.7 years younger. Although no one knows precisely how omega-3 fatty acids work to prevent heart attacks, some experts believe that these substances prevent the buildup of plaque along arterial walls. Others suggest that omega-3s help stabilize a person's heartbeat, cutting down on the irregular heart rhythms associated with heart attacks. Omega-3s also appear to make platelets less sticky, decreasing the risk of clotting. Recent data showed a 52 percent decrease in sudden death when fish was consumed at least once a week. Omega-3s may also reduce blood pressure. Although you can buy fish-oil supplements at the health-food store, it's best to eat fish itself.

Shellfish contain omega-3s, but not as much as fish. Although high in cholesterol, shellfish are low in fat and therefore make a good diet option. Finally, be careful about eating raw seafood, which is more likely to carry disease-causing germs than cooked seafood.

12. Make Substitutions

Eating habits learned over a lifetime can be hard to break. Learn how to substitute healthy ingredients into recipes that have always been unhealthy. When a recipe calls for butter, ask yourself, "Does the recipe really need all that saturated fat? Could I use something else? Could I substitute orange juice and ginger? What about a teaspoon of olive oil?" Garlic, ginger, vinegar, and spicy ingredients can often make up for the lack of saturated fat in a dish. My mother used to make mashed potatoes with lots of milk and butter, but I roast a head of garlic and mix the cloves in with the potatoes while mashing them. Roasting gives the garlic a mellow flavor, and the individual cloves take on the consistency of butter. Fruit butters, such as apple butter, contain no fats and are a good substitute for real butter. Use them as a spread for bread or mix them in with other foods.

If you're roasting a chicken or other meat, put it on a rack so all the fat drips down. Cook tomato sauce and balsamic vinegar and add some spices and herbs to make a tasty sauce for everything from chicken breasts to eggplant to pasta. Baste your meats with fruit juice, not drippings from the pan. Make sauces out of vegetable purees or wine instead of cream. Soups can be just as creamy when you substitute potato-chicken broth puree for the cups of whipping cream. Every time you use a recipe that calls for saturated fats or trans fats, ask yourself, "How can I cook this so I maximize the nutrients and minimize the fats?"

13. Be Aware of Hidden Fats and Calories

Most saturated fats, trans fats, and sugars enter the diet in the form of "hidden" ingredients in many processed foods, and the package labels may provide the clues you need. For example, many commercial brands of cereal and most processed breads contain a great deal of added fats and sugars. In addition, canned soups and vegetables and even granola are often high in both sugars and saturated fats or trans fats. By becoming a label reader, you won't consume needless calories that you didn't know were there.

Remember, "fat-free" doesn't mean "not fattening." Many "fat-free" products are good for you and will form part of an Age Reduction diet, but that is not always the case. Fat-free cookies and fat-free ice cream may be "fat-free," but they are usually full of calories yet low on nutritional value.

14. Cut Back on Cholesterol and Salt

Cut dietary cholesterol intake to less than 300 mg a day (see the cholesterol section later in this chapter). Limit sodium intake to 2,400 mg a day, preferably 1,600 mg or about a teaspoon of salt (see Chapter 7).

15. Eat Regularly Throughout the Day

Many people believe they will lose weight if they starve themselves all day, waiting until dinner to eat, at which time they gorge. This habit adversely affects overall body metabolism. More important, most people cheat, sneaking a cookie here or a candy bar there sometime in the mid-afternoon. Make sure to eat regular meals and don't skip breakfast (see Chapter 10). Many experts recommend "grazing"—eating a number of small meals throughout the day, rather than just two or three large ones. That way, your body metabolizes food on a regular basis, not going through long periods without fuel, followed by intense periods of excess. See if eating this way helps you eat more nutritious food and lose weight.

16. Don't Forget the Water

Because your body is approximately 80 percent water, you need lots of fluid (at least eight glasses a day) to keep it running right. Water is best, although juices, soups, and skim milk can also rehydrate you. Make sure you drink extra water to keep yourself properly hydrated, especially if you are exercising or the weather is hot. What's the best kind of water? We don't know. But most experts agree that as long as your town treats its water, tap water is just fine.

17. Think "Healthy" at the Grocery Store

Think about the control you have over your diet when you go shopping for food. If you don't buy food that's bad for you, you won't eat food that's bad for you. Before you put any item in your cart, ask yourself, first, "Why am I eating this?" And, second, "Will it help keep me young?" If the answer to the first question is "Because it's quick," and the answer to the second question is "No," get it out of your cart. Fast!

Become a label reader. Look out for saturated fats and trans fats and see what you can do to buy foods with the most nutrients. Even similar products may have different ingredients. For example, I remember trying to buy a can of refried beans for a Mexican dish. One brand contained partially hydrogenated oil, while another had canola oil, and the third had no oil at all. Although they all looked the same, their calorie and fat content were very different. The first was unhealthy, the second was moderately healthy, and the third was very healthy. If I hadn't bothered to look, I wouldn't have known.

18. Age-Proof Your Kitchen

Get rid of staples that will surreptitiously make you age faster than you want. Then make substitutions. Throw out all those cooking implements—ice cream makers and deep-fat fryers—that will entice you to eat foods that age you. Clear out your recipe files, banishing recipes that call for a lot of cream or butter. While you're at it, throw out any take-out menus for places that serve unhealthy food. Keep the menu from the Vietnamese restaurant and toss the one from the fried chicken joint. That way, you won't be tempted.

19. Don't Let Situations You Can't Control Stop You from Making Smart Food Choices

At home, it is relatively easy to develop a diet plan and stick with it. When you're out on the town it's a different story. Many people find it hard to keep eating right when they go out for meals or have to travel. Learn how to make the situations in which you have less control more manageable for you. For example, when you go out to eat, look for low-fat options on the menu. If you don't see anything, try to modify an existing dish by asking the waiter to have it baked or broiled without fat. Ask to have sauces served on the side, or request that your omelet be made with just egg whites. Most restaurants prove extremely accommodating. (I remember eating in a restaurant with nutrition expert Dr. Jerry Stamler and being amazed at how he changed the menu, asking the chef to modify dishes to suit his dietary requirements.) The answer is usually YES, and the food delicious.

Also, if you're invited to a party and think that everything's going to be calorie laden and heavy, eat before you arrive and then eat less when you get there. Just smile and say, "It's fabulous but just so filling." If you travel frequently on airplanes, pack your own snacks. Or call ahead to see if you can order a special meal. Most airlines offer vegetarian food or heart-healthy selections, and these meals are generally tastier, more nutritious, and lower in saturated fats and trans fats than their usual entrées. Wherever you are, don't hesitate to take a low-fat snack pack with you when you're on the run—at work or at play. It will help you keep the years away.

20. Finally—and Most Important— Make Healthy Eating Fun

You are making changes for a lifetime—changes for a younger lifetime. This shouldn't be hard work. Healthy eating should be part of enjoying all those years of added youth. Buy a low-fat cookbook. Try out a new recipe three nights a week or every Sunday. If you live with someone who shares cooking, make it a game. See who can make the best-tasting low-fat dishes. Be inventive. If you haven't a clue what to do with that funny new vegetable (like kohlrabi), figure something out. Dare to be bold and adventurous. If you always eat a certain style of food, break the mold. Try new options: Thai food, Italian, or vegetarian. Make low-saturated-fat eating an adventure, not a chore.

These are general guidelines for Age Reduction eating. It may take a while to adjust to the changes. Stick with it for a couple of months and see how you do. If you have questions regarding serving sizes or the nutrient content of foods, I suggest you buy a nutritional information book. Many good books list the calories and nutrients in a whole range of foods. (I love the tables in Roy L. Walford's *The 120-Year Diet*, Pocket Books, 1988.) The better informed you are about what you eat, the better food choices you will make, and the younger you will stay.

Now let's consider three food concerns we all have and about which you will want more information: fat consumption, cholesterol intake, and weight maintenance.

CUT THE FAT: KEEP THE TASTE

One of the best things I ever learned about eating, I learned from my daughter—by accident. To ensure that we spend time together in spite of our busy schedules, Jennifer and I arrange father-daughter evenings during which we do something fun together—watch a movie, see an exhibit, set off on some kind of adventure—and then we go out to dinner, just the two of us. One Saturday, when Jennifer was about eleven, we spent the early evening playing squash together. By the time we'd finished the game, Jennifer was hungry. By the time we got to the restaurant, she was famished. She just couldn't wait for an entrée. Trying to come up with a quick solution, I suggested, "Let's eat dessert first." Jennifer couldn't believe it. Here was Dad suggesting what she'd always dreamed of. "Really?" she said, "Can we?"

"If you don't tell mom." Then, to cover my tracks, I added, "They'll bring it to us quickly. We'll eat a small amount of dessert first, getting us lots of calories, sugars, and fats, so you won't feel so hungry, and then we can take our time with the rest of the meal and eat right."

Jennifer thought I'd lost it, but she didn't complain. And, in what was to become a tradition for father-daughter evenings, we shared a dessert first. Only later did I learn that not only was it fun, it was good for us!

Cutting back on fats, especially saturated and trans fats, is one of the most difficult things we face when trying to improve our diet. We all need some fat in our diets, but most Americans get much more than they need. One way to cut back on fats and calories is to time when you eat them. Eating a little bit of fat at the beginning of the meal helps you feel full faster, and that means you end up eating fewer total calories. The little bit of fat prevents your stomach from emptying (see Figure 8.1 in the previous section).

Fat is by far the most complicated food choice you have to make when it comes to diet. First, *fat* can mean two things: body fat, the fat you have on your body, and dietary fat, the fat you eat. Fat is a chemical compound found in most living organisms, plants and animals alike.

Although we need to eat less fat, fat is essential for you. The body cannot manufacture the three essential fatty acids contained in dietary fat, so you must get them from food. Also, you need to eat some fat to be able to absorb vitamins A, D, E, and K and antioxidant Age Reducing substances, such as lycopene. The problem is not so much that we eat fat, but that we eat too much fat and too much of the wrong kinds of fat.

There are four major types of fat: saturated, polyunsaturated, monounsaturated, and trans fats. The first three occur naturally. Trans fat is an artificially created imitation of saturated fat. Although all four kinds of fat have the same number of calories per serving (120 per tablespoon or 9 per gram), each type can affect your body differently. Saturated and trans fats cause aging of the arteries and accelerate aging of the immune system. Polyunsaturated fats, except for their high calorie count, do not seem to have any aging effects *per se*. Monounsaturated fats actually appear to make you younger, helping to boost the levels of HDL (healthy) cholesterol in your blood, but they are high in calories.

No matter what kind of fat you eat, remember that fats are "fattening." Fats, whether in our bodies or in the plants and animals we eat, are energy stores and loaded with calories. Fat contains more calories, per gram, than either protein or carbohydrate. All fats, whether unsaturated or saturated, contain 9 calories per gram, whereas carbohydrates and proteins contain only 4 calories per gram.

The average American consumes 90 grams of fat a day, which is about 40 percent of his or her total calories. I recommend that you limit your total fat intake to no more than 30 percent of your total dietary consumption. Better still, cut back to 25 percent. Diet specialist Dean Ornish believes the level should be as low as 10 percent. In any case, make sure *saturated* fats and *trans* fats make up no more than 10 percent of your total calories, especially if you are at a special risk of arterial aging. Active women who do not need to lose weight and have no fat-associated risks should try to eat no more than 50 grams of fat a day. Healthy, active men should aim for 55 grams or less.

Saturated Fats

Of all the fats, saturated fat is the worst. Just remember "s" for "stay away." Saturated fat is found in red meats; whole-fat dairy products; palm or coconut oil; and, to a lesser extent, poultry and other animal products.

No food element has been more closely linked to arterial aging than saturated fats and their cousins, trans fats. This relationship was confirmed by a twenty-five-year study that evaluated the long-term risk of death and the development of coronary heart disease. Studies have repeatedly found a strong correlation between cardiovascular disease and the consumption of saturated fats.

Foods high in saturated fats promote the plaque buildup along the arterial wall, the first stage of cardiovascular disease and arterial aging. Saturated fats facilitate the mechanism that increases LDL cholesterol in the bloodstream. Only 20 percent of cholesterol is absorbed from food. The liver manufactures the rest from saturated and trans fats. Consumption of saturated fat, not cholesterol, is the biggest dietary factor contributing to elevated levels of cholesterol in the blood. Excess saturated fat consumption is also linked to elevated triglyceride levels, a reading of the fat ratio in the blood. Elevated triglyceride levels have been strongly linked to arterial aging.

Does eating saturated fat cause your body to age in other ways? Yes. Although the link between fat consumption and cancers remains nebulous, several studies have shown strong correlations. Some experts estimate that as many as one-third of all cancers may be provoked by the dietary choices we make. And saturated fat appears to be a leading culprit. A recent study, the Iowa Women's Health Study, indicated that postmenopausal women who have been diagnosed with breast cancer have a better survival rate if they keep their weight down and consume a diet low in saturated fats. Other studies have noted a connection between fat intake and higher incidences of other types of cancers (including lung cancer, lymphomas, and ovarian and prostate cancer).

The Food and Drug Administration (FDA) mandates that product labels list the percentages of saturated fats. Companies now advertise their products as being "low in saturated fat." But as bad as saturated fats are, there is another kind of fat that is just as bad, if not worse: trans fat.

Trans Fat

Recent research suggests that trans fats are at least as dangerous as saturated fats. Trans fat—also called trans fatty acid—is created when unsaturated fats are hydrogenated (combined with hydrogen), a chemical process that causes fats that would normally be liquid at room temperature to become solid at room temperature. Any fat we usually eat that is liquid when heated but that hardens when cooled to room temperature is made either of saturated or trans fat. Here's a good test for deciding if a fat is good for you: If it's solid, it will age you. Stick margarine is a trans fat. So is the fat in donut glaze. Trans fats, like saturated fats, alter basic metabolic pathways, causing a rise in overall cholesterol levels, particularly increasing the amount of LDL (lousy) cholesterol in your bloodstream.

Studies have shown that the more trans fat a person consumes, the faster the cardiovascular system ages. In one study of more than eighty-five thousand participants, women who consumed more than four teaspoons of margarine a day had a 70 percent higher risk of cardiovascular disease than those who rarely consumed margarine. Thus, in RealAge terms, the fifty-five-year-old woman who uses stick margarine is 2.7 years older than the woman who uses olive oil. Some researchers have attributed as many as thirty thousand deaths a year to the consumption of trans fats.

Because food producers are not required to list trans fats on their nutrition labels, trans fats are called "the hidden fats." Many packaged foods—cookies, crackers, and potato chips—contain these oils because they give food a longer shelf life. A lot of cookies and crackers claim to be "baked, not fried" or to contain "no cholesterol," implying that they are low in fat, when they are, in fact, chock-full of trans fat. It doesn't matter if a food is "cholesterol-free"; if it contains trans fat, it will damage your arteries.

Many fast-food restaurants cook food in trans fat to produce the flavor of food cooked in lard, the ingredient used before consumers became concerned about saturated fats. Most french fries at your local burger stand contain as much or more artery-clogging fat as if they had been fried in lard. Even the chicken at most fast-food restaurants, an option you might think would be healthier than a burger, is almost always high in fat, often containing more fat than a full steak dinner.

How do you know if a food contains trans fat? You don't. As of 1998, food producers aren't required to list trans fats on nutrition-information labels, although the FDA is considering changing this requirement. When looking at a nutrition information label, check the total fat content. Then look at the saturated fat content. Subtract the saturated fat from the total fat. This leaves both unsaturated fat and trans fat. If the ingredient label lists hydrogenated or partially hydrogenated oils before polyunsaturated or monounsaturated oils, you know that the product contains lots of trans fat. A food label must list the ingredients in order of quantity, from most to least. The fats listed first are in greater quantity than those listed later. If the label lists unsaturated or monounsaturated oils, olive oil, or canola oil first, you know that the fats are probably okay. Some experts contend that trans fats constitute 25–60 percent of all fats contained in processed foods, making up 15–30 percent of the total intake of dietary fat. Others disagree, saying the proportions are much lower.

The full effects of trans fats are still not understood. Some scientists believe that the artificial molecular structure of trans fat actually causes more harm than naturally occurring molecules of saturated fat. Stick margarine *might* be even worse for you than butter. We can't say for sure; the research still needs to be completed.

The best advice is to cut out as much saturated fat and trans fat from your diet as possible. Use liquid vegetable oils in recipes that call for butter or margarine. Make substitutions. If you decide to eat margarine, buy liquid or tub margarine. The first ingredient listed in the fine print should be water, vegetable oil, or vegetable oil blend.

Unsaturated Fats

The other two types of fats are the unsaturated fats—monounsaturated and polyunsaturated fats—which are found in vegetable and fruit oils. These fats remain liquid at room temperatureare because they unsaturated. The prefixes *poly* and *mono* refer to their chemical structure. Unsaturated fats are found exclusively in plants. We consume them largely as vegetable oils.

Polyunsaturated fats appear neither to promote nor prevent premature aging, although some very preliminary studies have questioned whether these fats might be linked to the onset of certain cancers. I rate them a "p" for "passable": They're okay but not great. Monounsaturated fats may actually be good for you. Monounsaturated fats—in contrast to saturated fats—help reduce the amount of bad cholesterol in the blood and boost the amount of good cholesterol, causing LDL levels to sink and HDL levels to rise. The exact mechanism remains unknown.

All oils contain some of each kind of fat—polyunsaturated, monounsaturated, and saturated—but in varying proportions. For example, olive oil is higher in monounsaturated fats than almost any other oil but still contains some saturated and polyunsaturated fats, too. At the other end of the scale are palm and coconut oils, which contain a small amount of unsaturated fats yet have more saturated fat per gram than red meat. In between are corn, vegetable, and soybean oils, which are predominately polyunsaturated fats. The oil with the highest ratio of unsaturated fat to saturated fat is canola oil. Aside from olive oil, canola oil has the most monounsaturated fat per ounce than any other oil and is the lowest in saturated fats of any oil.

Olives and olive oil are a key source of monounsaturated fats. Avocados represent another food that is rich in monounsaturated fats, high in fiber, beta carotene, and potassium; and one of the few dietary sources of vitamin E. If you wish to eat fat, an avocado is a good choice. Remember that one avocado can be as much as one-third of your daily fat allowance, since each one contains nearly 20 grams of fat. For aficionados, Florida avocados—although not as creamy tasting as California avocados—contain significantly less fat. When you buy oil, buy either canola or olive oil. Still, use each sparingly because, like all fats, they are fattening (if the "s" in saturated stands for "stay away," the "t" in trans fat is "terrible," and the "p" in polyunsaturated is "passable," then the "m" in monounsaturated means "in moderation").

CHOLESTEROL:
THE FACTS BEHIND THE HYPE

Remember when almost every health story featured cholesterol as its subject, and everyone you knew was rushing out to have his or her cholesterol levels checked? Even as recently as a few years ago, we thought that having a low cholesterol level ensured long-term arterial health. We now know the story is more complex. Sure, it's generally good to have a low total cholesterol level, but many other factors are more important to aging than cholesterol. In fact, most people who have cardiovascular disease have cholesterol levels below the "high" marker of 240 mg/dl (milligrams per deciliter). Although high levels of total cholesterol and/or LDL (lousy) cholesterol can contribute to arterial aging, other factors contribute even more: high blood pressure; cigar, cigarette, or passive smoking; not exercising; high levels of homocysteine; diabetes; and a diet that is heavy in saturated fats and trans fats and poor in nutrients. Nevertheless, you should keep in mind that high cholesterol levels *can* affect your rate of aging.

What Does "High Cholesterol" Mean?

Cholesterol is a type of lipid (a fat soluble molecule) found in three places: in our cells, in our food ("dietary" cholesterol), and in our blood. As much as we fear cholesterol, it is a vital component of our bodies. Cholesterol is required for the body to manufacture hormones, build cell walls, and produce bile acids, which are essential for the breakdown and digestion of fats. In some areas of the body, cholesterol levels are high. For example, skin cells contain a lot of cholesterol, making them highly water resistant. This water resistance protects the body from dehydration by reducing the evaporation of water. The brain also has high concentrations of cholesterol.

When we measure cholesterol, we measure the amount of cholesterol circulating in the blood. Problems develop not from having cholesterol in the blood, but from having too much cholesterol *and* too much of the wrong type of cholesterol in our blood, where it can cause damage to our arteries. In general, having a high total cholesterol level is bad: Excess cholesterol can promote arterial aging. However, even among such high-risk populations as middle-aged men, only 9–12 percent of those with total cholesterol readings of over 240 mg/dl will actually have symptomatic cardiovascular disease as a direct result of cholesterol. For each 1 percent increase in the overall cholesterol reading in middle-aged men (for example, for 202 versus 200 mg/dl), the risk of developing cardiovascular disease increases by 2 percent. High cholesterol levels affect different population groups disproportionately. For example, high cholesterol seems to have a significant aging effect on young and middle-aged men, but a much less significant effect on older men and women of all ages. The female sex hormone estrogen generally decreases the presence of cholesterol in the blood, whereas androgens— the male sex hormones—increase blood cholesterol. Premenopausal women rarely have to worry about their cholesterol levels.

The Ratio of LDL to HDL

Far more important than a person's total cholesterol reading is the ratio of his or her LDL to HDL. There are three basic types of cholesterol in your body: low-density lipoproteins (LDL), high-density lipoproteins (HDL), and very-low-density lipoproteins (VLDL). Because the VLDL level is rarely measured directly, in general, cholesterol tests measure total cholesterol, LDL, and HDL cholesterol. (LDL is calculated by subtracting HDL from total cholesterol.) LDL cholesterol causes aging of the arteries; HDL cholesterol prevents it. (Recall that I remember the "L" of LDL as "lousy" and the "H" of HDL as "healthy.")

In general, a total cholesterol reading of 240 mg/dl is too high and can cause arterial aging. In the most rigorous study on cholesterol, the Framingham Study, individuals with a cholesterol reading lower than 200 mg/dl had a 10 percent risk of coronary artery disease over a twenty-year period. Those with a total cholesterol reading above 240 mg/dl had about twice as much chance (20 percent) of developing the disease.

Most people who have high cholesterol also have high levels of LDL cholesterol, which causes arterial aging. LDL molecules deliver cholesterol to the cells in the body. When cholesterol rises, excess LDL molecules in the bloodstream can attach to small ruptures or lesions in the arterial wall, the endothelium, and trigger a process that can lead to the development of arterial plaques and cardiovascular aging.

It is interesting to note that some people with very high cholesterol levels have arteries that are in better condition than those of other individuals who have low cholesterol levels. These lucky people have high levels of HDL cholesterol and low levels of LDL cholesterol. Since HDL molecules remove excess cholesterol from the arteries, the more HDL you have, the less excess LDL cholesterol you have and the less arterial aging you will undergo. Unfortunately, these people are the exception, not the rule.

When you get your cholesterol levels tested, make sure to ask not just for your total cholesterol level but for your total/HDL ratio. The lower the ratio, the better. The average ratio for middle-aged Americans is 5. It is calculated by dividing the number for total cholesterol by the number for HDL. For example, if you have a total blood cholesterol of 200 and your HDL is 40, the ratio is 5 (200/40). On the other hand, if your total blood cholesterol is 200 but your HDL is 57, your ratio is 3.5. A fifty-five-year-old man with a ratio of 3.5 would have only about half the risk of arterial aging as the average man in his age group; his RealAge would be eight years younger. In contrast, if that man had a ratio of 9 (for example, 270 total/30 HDL), he would have more than five times the risk of arterial aging as the average man in his age group; his

RealAge would be twelve years older than average. Similarly, having either high LDL or a high LDL/HDL ratio can cause arterial aging.

As mentioned, having a total cholesterol of over 240 mg/dl suggests a high risk of aging. Likewise, a level of LDL cholesterol above 160 mg/dl or an HDL reading below 35 mg/dl correlates with an increased rate of arterial aging. If your total cholesterol is more than 240, if your LDL cholesterol is higher than 160, or if your HDL cholesterol is lower than 35, you should talk seriously with your doctor about improving your cholesterol levels to retard arterial aging. Having either high LDL levels or low HDL levels can make your RealAge anywhere from three to six years older. Having both high total LDL and a high LDL-to-HDL ratio can make your RealAge anywhere from six to eighteen years older, depending on the ratio. Even if your cholesterol status is more moderate—LDL levels above 100 but below 160 or HDL levels less than 55 but above 36—you should also consider taking steps to reduce your LDL cholesterol and increase your HDL levels.

Despite all the buzz about cholesterol-free foods, cholesterol is one factor that is largely determined by genetics. Genetics determine whether you have a tendency toward high LDL levels, and genetics largely determine your LDL-to-HDL ratio. That means that genetic factors greatly determine how seriously you will be affected by arterial aging caused by elevated LDL cholesterol levels if you don't adopt Age Reduction activities that are specifically targeted toward preventing arterial aging. For example, if you are a man with a high LDL cholesterol level or a high LDL-to-HDL ratio and a number of your close male relatives died early from heart disease, you are at a high risk of the premature onset of cardiovascular disease (see Table 8.2).

As I mentioned, an HDL level above 60 mg/dl appears to provide tremendous protection against arterial aging. Although some medications will help increase HDL levels, drugs are not the most effective way of improving your cholesterol ratio. In fact, no techniques have been proven to work for everyone. Exercise is one of the best ways to improve your HDL reading. Women tend to have higher HDL levels than men, and women are able to improve their HDL levels with exercise to a greater extent than men. A recent North Carolina study found that aerobic exercise increased HDL by 20 percent in female patients but by only 5 percent in male patients. Also, a glass of alcohol a night (half a glass for women) may increase your HDL level (see Chapter 10). For many people, losing excess weight improves their HDL readouts. Although the interaction between weight gain and cholesterol levels is still not well understood, the correlation between the two is strong.

In contrast, if you have low LDL cholesterol, your genetics are protecting you from arterial aging. Finally, there are a lucky few who have high total

TABLE 8.2

The RealAge Effect of Blood Cholesterol Levels

FOR MEN

| Calendar Age | Total Cholesterol Below 160 mg/dl and HDL of | | |
| | More than 59 mg/dl | 35 to 59 mg/dl | Less than 35 mg/dl |
	RealAge		
35	32.9	34	35.3
55	51.7	53.2	57.2
70	66	66.9	70

| Calendar Age | Total Cholesterol of 160–200 mg/dl and HDL of | | |
| | More than 59 mg/dl | 35 to 59 mg/dl | Less than 35 mg/dl |
	RealAge		
35	33.9	34.6	35.9
55	52.1	54.2	57.5
70	66.9	66.4	71.6

| Calendar Age | Total Cholesterol of 200–240 mg/dl and HDL of | | |
| | More than 59 mg/dl | 35 to 59 mg/dl | Less than 35 mg/dl |
	RealAge		
35	34.1	35.1	36.1
55	52.3	55	58.3
70	67.6	70.3	72.3

| Calendar Age | Total Cholesterol Over 240 mg/dl and HDL of | | |
| | More than 59 mg/dl | 35 to 59 mg/dl | Less than 35 mg/dl |
	RealAge		
35	35.8	37.4	38.7
55	56.7	58	58.8
70	70	70.7	72.5

FOR WOMEN

| Calendar Age | Total Cholesterol Below 160 mg/dl and HDL of | | |
| | More than 59 mg/dl | 35 to 59 mg/dl | Less than 35 mg/dl |
	RealAge		
35	33.7	34.6	35.3
55	52.6	53.2	56.4
70	68.5	68.5	71.8

| Calendar Age | Total Cholesterol of 160–200 mg/dl and HDL of | | |
| | More than 59 mg/dl | 35 to 59 mg/dl | Less than 35 mg/dl |
	RealAge		
35	34	34.6	35.6
55	52.8	53.4	56.5
70	68.5	68.5	71.8

| Calendar Age | Total Cholesterol of 200–240 mg/dl and HDL of | | |
| | More than 59 mg/dl | 35 to 59 mg/dl | Less than 35 mg/dl |
	RealAge		
35	34	35.1	35.6
55	52.8	54.7	56.4
70	68.5	68.5	71.8

| Calendar Age | Total Cholesterol Over 240 mg/dl and HDL of | | |
| | More than 59 mg/dl | 35 to 59 mg/dl | Less than 35 mg/dl |
	RealAge		
35	36.6	36.9	37.3
55	55.3	55.6	57.4
70	68.5	69.4	71.8

Soybeans as Youth Beans

Recent studies have linked soy protein to a reduction in levels of LDL cholesterol. People who regularly consume soy products—soy milk, tofu, and soy beans (and that doesn't mean soy sauce!)—have LDL cholesterol levels that are, on average, 13 percent lower than those who don't. Try substituting soy-based products for animal protein in your diet. The consumption of soy products may have a particularly big impact on those with very high cholesterol levels. It is not clearly understood why or how soy protein helps reduce cholesterol levels, although some experts theorize that the soy works as an antioxidant on cholesterol. Others think that soy may interfere with the formation of plaque. To make a substantial difference in cholesterol, you would need 31 to 47 grams of soy protein a day. Soy also contains a natural estrogen that has been shown to reduce the risk of both breast and prostate cancers and to provide extra protection for aging of the bones.

cholesterol and high HDL cholesterol. These people have a genetic trump. All that HDL cholesterol helps protect them from arterial aging. They can have a RealAge as much as twenty-six years younger than their cohorts.

How to Reduce Cholesterol Levels

Since there has been so much focus in the media on eating a "low-cholesterol" diet, it is surprising to learn that eating a low-cholesterol diet is not an especially effective way to reduce LDL cholesterol. Cholesterol consumed in food will cause a rise in cholesterol levels for some people and will have no effect on other people. Only 15 percent (one in seven individuals) who try a low-cholesterol diet get a significant antiaging effect from doing so. Again, genetics play a role: Genetic factors largely determine your sensitivity to dietary cholesterol, and people can range from extreme sensitivity to complete insensitivity. A person who has a genetic insensitivity may consume as much as 1,000 mg of cholesterol daily without negative consequences. In general, though, it is recommended that you consume less than 300 mg of cholesterol a day. People who show a particular sensitivity to dietary cholesterol should eat even less than that to retard or reverse arterial aging. How do you know your responsiveness to dietary restriction of cholesterol? Only by measuring blood levels before and after restricting dietary cholesterol. A dramatic decline suggests that you are sensitive. A more modest decrease of 10–15 percent suggests that you are not.

For most of us, consumption of fat influences our levels of cholesterol in the blood far more than consumption of cholesterol itself. Unless you are especially sensitive to dietary cholesterol, your body produces almost all the cholesterol that exists in the bloodstream. The liver manufactures cholesterol from the saturated and trans fats you consume. This is yet another reason why it is important to eat a diet low in saturated and trans fats.

The best way to reduce high LDL cholesterol is to choose foods that are low in cholesterol, saturated fat, and trans fat. If you have high LDL cholesterol, you may want to consider taking medicine to reduce those levels. Talk to your doctor about getting a more extensive lipid evaluation and about the pros and cons of medication for improving either your overall cholesterol level or your LDL-to-HDL ratio. The latest and most effective drugs for reducing LDL cholesterol levels are the so-called statin drugs (such as pravastatin, Pravachol). They lower LDL and increase HDL more effectively than the older generation of drugs and have better tolerability and acceptance. Since these drugs are so new, we still do not know whether they might have negative effects—that is, they might accelerate aging—when used over a long period. The longest-running study lasted only six years. However, the data strongly suggest that these drugs greatly retard arterial aging.

Triglyceride Levels

Triglycerides are lipids (fats) that circulate in the bloodstream. Triglyceride measurements are usually taken after an overnight fast and when cholesterol levels are analyzed. The average fasting triglyceride level is 120–125 mg/dl. Levels above 200 mg/dl are associated with significant arterial aging, especially with plaque buildup along the arterial wall. Since triglyceride levels fluctuate a fair amount, people with high levels (above 190 mg/dl) will want to have their blood analyzed several times to get an accurate estimate. If your fasting triglyceride level is above 200 mg/dl, reduce total fat intake. Cutting saturated and trans fats to less than 7 percent of your total caloric intake, eating fish rich in omega-3 fish oils at least three times a week or more, and increasing your physical activity are all actions to choose before considering possible drug therapies (see Table 8.3).

Low Cholesterol Levels

With all this talk about high LDL cholesterol, do we have to worry about the other side of the spectrum? Can your cholesterol level dip too low?

TABLE 8.3

The RealAge Effect of Triglycerides

FOR MEN

| Calendar Age | Concentration of Triglycerides in the Blood (mg/dl) | | | |
	Less than 90	90–123	124–209	More than 209
	RealAge			
35	33.2	35.3	35.3	35.7
55	41.6	55.7	55.7	60.9
70	65.7	71	71	78.2

FOR WOMEN

| Calendar Age | Concentration of Triglycerides in the Blood (mg/dl) | | | |
	Less than 90	90–123	124–209	More than 209
	RealAge			
35	33.9	35.2	35.2	35.5
55	50.1	55.5	55.5	65.9
70	66.8	70.7	70.7	74.8

Apparently, yes, although we know far less about ultra-low cholesterol than high cholesterol, as very few people without an acute disease or chronic malnutrition have cholesterol levels low enough to be of concern. In a few but not all studies, people with low total cholesterol levels appeared to have a higher incidence of cancers and, curious to note, suicides. Although very few studies have been done on this subject, and we still cannot say with any certainty how low "too low" is, it appears there is some risk. A possible explanation for the relationship to cancer may be that cholesterols are necessary components of vitamin D_3, a proven cancer fighter (see Chapter 7). As for the suicides, no one really knows. Cholesterols are important in the functioning of brain cells and the production of hormones, so an ultra-low level of cholesterol may affect these two functions.

SLIMMING DOWN

How Shedding Pounds Amounts to Shedding Years

Perhaps no health issue is more emotionally charged than weight gain. We need only to look at the plethora of diet books and the news stories about eating disorders to sense the concern. Ironically, in spite of the abundance of information on diet, nutrition, and the health problems associated with being overweight, the American population has been getting progressively heavier.

Being overweight can provoke many conditions that age your body. It causes high blood pressure, inhibits exercise, and promotes chronic diseases like diabetes. Excess weight is associated with accelerated arterial aging and the onset of cardiovascular disease; aging of the bones and joints; diseases of aging, such as gallbladder disease and gout; increased levels of depression; and increased incidence of cancers, especially breast, uterine, and prostate cancers. Being overweight can make your RealAge as much as ten years older.

Fad diets are not the solution. Losing weight—and keeping it off—is no easy trick. The only way to do it is to change behaviors at the most fundamental level: Weight loss and maintenance of the ideal weight are always tied to healthy eating and exercise behaviors that are practiced for a lifetime. Repeatedly losing weight and gaining it back stresses your body and actually accelerates aging.

The customary way of calculating your ideal weight is to determine your body mass index (BMI), or your weight-to-height ratio (see Table 8.4). The BMI reading is one of the best tools for assessing whether a person weighs too much because it accounts for variances in body size, giving a standard for evaluating people at a range of heights. (Although BMI is not the best measure of body fat, for most people, it provides a good general estimate and can easily be calculated at home.)

The average BMI for Americans is 26.3 kg/m^2 (kilograms per meter squared). In terms of Age Reduction, the ideal BMI is 23 or less. As long as your weight is not abnormally low because of some health complication, such as a chronic disease, if you have a BMI of 23 or less, you can expect your RealAge to be as much as eight years younger than if your BMI were at the national average of 26.3.

If your BMI is over 25, you will probably want to consider a moderate weight-loss program that includes boosting exercise and cutting caloric intake. If your BMI is over 27, excess weight is causing unnecessary aging (see Table 8.5), and, again, you should consider a safe and gradual weight-loss

TABLE 8.4

What Is Your Body Mass Index?

	Body Mass Index (kg/m²)*													
	19	20	21	22	23	24	25	26	27	28	29	30	35	40
Height (inches)	Body Weight in Pounds													
58	91	96	100	105	110	115	119	124	129	134	138	143	167	191
59	94	99	04	109	114	119	124	128	133	138	143	148	173	198
60	97	102	107	112	118	123	128	133	138	143	148	153	179	204
61	100	106	111	116	122	127	132	137	143	148	153	158	183	211
62	104	109	115	120	126	131	136	142	147	153	158	164	191	218
63	107	113	118	124	130	135	141	146	152	158	163	169	197	225
64	110	116	122	128	134	140	145	151	157	163	169	174	204	232
65	114	120	126	132	138	144	150	156	162	168	174	180	210	240
66	118	124	130	136	142	148	153	161	167	173	179	186	216	247
67	121	127	134	140	146	153	159	166	172	178	185	191	223	255
68	125	131	138	144	151	158	164	171	177	184	190	197	230	262
69	128	135	142	149	153	162	169	176	182	189	196	203	236	270
70	132	139	146	153	160	167	174	181	188	195	202	207	243	278
71	136	143	150	157	165	172	179	186	193	200	208	215	250	286
72	140	147	154	162	169	177	184	191	199	206	213	221	258	294
73	144	151	159	166	174	182	189	197	204	212	219	227	265	302
74	148	155	163	171	179	186	194	202	210	218	225	233	272	311
75	152	160	168	176	184	192	200	208	216	224	232	240	279	319
76	156	164	172	180	189	197	205	213	221	230	238	246	287	328

*To use the table, find your height in the left-hand column. Move across the row to your weight. The number at the top of the column is the body mass index for your height and weight.

If your BMI—the ratio of weight to height expressed in units of kilograms per meter squared (kg/m²)—is not on the chart, or if you want to calculate your BMI more precisely, the formula for doing so is relatively easy:

1. Convert your weight in pounds to your weight in kilograms by dividing your weight in pounds by 2.2.

2. Convert your height in inches to your height in meters by multiplying your height in inches—not feet—by 0.0254. (If you are 5 feet tall, your height is 60 inches, or 1.52 meters. If you are 6 feet tall, your height is 72 inches, or 1.83 meters.)

3. Square your height in meters (that is, multiply your height in meters by itself).

4. Divide your weight in kilograms (the number you obtained in item 1) by the number you obtained in item 3.

TABLE 8.5

The RealAge Effect of Weight

FOR MEN

	Of Having a Body Mass Index of							
	18.5 or less	*18.6– 21.9*	*22– 24.1*	*24.2– 26.4*	*26.5– 28.7*	*28.8– 31.0*	*31.1– 33.3*	*33.4– 35.7*	*Greater than 35.7*
Calendar Age	RealAge								
35	35.2	34.7	35	35.4	35.8	36.1	36.1	36.2	36.3
55	55.3	54.3	55	56	57	58.2	58.2	58.5	58.6
70	70.5	69	70	71.4	72.8	74.7	74.7	75.3	75.4

FOR WOMEN

	Of Having a Body Mass Index of							
	18.5 or less	*18.6– 21.9*	*22– 24.1*	*24.2– 26.4*	*26.5– 28.7*	*28.8– 31.0*	*31.1– 33.3*	*33.4– 35.7*	*Greater than 35.7*
Calendar Age	RealAge								
35	34.9	34.6	35	35.5	36	36.6	37.1	37.5	37.6
55	54.9	54.4	55	55.8	56.6	57.6	58.6	59.6	60.0
70	69.9	69.2	70	71.0	72.1	73.4	75.0	76.1	76.7

plan involving exercise and cutting calories. People with BMIs over 30 should consult a physician or weight-loss professional before beginning any diet, to establish a safe and practical weight-loss plan.

Despite the well-publicized health problems from obesity, more than 40 percent of all men over age fifty are significantly overweight. That is, they are 20 percent or more above their desirable weight and have a BMI over 27.8. Fifty-two percent of women in their fifties and 41 percent of women age sixty and over are significantly overweight: they are 20 percent or more above their desirable weight and have a BMI over 27.3. In 1960, fewer than one-quarter of all Americans were significantly overweight; now more than one-third are. From 1980 to 1990, the weight (adjusted for height) of the average American increased by eight pounds.

What is the major factor causing this increase in weight? Some scientists argue that obesity stems largely from our food choices. We choose to eat a calorically dense diet, one that is high in saturated fats and trans fats, rich in sugar, and low in both fiber and nutrients. Others argue that we are genetically predisposed to obesity. Yet others believe that in our sedentary society, obesity is due to the abundance, variety, availability, and palatability of the food we can eat. That is, we overeat. I say it's double trouble; even when genetic factors are taken into account, we eat too much, and we eat the wrong things. In addition, we don't get enough exercise, especially strength-building exercise.

The best way to lose weight and to get younger by doing so is to eat less food and get more exercise. Approximately three hundred thousand people die a year because of weight-related illnesses. Indeed, our society's tendency to correlate thinness with beauty has done incredible harm. Instead of learning healthy eating practices, we crash diet to lose pounds and, in the process, do incredible damage to our bodies. Or else we give up, thinking that because we will never be supermodel thin, we may as well not bother losing weight at all.

How to Spot a Fad Diet

Every year there are new diet plans and lots of hype accompanying them. One year it is the grapefruit diet, the next year the cabbage soup diet. Some of these plans contain reasonable and healthful information. Others encourage bad diet habits or contain information that is just plain wrong—information that can either do nothing for you or, in some cases, cause real harm. The Food and Nutrition Science Alliance gives good advice on how to spot a bad diet fad:

1. If it sounds too good to be true, it probably is.
2. Don't believe in the quick fix. When it comes to food, there are no overnight miracles.
3. Dire warnings—or raves—about one ingredient or regimen are not the answer. The all-tofu diet isn't going to keep your weight down.
4. Don't be tricked by simplistic conclusions drawn from complex studies. View what you read with a critical eye. Look for informed commentary in the health-minded press.
5. Recommendations based on single studies should not be believed. Wait for confirmation.
6. Dramatic claims that are disputed by other experts in the field are a clear warning sign. Try to evaluate who is correct.

In most of the discussions about weight, what is forgotten is the relationship between weight maintenance and good health. The point is not to be the skinniest person around, but to be the right weight for your height and build. So far, there are no good and lasting quick fixes. If you are just a bit overweight, you can probably increase your exercise levels or reduce your caloric intake and lose the weight.

Recent studies, such as one just completed at the University of Chicago, have found that the best way to lose weight is to increase exercise. In the University of Chicago's research on overweight women, not only did exercise burn calories, it also boosted the overall metabolic rate. When you exercise regularly, the body burns more calories per minute even when you are not exercising. Strength exercises are especially important because they build muscle, which burns more calories per minute than other kinds of body tissue (see Chapter 9).

New evidence shows that weight gain between the ages of eighteen (for women) or twenty-one (for men) and forty is particularly dangerous. Weight gain during these years can make your RealAge six months to one year older for every 10 percent gain in the BMI. Furthermore, every 10 percent increase in relative weight is associated with a 6.5 mm rise in systolic blood pressure, and high blood pressure is one of the major factors affecting aging.

Why are some people more prone to being overweight than others? Two factors that contribute are genetics and behaviors. Certainly, one key factor is heredity. Some of us are born thin, and some of us aren't. Our genes determine all kinds of influences on height, body weight, and metabolic rate, and these influences vary widely from person to person. The study of genetic factors affecting weight gain is a burgeoning field, and scientists have already discovered some genes and gene products that are tied to weight gain. For example, in 1994 and 1995, one of the first hormones tied to fat regulation—leptin—was characterized in the now-famous studies of "fat mice": Mice with genetically caused obesity were given injections of leptin and lost weight. Despite the initial belief that a magical new weight-loss drug had been found, the discovery of leptin proved how complicated the genetics of food metabolism and weight gain are. Subsequent investigations showed that leptin is just one hormone of many involved in a complicated metabolic pathway. Some people with genetically caused weight problems have leptin-related disorders, but others don't. Weight regulation is a complex genetic trait: Many different genes and proteins interact to determine body size. We are still years from understanding the interactions. Fortunately, heredity isn't everything.

What should you do to shed extra pounds? First, review this chapter, which contains tips on eating an Age Reduction diet. Then read the next chapter, in which you will learn how to develop an Age Reduction physical activity plan.

Second, don't torture yourself. The dieter's mentality of sacrifice and denial leads to failure. Don't punish yourself for occasional slipups. Instead, try to establish good eating behaviors that will last a lifetime. It makes no sense to go on a diet for six weeks. Instead, you need to establish routines that will help you keep the weight off for the long term. Don't do anything dramatic or extreme. Use common sense and talk to your doctor. Remember, your food choices are for life: You can keep young by choosing to eat well.

Third, don't go it alone. It's too easy to lose your willpower. Find someone who has a common goal and try to lose weight together. Encourage your spouse or partner, friends, and colleagues to support you or join you. Although a diet sounds like the least entertaining thing imaginable, there are ways of making weight loss fun. For eleven years, I had a running bet with a group of friends. We agreed to lose two to three pounds a month—an achievable goal. Once a month we met for a weigh-in. Anyone who weighed in higher than his or her goal had to pay each of the others a hundred dollars for every pound he or she was over the target weight. Having the penalty be that high gave all of us an extra incentive to meet our goal. In eleven years and 132 weigh-ins, only one of us ever missed our target weight.

Fourth, if you're on a diet, reward yourself. When you lose the pounds you want, treat yourself to a new outfit, a night on the town, exercise clothes, a massage, or whatever makes you feel good—anything except an ice cream sundae! If you know a dieter, help celebrate when his or her weight-loss goal is reached.

Finally, you may want to have professional support. Joining a responsible weight-loss clinic or participating in a program such as Weight Watchers can help you lose extra pounds. These diet clinics and programs can teach you simple tricks for eating healthier, choosing foods that are good for you, and consuming fewer calories. They provide handy tips like what to order in a restaurant when no low-fat options are obvious and how to avoid empty-calorie foods. Also, the social environment really appears to pay off. It encourages a "we're-all-in-this-together" kind of attitude as you learn how to motivate each other and make healthy food choices together. These groups help you celebrate those pounds-off victories.

9
Fit for Youth

AGE REDUCTION EXERCISE MADE EASY

So you think you don't have time to exercise? You don't have time not to. Time spent exercising actually gives you more time. It not only increases longevity, making your RealAge years younger, but it also gives you more energy so that (like other Age Reduction choices) you actually feel years younger, too. By adopting a three-pronged approach for boosting your physical activity, you can reduce your RealAge by 8.1 years. A moderate and balanced exercise routine is an integral piece of your overall Age Reduction Plan, and it's easier than you think to integrate into your everyday life.

- Boost physical activity. You don't have to run marathons to benefit from exercise. Just taking a twenty-minute walk every day can reduce your risk of a heart attack or stroke by 15–30 percent in just twenty weeks. And it makes your RealAge one year younger. Make physical activity—walking to work, taking an evening stroll, or pedaling the exercise bike while watching the evening news—part of your daily life, slowly building up to a goal of expending 3,500 kcal (kilocalories) a week. It will make your RealAge 3.2 years younger.

  Difficulty rating: Moderately difficult

- Build stamina. Through vigorous exercise—whether it's aerobics classes, swimming, jogging, tennis, or anything else that makes you break into a sweat and causes your heart to beat faster—you can reduce your RealAge. Exercise strengthens your heart, arteries, and lungs and delays—and may even reverse—arterial and immune system aging. Exercises that cause you to sweat have a double benefit: They not only count toward the sixty minutes of stamina exercise required per week for optimum Age Reduction, but also burn extra calories toward your 3,500-kcal-per-week goal. Stamina exercises can make your RealAge as much as 6.4 years younger.

Difficulty rating: Moderately difficult

• Build strength and flexibility. Keeping your body strong and flexible helps fend off the wear and tear that make us older. Doing strength and flexibility exercises three times a week keeps your muscles supple and strong. Stretching, weight lifting, and yoga all promote a younger body. You don't need to invest that much time to benefit: Lifting weights for ten minutes just three times a week makes you 1.7 years younger.

Difficulty rating: Moderately difficult

When it comes to fitness, remember the number three. There are three basic types of physical activity that make you younger—general physical activity, stamina-building activities, and strength and flexibility exercises—and each affects your aging process differently. To get the maximum Age Reduction effect from your fitness plan, you need all three.

First, there is just general physical activity—walking, gardening, bringing in the groceries—anything that uses your muscles, no matter what it is. Just boosting your overall activity level—not even breaking a sweat—can earn you 40 percent of the Age Reducing effect normally attributed to exercise. Raising your overall caloric expenditure to 3,500 kcal a week makes your RealAge 3.2 years younger. A kcal is the same amount of energy as a calorie, except that, for some reason, the custom is to use the term *calories* when we're talking about food and *kcal* for the same amount of energy when we're talking about exercise. Therefore, a donut is said to contain about 400 calories, and swimming is said to burn 400 to 600 kcal an hour.

Second, there are activities that raise your heart rate—the so-called stamina activities. This is what most of us think of when we think "exercise"—jogging, biking, swimming, aerobics, a "workout." This kind of exercise contributes another 40 percent to the Age Reduction that can be tied to physical fitness.

Third, there are strength and flexibility exercises. Building and strengthening muscles and keeping them in top form through weight lifting, stretching exercises, or other activities contribute just 20 percent to the overall Age Reduction effect of exercise. But don't be fooled; it's a critical 20 percent. These activities provide a kind of insurance policy for the body, helping you to avoid injury and skeletal weakening and allowing you to continue your overall exercise routine without the disruptions caused by pulled muscles or broken bones. Strengthening exercises are especially important for women. To protect bone mass and density, women need to lift weights even more than men. Lifting weights for just thirty minutes a week makes your RealAge 1.7 years younger.

The best fitness plan is one that builds on all three components. One without the other two will provide some, but not the maximum, Age Reduction effect.

EXERCISE AND LONGEVITY: THE BASIC FACTS

How many times have you told yourself, "I will start exercising"? How many times have you finished that sentence with "tomorrow"? Although more than 90 percent of Americans agree that exercise is an important part of healthy living, only 15 percent get as much exercise as they should. More than 76 percent fail to do even one vigorous activity a week. Over two hundred fifty thousand deaths a year, 12 percent of the national total, are attributable to the lack of regular physical activity. Despite the sports fashion boom of the 1980s, Americans seem to be exercising less and less. As a nation, our fitness level is declining. Fewer people are fit in the 1990s than they were in the 1980s, and fewer people in the 1980s were fit than in the 1970s. Although Americans spent more than $40 billion on fitness equipment in 1995, much of that equipment is gathering dust in the basement.

Even modest physical activity can make your RealAge younger—substantially younger. A study published in the *Journal of the American Medical Association* found that one of the key reasons Americans don't exercise is the common misconception that a person needs to do taxing and rigorous workouts to reap benefits. That's simply not true. Almost all of us would benefit greatly by just boosting our overall physical activity. In fact, a recent policy statement from the Centers for Disease Control and the American College of Sports Medicine suggested that getting just half an hour a day of moderately intense activity, such as walking, gardening, or housecleaning—that is, burning just 200 kcal a day (or 1,400 kcal a week) beyond the "resting metabolic rate"—can provide many of the health benefits attributed to exercise. Even getting just 750 kcal a week of physical activity—that means about two ten-minute walks a day—makes your RealAge 0.9 to 1.7 years younger than if you did nothing. If you get an hour's worth of physical activity a day—and that includes such things as walking up the stairs or taking a couple of ten-minute strolls—you can reduce your RealAge two to five years. That doesn't mean hard-sweat exercise, just anything that uses your muscles. In fact, I often don't even use the term *exercise,* preferring the term *physical activity.* Physical activity—just boosting your overall activity level—is a key component of Age Reduction.

Who should exercise? Everyone. Who can exercise? Everyone who is not seriously incapacitated. Just two decades ago, many doctors and scientists believed that heredity determined your ability to do exercise and to benefit from it. More recent studies have indicated that choices and habits—that is, your own desire and resolve to stay in shape—determine, by more than 70 percent, your ability to achieve and maintain physical fitness. The first step is changing your frame of mind.

Even if you have a health problem—especially if you have a health problem—you should integrate exercise into your life. Exercise makes the RealAge of those who are at a higher risk of cardiovascular disease and other chronic illnesses disproportionately younger. You get the biggest benefit if you begin exercising before you have a major health problem or, as I like to think of it, an aging event.

People who start exercising or doing even moderate physical activity in midlife have a decreased rate of aging. In fact, you are never too old to begin. Fitness researchers have even found that encouraging the frailest nursing home residents—people already in their nineties and even as old as one hundred—to lift weights actually makes an astounding difference in the quality of their lives, enabling some to move out of their wheelchairs and back on their feet. In fact, I've been told that the nursing home where these studies were done had to close a wing after the studies were finished because so many of their residents got well enough to go back home. No matter what your age or physical condition, exercise almost always makes you younger. What is most important about fitness is that you continue to exercise. Studies have found that within five years of giving up their sports and exercise, college athletes were no more fit—and no younger—than those who had never exercised. Exercise keeps you young only as long as you keep doing it.

EXERCISE AND DISEASE:
LOWERING RISK, GETTING YOUNGER

Exercise is a whole-body phenomenon. It doesn't just make your muscles stronger, it slows down the aging of your entire body. Exercise affects everything: your cardiovascular system, your immune system, your musculoskeletal system, and your emotional well-being. It affects you all the way down to your cells. Let's consider the scientific research on exercise as it pertains to various health conditions.

- Coronary and arterial aging. People who exercise regularly have significantly less cardiovascular aging and are at a far lower risk of heart attacks and strokes, regardless of their genetic background. Exercise lowers blood pressure, raises the levels of protective HDL cholesterol, stimulates weight loss, and helps prevent blood clots. The Harvard Alumni Study found that the incidence of heart attack was inversely proportional to the amount of exercise performed: Men who exercised less than 2,000 kcal a week had a 64 percent higher risk of heart attack than those who exercised more than that. Studies have also shown that a three-month period of intensive activity, like that experienced by military recruits, can result in an increase in HDL ("healthy") cholesterol of as much as 33 percent and a decrease in LDL ("lousy") cholesterol of 9 percent. Even moderate amounts of physical activity are shown to lower total cholesterol rates and to lower LDL/HDL ratios, although the results are not as dramatic. Exercise is a way to control cholesterol without medication and to make your RealAge younger.

- Immune system aging. Physical activity affects you even at the cellular level. It reduces the rate at which your cells age, meaning that you are less likely to develop cancers and that microscopic cancers that do exist are less likely to spread. Exercise also improves the overall functioning of the immune system, increasing the production of "watchdog" cells that seek and destroy invading disease cells and cancer cells. Those who are physically fit have fewer colds and other illnesses.

- Colon cancer. The rate of colon cancer is significantly higher in highly industrialized, affluent societies. Why? Researchers blame our fatty diets and sedentary lifestyles. Several studies have shown that individuals who are physically active have much lower rates of colon cancers; a study in Sweden found that those with low levels of activity were three times more likely to get colon cancer.

- Breast cancer. Preliminary studies show that women who exercise regularly have an incidence of breast cancer that is almost one-third lower than that of women who do not exercise regularly. One Norwegian study found that among women who exercised, the risk was reduced by 37 percent. Unfortunately, many questions still exist about the relationship between breast cancer and exercise. Some scientists hypothesize that women who exercise more have lower fat stores and, hence, less long-term exposure to impurities stored in fat cells. Others hypothesize that endurance training helps increase the number of immune system cells that are known to kill off potential cancer cells.

- Prostate cancer. Prostate cancer is linked to elevated testosterone levels, and regular vigorous exercise reduces such levels. Men who exercise consistently have much lower rates of prostate cancer. The Harvard Alumni Study found a significantly reduced risk of prostate cancer among men who exercised more than 4,000 kcal a week and an increased risk for men who expended less than 1,000 kcal a week. The risk was nearly 50 percent lower for men over age seventy and more than 80 percent lower for men under age seventy. Although other studies have confirmed the link, there is still debate over the exact relationship between exercise and prostate cancer.

- Arthritis. Practically everyone over age sixty-five begins to show some sort of arthritic symptoms. A study recently published in the *Journal of the American Medical Association* found that people who had osteoarthritis can and should exercise. Moderate to vigorous exercise, in conjunction with strengthening exercise, eliminated many of their symptoms and made their joints younger.

- Weight management. By burning calories and increasing your metabolic rate, exercise helps you lose weight and replace fat with muscle. The more muscle you have, the more calories you burn, even when you're not exercising. Strengthening exercises are particularly important because they build muscle.

- Diabetes. Exercise helps increase the body's sensitivity to insulin. This increased sensitivity to insulin, in turn, lowers blood sugar levels and decreases insulin production. Active people, even if they have a genetic predisposition to the disease, are much less likely to develop adult-onset (Type II) diabetes. Furthermore, if symptoms do occur, exercise helps diminish their aging effect.

- Osteoporosis and loss of bone density. Any resistance activity—walking up a hill or lifting groceries—strengthens muscles and, just as important, increases bone density, making bones stronger and less likely to fracture. Indeed, resistance activity actually increases the calcium content of bones. Although strengthening—or weight-bearing—exercises are the best for improving bone strength, new evidence shows that exercises such as riding a stationary bicycle and water aerobics may also increase bone density. Take note, however: Some new studies warn that people who exercise vigorously need to get proper amounts of calcium—1,000 to

1,200 mg a day—to ensure that enough calcium is available for the bones to build density. During intense training, large amounts of calcium are lost through perspiration.

- Falls and broken bones. Each year, approximately 30 percent of people over age sixty-five fall down, and 15 percent of those who fall suffer serious injuries. More than 6 percent of all medical care dollars spent on people over age sixty-five involve fall-related injuries. Hip fractures and other bone breaks age a person significantly. It's not just the bone breaks that age, but the long periods of immobility that often follow. Studies of the elderly population have found that those who exercised, particularly those who did balance-building exercises, such as tai chi chuan, were much less likely to fall or to sustain fall-related injuries.

- Sleep-related disorders. Studies done at both Stanford and Emory Universities found that adults who exercised fell asleep more quickly and slept better than their sedentary counterparts.

- Depression and anxiety. Exercise has significant emotional benefits: It helps ease depression, anxiety, and other psychological disorders. Depression is a widespread, though often undiagnosed, problem among older people. Doctors have known for years that exercise, particularly when done in a social environment, helps relieve clinical depression. Exercise also reduces anxiety disorders and improves mental health in other ways. Even for those who have not been diagnosed as having a psychological illness, exercise is a known mood lifter, helping them feel happier and more upbeat.

- Stress management. Regular exercise decreases the stress response, meaning that you are more relaxed, feel better, and are better prepared to cope with life's stressful events. We all have stresses, but by staying fit, we are better equipped to avoid their aging effects.

- Long-term memory. Exercise helps improve long-term memory and brain function. It helps prevent the arterial aging that contributes to the early onset of Alzheimer's disease.

- Tobacco use. Increasing exercise levels helps people quit smoking. Regular exercise diminishes nicotine cravings.

As this list shows, exercise clearly helps us stay young. But how are we to motivate ourselves to take on a real exercise regimen?

THE EXERCISE BASICS

Cynthia W. was forty-three when she became my patient. At 5 feet 5 inches, she was eighty pounds heavier than she had been at age eighteen. Her body mass index was 38, well over the cutoff point for being considered overweight. The managing editor of a business magazine, she had a high-stress job. She spent every day sleuthing stories, answering phone calls, and making sure that the news got out on time. When deadlines neared, she worked around the clock, living on take-out food. By the time she became my patient, she had had a heart scare that brought her in for an electrocardiogram. She realized it was time to start taking care of herself.

When I tried gently to bring up the matter of her weight, she said, "Dr. Roizen, don't beat around the bush. I know I need to lose weight. And," she smiled, "you're the one who's going to help me do it." After fighting with issues of body image and beauty for a long time, her recent heart scare made Cynthia realize that weight loss wasn't about looking good—it was about being healthy.

She told me, "All of sudden, I woke up one day, and I was five times the size I always thought I was. I just never made the time to take care of myself. But I don't want to haul all this weight around anymore. Tell me what I can do."

"Eat less and," I paused, "exercise."

"Damn. I thought you'd say that."

"Sorry, but what else can I say? Let's develop a plan you can stick to."

Cynthia started her first "workout" that day. She walked from her house to the end of the block and back. That was it: short, sweet, and slow. The next day, she did it again. By the end of the next week, she was walking all the way around the block. Within three weeks, she was walking eight city blocks—the equivalent of a mile—each day. Then she began timing herself, increasing her pace a little bit each time. Within three months, she was walking half an hour each day. On weekends she would walk for a full hour. "Mike," she said to me one day, "I never thought I'd say this, but I actually find myself craving my daily walk. Me, the living paperweight, actually wanting to exercise! I'll be at the office, the phones will be ringing off the hook, and all I can think is, 'Gee, I really want to take a walk.'"

She had discovered that exercise doesn't have to be painful or exhausting. It can be something to look forward to, a reward. Soon Cynthia set a goal to walk in a five-kilometer walk-run race, just over three miles. And she did it, even jogging part of the way.

Within two years, she has lost more than forty-five pounds. Her blood pressure has dropped, and she feels a whole lot better. "I have more energy, and I actually like the way my body looks and feels," she laughed. Cynthia still hasn't reached her goal of getting back to the weight she was at eighteen, but she's getting closer every day.

Cynthia's doing it the easy way, remembering that health should play an important part of every day. She's working up gradually, aiming to meet her own goal of eight years younger. Cynthia started with the goal of just boosting her overall level of physical activity, aiming to get half an hour a day of moderate activity. Then she moved on to building up stamina, strengthening her heart, lungs, and arteries and to increasing her overall endurance. She has gone from getting less than 500 kcal of activity a week to reaching the ideal goal of 3,500 kcal a week. She still isn't doing lots of vigorous exercise, but she did buy an exercise bike and, on it, she reaches her goal of 65 percent of her maximum heart rate for twenty minutes or so at least three times a week. She is aiming to bring it up to 80 percent of the maximum. She still needs to do some strengthening and flexibility exercises, especially as she builds more stamina, to prevent injuries.

If you want to start exercising, how should you start? Like Cynthia, you should start slowly. A behavior change that can last a lifetime takes effort. Don't try to fit a year's worth of workouts into the first week. You'll just get discouraged.

The most common reason for not exercising is "I don't have the time." Yet, exercising doesn't use up time; it makes more of it. If you invest a little time each day, you will become younger in the here and now. In just ninety days, the effects will be measurable. You will feel better and more energetic, and your body will be healthier and more efficient. When people say they don't have time to exercise, I remember a clearly out-of-shape comedian who said, "All the time I gain from exercising, I spend exercising." Funny but, thankfully, not true. Just twenty minutes a day of physical activity will make your body younger and more efficient for all the other minutes of the day. In fact, most of my patients who have adopted the three-pronged RealAge physical activity plan tell me that they save more than an hour a day when they exercise. They are more energetic and more efficient in all the other things they do. No wonder. They are 8.1 years younger.

PHYSICAL ACTIVITY: THE ANTIAGER

The first goal of any fitness plan is to figure out how to boost your overall level of activity. Most of us lead sedentary lives. We sit at desks all day at work, watch TV when we get home, and drive too much. Future archeologists will label us "The-Sit-Around-and-Get-Round-Society." The decision to get in shape is a big decision, but it's the small steps that really matter. Like deciding to walk to the neighborhood grocery instead of driving. Pedaling an exercise bike while watching the football game. Lifting weights instead of chips during the commercials. Actually walking the dog, instead of just tossing or shoving him out into the backyard. Every movement you make improves your physical fitness level. Housework, gardening, and mowing the lawn—not to mention fun things, like dancing and sex—are all activities that burn extra calories. The point is to get your muscles moving. The more active you are, the younger you are.

At rest, your body burns 1,400 to 1,900 kcal a day. This is your "resting metabolic rate." This is the energy your body spends just keeping you alive—the energy it uses to keep your heart beating, to keep your blood flowing, to digest your food, and to breathe. Your resting metabolic rate is approximately 1 kcal per kilogram of body weight per hour. (To get your weight in kilograms, divide your weight in pounds by 2.2.) If you weigh 132 pounds, or 60 kilograms, you will burn 60 kcal an hour. Then multiply this hourly number by 24 hours to get your expenditure per day. A person weighing 60 kilograms would burn 1,440 kcal a day even doing nothing. Likewise, a person weighing 90 kilograms, just about 200 pounds, would burn 90 kcal an hour and 2,160 kcal a day. Ideally, you should expend 3,500 kcal of energy a week in exercise above and beyond your resting metabolic rate. Getting that much physical activity gives you the maximum health benefit with none of the drawbacks of overexercising. Just as examples, brisk walking burns 300 kcal an hour, and jogging burns 400 to 500 kcal an hour (see Table 9.1).

Think about your daily routine. How and where can you integrate more activity into your routine? At work, take the stairs instead of the elevator (each flight burns 5 kcal). Take a walk at lunchtime, or ride your bike to work instead of driving. In the middle of the afternoon, take a ten-minute break and, instead of having another coffee, walk around the block. It will give you an energy burst without the caffeine. You can even plan a meeting around a walk. I call it the "walk-and-talk." Walking a city block burns up 9 kcal. Walk short distances instead of driving. Instead of spending ten minutes looking for the perfect parking spot, park a bit farther and use those ten minutes to walk to your destination. Buy a stationary bicycle, treadmill, or rowing machine and

220   REALAGE

TABLE 9.1

How Many Kilocalories (kcal) Each Activity Uses

Activity	Kcal Used Per Minute
Walking for pleasure	3.5
Bicycling for pleasure	4
Swimming, slow treading	4
Conditioning exercises, slow stretching	4
Home care, carpet sweeping	4
Raking lawn	4
Walking briskly	4–5
Home repair, painting	4.5
Mowing lawn, walking behind power mower	4.5
Racket sports, table tennis, doubles tennis	5
Golf, pulling cart or carrying clubs	5.5
Conditioning exercise, general calisthenics	6
Fishing in stream	6
Ice (or roller in-line) skating	7
Soccer	7
Moving furniture	7
Conditioning exercise, stair stepper, ski machine	7
Singles tennis, raquetball	7–8
Running	8
Basketball—game play	8
Cycling, fast or racing	10
Squash	12
Canoeing or rowing in competition	12

Modified from Ainsworth, B. E., et al., "Compendium of Physical Activities: Classification of Energy Costs of Human Physical Activities." *Medicine & Science in Sports and Medicine,* 1993; 25: 71–80.

put it in front of your TV. That way, you can catch the evening news, expand your mind, and burn 300 to 600 kcal in an hour.

Getting just thirty minutes of physical activity a day, done in eight- to ten-minute bursts, not only leads to measurable changes in physical fitness levels but has positive emotional effects. It makes you feel younger and more vigorous. Exercise provides a "dose-response" relationship. The more exercise you get, the better you feel. The benefit of exercise reaches its maximum at about 3,500 kcal a week. Above that, the benefit is more or less the same until you reach 6,400 kcal a week, at which point you may be overexercising and causing aging.

Some good news: Every little bit of physical activity matters. Studies have found that people who begin exercise programs doing several small segments in a day are more likely to stay with the program than those who try to do an extensive workout all at once. If you are now relatively sedentary, burning just 750 kcal a week beyond your daily average can make you one year younger.

Although everyone needs exercise, exercise is even more important for those already at elevated risk of cardiovascular disease and other kinds of chronic disease. A famous study done by fitness researcher Steven Blair at the Cooper Center in Dallas showed that people who were physically fit, and even those who achieved physical fitness later in life, had significantly lower death rates no matter what the cause of death and regardless of any other risk factors, such as a family history of cardiovascular disease or previous heart attacks. The Harvard Alumni Study found that people who smoked, had high blood pressure, and didn't exercise had more than seven times the chance of having a heart attack. Having two of these three factors meant that a person's risk was only twice as high as the norm. If you are a smoker, have high blood pressure, or any other major risk factor that ages your arteries, exercise is especially important to retard or reverse aging.

Family support is an important part of being able to maintain an exercise routine. Talk to your spouse or partner about the need to get in shape and about how important it is for both of you. Each of you should set exercise goals. When one of you reaches a goal, have the other one cook a special saturated-fat-free celebratory meal or give some other reward. It may be corny, but encouraging someone to stay in shape is the best way to say "I love you." It means you want to have that person around for a long time. Use exercise as a way to find time in your busy schedules to get together. You can fill each other in about the day's events just as easily when you're on exercise bikes at the gym as you can in front of the TV at home.

Another problem many of us face when beginning an exercise plan is that we're literally fair-weather friends. Many people begin an exercise regimen in the spring, work out in the summer, reach their fitness peak in the fall, and then give up altogether as winter approaches,. Then they start from scratch all over again the next spring. Instead, plan for the cold weather. Join a gym or a club with an indoor pool. Even shopping malls provide indoor walking routes. More than 3 million Americans over calendar age sixty-five now mall-walk

Starting to Exercise

Here's how I recommend that my patients start Age Reduction exercising:

1. Start slowly. Don't overdo it. Just go for five or ten minutes at the beginning. Even a walk around the block is a place to begin.

2. Do a bit more each week. Try to build your workout by a couple of minutes each week. Aim to increase your workout by 10 percent a week.

3. Warm up first, then stretch, and stretch again afterward. Save your muscles from pulls and tears and notice how good your body feels when your muscles are warm and stretched.

4. Visualize. Imagine yourself doing your sport. Make a picture in your mind of hitting the perfect shot or running in perfect form. Imagine how your body would move.

5. Treat yourself right. If it hurts, slow down. If it feels good, do more than you planned.

6. Cross-train. Try to plan your workout schedule around a number of different activities, such as walking, biking, and swimming. Rotate your activities on different days.

7. Reward yourself. Set goals and when you achieve them, treat yourself. Buy a new pair of shoes or get a massage. Celebrate your Age Reduction!

8. Drink water. Every ten or twenty minutes, take a break and drink half a cup or more of water. Don't let yourself get dehydrated.

9. Find an accomplice. Exercise with a friend. You'll encourage each other and push yourselves to meet your goals. Get the whole family involved.

10. Take a lesson. Even if you don't normally work out with a trainer or a pro, treat yourself to an hour with an expert who can show you how to maximize your workout and avoid needless injuries. It's a great way to get started.

11. Vary your workout pace. Do more on some days and less on others.

12. Consider whether you need a pre-exercise medical exam. Most adults do not need to talk to a doctor before beginning an exercise plan of moderate intensity. If you have a chronic disease or some other kind of health problem, you should talk to your doctor. Also, if you are a man over forty or a woman over fifty and are planning to start an intensive fitness program, you might also want to ask your physician to help you design a workout routine. If you don't have a regular doctor, ask your clinic or health maintenance organization (HMO) if anyone on its staff specializes in fitness.

regularly to boost their physical activity. That reduces their RealAge by as much as five years!

If you really like being outdoors but get stopped cold by winter, learn how to dress for the weather. Wearing the proper gear can mean the difference between suffering through your workout and enjoying it. You can keep running right through the winter if you wear a hat and gloves. The advances in exercise wear in the past ten years have produced new fabrics, such as fleece and Lycra, that make exercise clothing both warm and lightweight. To make the most of the cold weather, learn a winter sport. There are few sports that provide the complete body workout of cross-country skiing. Ice skating, downhill skiing, and snowshoeing are all sports that can turn those gray winter months into something you actually look forward to.

Some people find that they miss their exercise routine when they travel or go on vacation. Plan for exercise. For example, I do a lot of traveling for work, and I always try to stay at hotels that offer fitness facilities. I find it's a great way to unwind after a long day of meetings or to start the morning off right. If I can't find a hotel with a gym, I pack a jump rope (some of my friends pack exercise bands). Twenty minutes of jumping rope—done in the right shoes and on a low-impact surface—is a great workout that you can do anywhere with a little bit of room. The ceilings in most hotel rooms are high enough. I often wonder what the person in the room below me thinks, but I know that I am not letting being away from home get in the way of keeping myself young.

Boosting your physical activity levels should be a starting point. It provides the first 40 percent of the Age Reduction benefit attributable to fitness (see Table 9.2). To get the next 40 percent, you have to move to the second phase: stamina exercise.

BUILDING STAMINA: GETTING FIT FOR THE LONG RUN

The second element of any exercise routine should be aerobic (stamina-building) exercises. These are exercises that raise your heart rate and make you sweat. Activities like jogging, swimming, biking, and even brisk walking provide a fundamental piece of your Age Reduction exercise plan. Realistically, if you plan to get 3,500 kcal of activity a week, you will need to do something that really gets you moving. You will want to start slowly and work your way up. Stamina building is a RealAge "two-for-one" special: Stamina exercises give you double RealAge credit. You get Age

TABLE 9.2

The RealAge Effect of Physical Activity

FOR MEN

	Kilocalories Expended Per Week				
	Less than 500	500– 2,000	2,000– 3,500	3,500– 6,500	More than 6,500
Calendar Age	RealAge				
35	36.7	35	33.1	31.4	32
55	57.7	55	53.3	51.6	52
70	72.9	70	69	66.7	68.2

FOR WOMEN

	Kilocalories Expended Per Week				
	Less than 500	500– 2,000	2,000– 3,500	3,500– 6,500	More than 6,500
Calendar Age	RealAge				
35	36.7	35	34.1	32.4	33
55	57.7	55	54.3	52	53
70	72.8	70	69	67.2	68.2

Reduction benefits for boosting your overall physical activity—burning kcalories—plus additional Age Reduction benefits for building stamina and aerobic capacity. In the Harvard Alumni Study of ten thousand subjects, those who expended 3,500 kcal a week had half the rate of aging for the period studied as the least active people. In RealAge terms, individuals who were fit—those who reached overall activity levels of 3,500 kcal a week and included stamina-building exercises in their weekly routines—were 6.4 years younger than those who were completely unfit.

Aerobic exercise increases the body's uptake of oxygen and boosts your overall metabolic rate, meaning that the more you exercise, the more calories you burn, even when you're sitting still. Elevating your heart rate to 60–90 percent of its maximum for twenty minutes or more three times a week will give you a stronger heart, arterial system, and lungs and will help your body attain a higher resting metabolic rate. You also will reach your 3,500-kcal-a-week goal in half the time.

In contrast to your overall fitness level, the goal of stamina exercises is not the expenditure of kilocalories, but an increase in "metabolic equivalent units," or METs—that is, a change in your metabolic rate, or the amount of oxygen that your muscles consume during exercise. One MET represents your metabolic rate at rest; 10 or 11 METs is the goal you should strive for when doing a vigorous workout. You will want to boost your metabolic rate to ten times its normal rate. Whereas kilocalories measure the total amount of energy burned, METs measure the intensity, or rate, at which you burn that energy. That is, the higher your metabolic rate (the higher your METs), the more kilocalories you burn in a shorter period. The goal of the second prong of your exercise plan—the stamina-building prong—should be to reach 10 METs for sixty minutes a week if you are a woman and 11 METs for sixty minutes a week if you are a man.

Now that you know what you're aiming for, how can you measure METs? Unfortunately, you can't, or at least not easily. METs can be measured accurately only at a sports medicine clinic or some other place equipped to monitor METs. There are three good substitute guidelines for measuring your metabolic rate: estimating the kilocalories burned per hour, estimating "sweat time," and determining your heart rate. Use these guidelines for measuring the intensity of your workouts. Look at "calories-per-hour rates" to get a rough guideline for your MET level (also see Table 9.1). If you walk briskly (300 kcal per hour), you will reach a metabolic rate of six to seven METs. If you do something that burns more than 600 kcal an hour, then you are somewhere close to 10 METs. You should try to exercise at this rate for at least twenty minutes three times a week. Another good way to estimate METs is by sweat time—try to sweat for twenty minutes or more three times a week. The amount of time you actually spend sweating is a relatively reliable indication you have reached 70 percent of your maximum heart rate and metabolic rate. The third way to estimate METs is by measuring your heart rate—the number of times your heart beats per minute. During bouts of vigorous exercise, your heart rate should get within 65–80 percent of the maximum.

How many beats per minute is that? First you need to calculate your maximum heart rate (the number of times your heart beats per minute when pushed to the limit). Calculate this by subtracting your calendar age from the number 220. If you are forty, your maximum heart rate should be about 180 beats per minute. If you are sixty, your ideal should be about 160 beats per minute. As

I've gotten more fit, I challenge myself by subtracting my RealAge from 220. When you first start on your exercise program, the goal is to raise your heart rate to at least 65 percent of the maximum for twenty consecutive minutes at least three times a week. As you get in better shape, you should try to reach 80 percent of that number. For example, if you are forty, you should try to raise your heart rate to 117 beats a minute for twenty consecutive minutes each time you do a stamina-building exercise. As you progress, try to increase that number to 144 beats a minute. If you are sixty and just beginning to exercise, you should raise your heart rate to 104 beats a minute and subsequently aim for 128 beats a minute (see Table 9.3).

These are general guidelines that describe ideal heart rates for the average person in a particular age range. Remember, however, that there are individual variations in heart rate.

How do you measure your heart rate? When you are well into your workout, stop your exercise for a few seconds. Place the finger of one hand on your opposite wrist and search for the pulse point. It lies on the spot of your wrist just below the base of your thumb. Feel around for it. Make sure to use a finger, not your thumb, to feel for the pulse, as the thumb itself has a pulse point that can distort your reading. Then count the number of heartbeats in fifteen seconds, subtract one, and multiply by four to get your heart rate for a minute. Remember, a heartbeat has two parts to it—an "in" and an "out." You should feel both. If you find it difficult to get this down, or if you want a more exact measure of your heart rate, buy a heart-rate monitor. These monitors are easily found at sporting goods stores but can be expensive. You can even get watches that have a heart-rate monitor in them.

As you start your new exercise program, begin slowly and build. Do as Cynthia did: Start with slow walks and gradually increase your workout each week by 10 percent. Soon you will start to sweat. When you begin a sport, it is more important to build stamina than intensity. Run farther but at a slower pace. Bike farther, rather than go all out for a short distance. Quantity matters most. Space your workouts during the week. Exercise every other day or switch between sports.

Forget the statement "No pain, no gain." Exercise shouldn't be painful. True pain is your body's way of telling you to back off. If you hurt, slow down or try a different regimen. The most common kind of pain you feel when you first start exercising is a slow, burning ache in the muscles and being out of breath. This feeling is normal because you are reaching your anaerobic threshold and are at the limit of your endurance. The pain is caused by the buildup of lactic acid in your muscles, which occurs when your muscles are not getting enough oxygen. This is not an indication of an injury but of reaching your

TABLE 9.3

Boosting Your Heart Rate

WHAT SHOULD YOU AIM FOR?

This table gives the range of heart beats per minute for each age group. To get a good aerobic, stamina-building workout, you should aim for 65–80 percent of your maximum heart rate.

Percentage of Maximum Heart Rate	Calendar Age (Years)								
	20	30	40	50	60	70	80	90	100
	Heart Beats Per Minute								
100	200	190	180	170	160	150	140	130	120
90	180	171	162	153	144	135	126	117	108
80	160	152	144	136	128	120	112	104	96
70	140	133	126	119	112	105	98	91	84
60	120	114	108	102	96	90	84	78	72
50	100	95	90	85	80	75	70	65	60
40	80	76	73	68	64	60	56	52	48

100 percent   Reaching your maximum possible heart rate is hard to do and impossible to maintain. Also, it may not be a safe thing to do.

90 percent   Only high-level athletes can achieve and maintain a heart rate this high.

80 percent   This should be your goal on the days you have a really strenuous workout.

70 percent   If you can get to this level and maintain it, you will be getting the benefit of a real stamina-building workout.

60 percent   This should be your goal when you first start working out. It's a good place to be.

50 percent or below   You're slacking off. If you want to get the benefits of stamina exercise, you need to boost your heart rate higher than this.

fitness limit. The more you work out, the higher your anaerobic threshold will go, and soon you will be able to work out for longer periods and at a more vigorous rate.

If you feel sore after a workout, especially the next day, don't worry. Unless something really hurts, it will probably go away within a day or two—eventually producing lean muscle where there used to be flab. That's why you should space your workouts and rotate between activities—so that different muscle groups are worked on different days, getting a day off in between.

As you do more of your workout, set new goals and try to meet them. Try to increase the length and intensity of your workouts. Start small but be consistent, and you will do wonders. Stamina-building exercise can give you 6.4 years of youth.

HITTING THE MAXIMUM: CAN YOU OVERDO IT?

How much exercise is enough? How much is too much? The odds are that you are not getting too much exercise. Since fewer than 15 percent of Americans exceed the 3,500-kcal mark that is the RealAge goal, most of us need not worry that we are overdoing it. As rare as it is, however, there is the possibility of too much of a good thing, and you can get older from exercising too much. For example, one of my patients, Mary, took up jogging in her early thirties. Within a few years, she was running road races and had even run several marathons. Her times were good. She often finished in the top twenty, and she began to take her training more seriously. Her goal was no longer to run a marathon but to win one. Soon she was running three ten-mile runs a week and a fifteen-mile run on Sundays. She was in fabulous aerobic shape. Yet the longer her runs, the more pressed she got for time. To run in the morning and still get to work on time, she began to shorten her warm-up time. She quit stretching and limbering up. And she did no strengthening exercises. (Running on a straight course—no hills—is an aerobic exercise but not a strength-building one.) Then the inevitable happened: She tore a ligament in her leg. She was on crutches for months and was never able to run seriously again. In the end, she gave up exercising altogether. Whereas at forty-five her RealAge had been close to thirty, one year later her RealAge was over forty. Needlessly.

Exercise fiends can make themselves older, particularly if they are not careful to maintain a well-balanced workout routine. Exercising too vigorously—that is, more than four hours a week at a top rate—can produce three major problems: antioxidant buildup and subsequent aging, destruction of muscle tissue, and injuries from overuse of tissues.

If you exercise more than 6,500 kcal a week or exert more than 800 kcal an hour for two hours in any one workout, you are overdoing it. This amount of exercise overwhelms your system and causes your metabolism to become less efficient during the workout. The body cannot dispose of free radicals fast enough, and they build up in your tissues. As I mentioned in the first chapter, the buildup of free radicals appears to be linked to accelerated aging. That is, exercise increases cellular metabolism and, hence, oxidation. And the buildup of oxidants can cause cellular damage, particularly to the DNA. Small-scale studies have shown that oxidation damage, and the aging it causes, is lessened in those who take vitamins C and E regularly. Although the findings are still preliminary, I recommend taking those two vitamins about an hour to two hours before you exercise, just as a precautionary measure. You should be taking C and E anyway (see Chapter 7). I also recommend taking an aspirin or another NSAID such as ibuprofen (for example, Motrin) one or two hours before exercising, to help prevent the swelling and inflammation that often result from exercise.

A second risk of overexercising is muscle damage. Overexercising usually means that certain muscle groups are getting used too much; they don't have time to repair themselves and rebuild after the workout. Optimal Age Reduction includes resting between workouts, plus cross-training (switching between activities on different days).

The third and most obvious problem associated with exercising is injury from the overuse of muscles and joints. The wear and tear that results can cause real problems.

AVOIDING INJURIES: BASIC GUIDELINES

What should you do to avoid exercise-related injuries? If you pull a muscle, don't stop exercising altogether. By staying in shape, you are more likely to avoid future injuries. Just lay off the sore muscle for a while. Try a different exercise that doesn't stress the pulled muscle. For example, if you injure a muscle in your leg, consider swimming, relying mainly on your arms to do the work. If your ankles or knees ache, try something with no impact—like a cross-country ski machine, an elliptical exercise machine, or a stationary bicycle. If your aerobics class has you hurting, consider taking a water aerobics class; you'll get the same workout with none of the impact.

If you tear a muscle or do something particularly damaging, you will know it. The pain will make it obvious. If you feel intense pain or notice swelling, remember "RICE"—rest, ice, compression, and elevation. In other words, don't use the muscle; ice the injury for twenty minutes every eight hours for forty-eight hours; wrap (and slightly compress) the injury with an Ace or similar bandage; and keep the injury elevated to reduce swelling. If the pain doesn't begin to subside or if you suspect a more significant injury, call your doctor.

Other sports injuries are more subtle: The tendon in your elbow aches or burns, but you keep on playing tennis every day anyway. You feel the throb in one knee, and so favor the other leg—upsetting your balance and doing more long-term damage. You keep running, despite the shin splints or the dull ache of the stress fracture. For any injury that bothers you for more than a few days or so, consult your doctor. Most clinics and health maintenance organizations now have doctors who specialize in sports medicine. Such doctors, in conjunction with the organization's team of physical therapists and other injury-rehabilitation staff, can help you when you do get injured, or when you want to devise a workout plan to stay in shape and keep from getting injured in the future.

If you haven't exercised in a long time, or if you are starting a new sport, consider having a session with a personal trainer or professional instructor—just a little time with someone who can teach you how to do the proper movements. Knowing what to do and what not to do, so as to get the most out of your workouts and to avoid injury-provoking mistakes, can save you days, if not weeks, of pain and grief.

Again, I cannot say it enough: If you are planning to make exercise part of your life—that is, if you plan to adopt an active lifestyle—there is no need to rush into it. You have time to work into it gradually. That way, you'll be less likely to have an injury and more likely to make it a manageable lifelong routine.

Here are some general guidelines to avoid getting hurt and to get the maximum Age Reducing benefits:

1. Vary your exercise pattern. Don't do the same activity every single day, and certainly not more than two days in a row. If you go jogging three days a week, consider swimming on the other two. Or rotate between the different aerobic machines at the gym: Do the StairMaster one day, the treadmill the next, and then the bicycle. Try to use all your muscles, working both the upper and lower body.

   Also, it is often better to do a variety of different exercises that complement a training routine, rather than just one activity. For example, when I trained to play in competitive squash tournaments, it took me years to learn that my squash game actually improved and that I was less prone to injury if I did a number of unrelated activities that built strength, flexibility, and stamina, rather than just play squash every day.

2. Add strength and flexibility exercises to your aerobic workouts. Combinations like biking and weight lifting, running and yoga, or aerobics and stretching exercises are mutually reinforcing. They help ensure against a damaging injury.

3. Warm up. Start by doing something that gets your muscles moving. Walk briskly or jog at a slow pace for a few minutes. Then stretch. Once your muscles are a little warm, your stretches will be much more effective. You will also be less likely to have an injury. Don't think that you will save time by skimping on the preworkout. Beginning a strenuous workout with tight, stiff muscles is the most likely way to damage or injure a muscle. You should do stretching and strengthening exercises for at least five minutes before you begin the vigorous portion of your stamina workout. Remember, too, to cool down by stretching your muscles at the end of each workout.

4. Use equipment designed for your sport. You don't need to go crazy buying sports equipment, but it is important to have equipment that is fitted to you and your particular activity. Wear shoes that are expressly made for your exercise program and replace them when they show signs of too much wear and tear (about every three hundred miles worth of workouts). You don't need expensive shoes (I never pay more than forty or fifty dollars for a pair), but they should provide good support for your feet and ankles. Be particularly careful about having good shoes if you do aerobics or any sport that involves lots of running, jumping, or bouncing because you will be more prone to ankle and leg injuries. Replace shoelaces frequently, as they get stretched out quickly and lose their support. If you bike, get a bike that fits you. Always wear a helmet (that keeps you younger, too!). Likewise, if you Rollerblade (in-line skate), make sure to wear a helmet, knee pads, shin guards, and wrist guards, especially if you are playing hockey or some other game on Rollerblades. Go to a specialty store and talk to the salespeople about the advantages of specific equipment and evaluate what you really need. The salespeople in small stores are often serious athletes themselves and can be extremely knowledgeable.

5. Avoid overexertion. Gradually increase your exercise time and do not increase it by more than 10 percent a week. Even if you are training to meet a goal like running in a marathon or playing in a tennis tournament, do not overdo it. More than 40 percent of marathoners who run over thirty miles a week develop injuries within the training year, the quickest way to put the dream of the race to rest.

STRENGTH AND FLEXIBILITY: STRETCH IT TO YOUR LIMITS

Strength and flexibility exercises are the important third prong of your Age Reduction exercise plan. We tend to think of stamina-building (aerobic) exercises as the most important kind of exercises, but such exercises do not build muscle or bone. Although the data on aging indicate that strength and flexibility exercises produce only 20 percent of the RealAge benefit attributable to exercise (1.7 years younger), these exercises help your body protect itself from such injuries as muscle tears or bone fractures. They also help retard aging of the bones and muscles, improve balance control, and help prevent fat gain and damage to joints, muscles, and tendons. These exercises keep your bones young and in this way prevent osteoporosis (the loss of bone density) and fractures. Strength and flexibility exercises increase the efficiency of oxygen use by your muscles, reduce arterial aging, and improve immune function, thus decreasing the risk of the early onset of chronic diseases, such as arthritis.

Although there have been fewer studies of the benefits of strength and flexibility exercises—in contrast to the extensive amount of research on aerobic exercise—the studies that have been done confirm that those who are strong and flexible are better able to perform everyday activities, are less likely to develop back pain, and are better able to retain mobility through old age. In 1995, a review in the *Journal of the American Medical Association* analyzed eight studies on the benefits of strength and flexibility exercises. Such exercises were important in preventing falls and increasing bone density. Some studies showed a RealAge benefit of 2.7 to 4 years with just ten weeks of strength and flexibility training. In general, keeping yourself strong and flexible can make your RealAge as much as 1.7 years younger (see Table 9.4).

Aging makes us more prone to stiffness and orthopedic injuries; muscles become stiffer, and tendons and joints are not as strong or elastic. Studies

TABLE 9.4

The RealAge Effect of Strength-Building Exercises

FOR MEN

| Calendar Age | Minutes Per Week Spent on Strength-Building Exercises | | | | |
	None	1–5	6 20	21–30	More than 30
			RealAge		
35	36.5	35	34.2	33.8	33.5
55	57.3	55	54.4	53.6	53.3
70	71.8	70	69.2	68.6	68.2

FOR WOMEN

| Calendar Age | Minutes Per Week Spent on Strength-Building Exercises | | | | |
	None	1–5	6–20	21–30	More than 30
			RealAge		
35	36.6	35	34.1	33.9	33.6
55	57.1	55	54.3	53.5	53.2
70	72	70	69.0	68.4	68.1

show that when people do strengthening exercises and become stronger, they are more likely to begin doing other exercises as well. We all lose muscle from our twenties on—that's one reason why we gain weight as we age. On average, a pound of muscle uses 150 kcal of energy per day, whereas a pound of fat uses 3 kcal of energy per day. Even marathoners lose muscle if they don't do strengthening exercises. If you do strengthening exercises regularly, you will counteract this attrition, and your body will burn more calories all day long, even when you're at rest. Stamina exercises, in contrast, don't build muscles. Doing just twelve weeks of strength and flexibility training six times a week for fifteen minutes at a time will increase the number of calories you burn by 15 percent.

You should always do flexibility exercises (stretches) before and after any vigorous workout—after warming up first, of course. You can do strengthening exercises either before or after your stamina workout or on the days in between.

There are many kinds of flexibility exercises. You can learn how to do stretching exercises at home. Many gyms offer stretch classes. And, of course, there is yoga. Although yoga is not any better than other stretching techniques, most yoga routines provide a comprehensive, full-body stretch of all the muscle groups in one workout.

Strength training involves working our muscles in opposition to a force of resistance, such as weights. One four-year study showed that lifting weights regularly led to increased bone density—up to one-third more than any other activity. Another study found that postmenopausal women who began weight training preserved bone density, gained muscle mass, and significantly improved their sense of balance. Within three months of starting a weight-lifting program, muscle strength can increase by as much as 20 percent, making you 0.9 years younger. Weight training can also help improve performance in other sports. For example, one study found that runners who began doing leg lifts regularly increased their speed by as much as 40 percent.

If you have never lifted weights or done any strengthening exercises, get instruction first. It is easy to get hurt from lifting weights incorrectly, and just a little guidance can ensure that you will get the most out of your weight-lifting time and avoid injury. One way of combining weight training and stamina training is to begin circuit training, in which you lift weights in rapid succession, walking briskly between sets. If you join a gym, it will probably have a Cybex or Nautilus circuit already set up for you. If you are going to buy weights to use at home, buy free weights. All-in-one weight machines are much more expensive and take a lot of time for readjustments between each maneuver, meaning you spend a lot of your workout time just fiddling with the machine. Also, many "aerobic" exercise machines allow you to set a particular level of resistance. On treadmills, you can raise the angle of the "track." Many stationary bicycles can be adjusted to increase the amount of force needed to pedal.

A Personal Trainer: The Benefits of Professional Instruction

Consider hiring a personal trainer for a few sessions. Although it may seem a luxury—the kind of thing we associate with Hollywood celebrities—using a trainer can provide a big payoff for not that much investment, and I strongly advocate it. When my daughter Jennifer needed rehabilitation for a knee injury, she initially refused to work with a trainer. I finally convinced her to try it, and once she started, she quickly realized the value. The trainer taught her how to focus on her workouts and how to visualize her muscles actually getting stronger. This process helped strengthen the muscles around the knee, so she recovered more quickly. She learned how different muscle groups worked and how best to strengthen them.

If you do decide to hire a trainer, how should you begin? Start with a number of sessions right in a row and then taper off. A good trainer will focus closely on technique, so you will learn how to do each exercise properly. Go several times in the first two weeks to reinforce what you learn, so you don't forget. After the first two weeks, go for a refresher session once a week for a month and then go once a month after that or as needed. If hiring a trainer seems like too much of a "splurge," consider a conditioning-training class. Even one lesson will help you improve your form and lessen the risk of injury.

One of the things Jennifer liked best about going to the trainer was that she learned several exercises for each muscle group. Now she can alternate between them or simply do the ones she likes best. "What my trainer really taught me is that you should do the exercises you love to do," she told me. "If you don't like something, there's usually another way to get the same effect."

Your basic exercise sequence should be this:

- Warm up
- Flexibility exercises
- Strength exercises
- Flexibility exercises again and cool down (same as the warm-up)

Flexibility Exercises: The Basics

When you begin to do flexibility exercises, remember that warm muscles respond better than cold ones. After you warm up your muscles by walking slowly for five to ten minutes, begin your stretching exercises. It is usually good to do your stretching exercises just before your stamina-building workouts, so you stretch before you do vigorous exercises. Even if you attend a stretch class, such as yoga, make sure to do these seven basic stretches before exercising. Each stretch should be done twice, with slow and gentle movements. Extend into each stretch, feeling the pull on your muscles, for thirty seconds. *Do not bounce* because bouncing can put you at risk of straining or tearing muscles. Even if you do stretching exercises before your stamina workout, as I recommend, you should do the whole sequence again at the end of your workout as well.

Joining a Gym

What You Need to Know

Joining a gym or health club can be a great investment, a time-saving and motivational way to get your body in shape. Or it can be a boondoggle: Only one of three people who join a gym works out more than one hundred days a year. Before sinking a lot of dollars into a membership, make sure that you will actually use the gym. Before you join a gym:

1. *Try it out*. Most reputable clubs will allow you to work out free at least once before joining. That way you can test the equipment and the atmosphere. Do your workout at the time of day that you normally plan to work out to see how crowded the club gets and how long you would have to wait for machines.

2. *Find out about classes*. Ask to see a class schedule and talk to some instructors. Find out if classes are free with your membership.

3. *Find out if there is someone regularly on staff to help answer questions about your workout*. Good gyms will have someone who will teach you how to use all the equipment properly for free. Also find out if your gym has personal trainers who can take you through your workout. (In most big-city clubs, the fee for a personal trainer is $25 to $50 an hour.) Although you might not want to use a trainer all the time, having a pro look at your workout once in a while can do wonders to improve your technique.

4. *Join a gym that is close to your home or work*. Fitness-club gurus have what they call the "twelve-week–twelve-mile" hypothesis: Most people who join gyms work out for only the first twelve weeks of their membership, and only if the club is less than twelve miles from their home or office. Find a place that's close and convenient.

5. *Consider the atmosphere*. Pick a gym where you feel comfortable. Look at the crowd that goes there and think about whether you would enjoy working out there. Perhaps working out with the "twenty-somethings" would make you strive for more. Or maybe you would prefer a place that offers classes designed particularly for people over sixty. Some clubs are geared to women, and others are geared to men. Shop around and decide what fits you best.

6. *Ask about hidden costs.* Before joining, read the contract carefully and ask about extra expenses that may be added. Remember, too, that if you sign a full-year contract, you will have to pay for the whole year, even if you don't use the gym.

7. *Ask if there are any special discounts for joining.* Gyms may have monthly deals or offer special rates to first-time members. Ask around for pricing specials at comparable gyms in the area. You might be able to get a lower price from the gym you want to join.

8. *Check out the equipment.* Does it look new? Is it of good quality? Is it what you need for your workout? Don't believe promises about new equipment that's coming in "next week."

9. *Determine your workout needs.* Some people like being pampered in upscale gyms that offer the most deluxe equipment and amenities, such as massages, juice bars, and day care. Others are happy in a concrete room with just a treadmill and a set of free weights. Decide what activities and frills you would like your gym to offer and which ones you are willing to pay for.

10. *Decide if it's the best option for you.* Local park departments may offer free or low-cost access to gyms and exercise equipment. Also, many YMCAs, YWCAs, and YM/YWHAs have gyms that cost less than commercial options. Check, though, to be sure that the membership does not include other services that you do not want to pay for.

- *Achilles tendon and calf stretch.* Face a wall. With both hands against the wall, place one foot well behind you and the other foot flat on the floor with the toes touching the wall. Keeping the rear leg straight, with your heel on the ground, slowly lean in toward the wall. Keep your back straight. Hold it. Then switch and do the other leg. This exercise stretches your lower leg and helps prevent damage to your Achilles tendon.

- *Gastrocnemius stretch.* Move the back leg closer to the wall and tilt the front foot upward along the wall, with the toes propped up against the wall. Lean in toward the wall. Repeat with the other leg. This exercise stretches your lower leg (calf) muscle.

- *Quadriceps stretch.* This exercise stretches the long muscle that runs down the front of your thigh. Face a wall. Put your left hand on the wall for balance. Bend your right leg backward. Then reach your right hand behind your back and grab your right ankle, pulling it gently toward your buttocks until you feel tension along the front of your thigh. Then alternate and do the same thing for the left leg; that is, place your right hand on the wall and grab your left ankle.

- *Hamstring stretch.* Stand on one leg. Prop the other leg straight out on a chair or table, so the top of the entire leg is parallel to the ground. Bend over so you bring your face over your knee. Slide both hands toward the propped-up ankle as far as they'll go. This exercise stretches the muscles running down the back of your thigh, as well as the muscles in your lower back.

- *Chest and triceps (back of the upper arm) stretch.* Find something taller than you that you can grab onto, such as the top of a door frame or an overhead pole designed for pull-ups or stretching. Reach both hands over your head and grab onto the door frame or pole. Lean forward and stretch out your upper torso.

- *Biceps (front of the upper arm) stretch.* Stand along a wall. Place your arm at shoulder height from the side nearest the wall outstretched to your side and slightly behind you with fingers and palm against the wall. Lean forward, so your arm is stretched out behind you.

- *Back and abdominal stretch.* Lay down on your back, facing the ceiling. Put a rolled-up towel in the small of your back. Place your arms on your stomach. Relax for five minutes.

Strengthening Exercises: The Basics

Focus on strengthening all the different muscle groups. Pay special attention to the biceps, triceps, abdominals, quadriceps, hamstrings, and calf muscles. These exercises are performed against some force of resistance, either a weight or the weight of your own body. At first, try eight to twelve repetitions for each exercise (one set). Then you should build your way up to three sets or more for each exercise. Start out with small amounts of weight. As you progress, you will find yourself increasing the weight limit.

- *Bent-knee push-ups.* Lie facedown on the floor with your feet together and the palms of your hands flat on the floor on either side of your chest. Support the weight of your upper body on your arms with your knees against the floor as you raise your body until your arms are straight. Keep your back as flat as you can. Lower your upper body until your nose almost touches the ground and then raise it again. This bent-knee push-up is much easier than the straight-knee version. This exercise strengthens the muscles of your arms, chest, shoulders, and back. By doing the bent-knee push-up eight to twelve times three times a week, you'll eventually develop the upper-body strength to do the much harder straight-knee version, in which the pivot point is your toes, not your knees. Try to build more and more repetitions. Your three-year goal: to do as many straight-knee push-ups as your RealAge (I use my calendar age; that way, I know that every year I get a little stronger).

- *Knee extensions and flexions.* Sit on a chair and place an ankle weight on each leg. (You can buy specially designed weights that have Velcro or an ankle wrap that has pockets into which you put progressively greater weight.) Extend one leg so it is straight out in front of you. Lower your leg back to its starting position. After eight to twelve repetitions, switch to the other leg.

- *Hip and knee extensions.* Stand up and grab the back of a straight-backed chair with both hands (you may not need to use a chair, but I did when I started doing this exercise). Stand up straight with your toes just wider than your hips and point your toes outward. From this position, bend your knees slightly, directing your body weight over your toes. Do *not* do a deep knee bend. Keep your heels on the floor because the strength benefits occur with only a partial dip. Return to the initial position. As you get stronger, you can wear a backpack and gradually increase the amount of weight in the backpack.

- *Chest and shoulder exercises.* Sit upright in a straight-back chair that has no arms. Your shoulders should be straight. Keep your arms at your sides. Hold a weight in each hand. (You can either buy free weights or make your own from milk or water jugs filled with liquid or sand.) Raise one arm slowly upward and outward, keeping the elbow straight. Stop when your arm is fully extended above your head. Slowly return your arm to its starting position. You can either buy heavier weights or increase the amount of water or sand in the jugs as you get stronger. Do the same exercises for the other arm.

- *Abdominal exercises.* Lie comfortably on your back with your hands resting on your chest or at your side. Bend your knees and put a pillow behind your knees. Slowly bend and bring your head and chest and abdomen as a unit straight upward toward your knees. Start with as many as you can easily do, and build by one of these "crunches" a week. After week five, add five crunches aimed at each knee laterally by slowly bending and bringing your head and chest and abdomen as a unit upward toward the outside aspect of each knee (first the right and then the left after going back to the starting position).

- *Abdominal exercises, advanced.* Lie comfortably on your back with your hands clasped behind your head. Lift both legs together. Hold for a count of six. Then move each leg up and down alternatively six times but do not touch the ground with either. Then do a scissors, moving the right leg left over the left leg, and vice versa, six times. Repeat the cycle three times before you put your legs on the floor again. Increase the count for each step as you get stronger.

Do three sets of these strengthening exercises after you do the flexibility exercises outlined above. Repeat the flexibility exercises at the end of the strength sequence. Again, these are just basic stretches and lifts that you can do at home without any elaborate equipment. As you progress, you may want to add more to your workout, increase the duration and intensity of your workout, or even take a class that integrates your strength and flexibility exercises into one circuit workout.

10

Young Every Day

HEALTH HABITS TO
KEEP YOU YOUNG

There are healthy habits that all of us can adopt to significantly reduce our rate of aging. Whether it's getting enough sleep, eating breakfast, drinking alcohol in moderation, or walking the dog, some daily routines and overall life strategies can help us live longer, healthier, and younger lives. Learn to incorporate these habits into your daily life.

- Often it's the simple things that matter most in Age Reduction. You think you don't have time to sleep seven or eight hours a night? You don't have time not to. Your body needs time to rest and regenerate, and getting enough ZZZZZs will make your waking hours more productive. Getting a full night's sleep can reduce your RealAge by as much as three years.

  Difficulty rating: Moderately easy to very difficult

- Once you've slept the whole night through, don't forget to start the day off right. Eating a low-fat, high-nutrient breakfast gives a power start to the day and helps keep you three years younger than those who never eat breakfast.

  Difficulty rating: Moderately easy

- Do you like to have a drink now and then? Well, moderate drinking—that is, one-half to one drink a day for women and one or two drinks a day for men—may help you stay younger longer. A little alcohol can help your heart and arteries keep their spring. Moderate drinkers may gain as much as a 1.9-years-younger RealAge benefit, but drinking too much and too often can be dangerous, even life threatening. Indeed, heavy drinkers may have a RealAge that is three years older than that of nondrinkers.

  Difficulty rating: Moderately easy (moderate alcohol consumption) to the most difficult (cutting back on excessive alcohol consumption)

- Fido owners, rejoice. People who own dogs actually stay younger longer. Think of your furry friend as an exercise-promoting stress-reducer. Sorry, cat owners, the greatest RealAge benefit of pet ownership has gone to the dogs: one year younger.

  Difficulty rating: Moderate

Humans are creatures of habit—bad habits, more often than not. It is so easy to slide into unhealthy behaviors that can make us age faster than we should. Pressed for time, we skimp on sleep. Feeling guilty about last night's bowl of double-chocolate fudge ice cream, we skip breakfast. But we can learn good habits, too, even some that we can look forward to. Drinking alcohol in moderation—one-half to one drink a day for women and one or two drinks a day for men—can help prevent arterial aging. ("One drink" is 12 oz of beer, 4 oz of wine, or 1.5 oz of 80-proof liquor.) One of the best habits is walking the dog. Why? More exercise. As the turn-of-the-century physician William Osler said, "Walk your dog. Even if you don't have one."

Maintaining the quality of your life affects the quantity of your life: The better you take care of yourself, the younger you stay. How many times have you heard, "Do everything in moderation" and "Achieve balance in life"? Until recently, those sayings were more folklore than science. When it comes to aging, research has confirmed that this commonsense folk wisdom is right. Let us now consider a few changes that are easy to do, simple to integrate into your life, and don't necessarily require the resolve that getting in shape or changing one's diet does.

BEAUTY REST:
WAKE UP YOUNGER IN THE MORNING

I was the worst offender. When I was training to become a doctor, interns and residents were expected to survive without sleep. As I continued my career and had a family, I found myself getting busier and busier, with less and less time to do all the things I wanted to do. I just kept cutting down on the hours I slept, learning to rely on five hours a night or less. I didn't realize I was making my RealAge older. And I was making all my waking hours less productive.

Several studies have evaluated the long-term health effects of getting regular sleep. The data, drawn from reports from around the world, show that sleeping seven to eight hours a night provides protection against needless aging. The best-known study on sleep patterns, the famous Alameda County, California, study, found that men who slept seven to eight hours a night and women who slept six to seven hours a night had a significantly lower mortality risk than those who did not. To translate that risk into RealAge terms, regular sleep patterns can make a three-year difference.

Our bodies aren't designed to accommodate the crazy schedules and hours that contemporary society demands of us. A hundred years ago, no one lived in a world lit by unnatural light. Life was largely shaped by the cycle of the day. Not so anymore. Our bodies evolved over thousands of years to adapt to the natural cycle of the day. Our natural rhythms follow this schedule, assisted by hormones, such as melatonin, serotonin, and cortisol, that are secreted at different times of the day to push us through our sleep-to-wake cycle. For example, as it begins to get dark, our bodies begin to secrete melatonin, a hormone that increases drowsiness. As the sun starts to rise, the adrenal gland begins producing cortisol, a hormone that gets us up and going. The less sleep we get and the less consistent we are about getting it, the more confused our body "clocks" become and the more tired we are.

More than 20 percent of American adults find themselves dozing off at inappropriate moments or during quiet and sedentary activities—a sign that, on the whole, we aren't getting enough sleep. When I was an intern, I woke up at a dinner party at my professor's house with pie à la mode on my face. After a night on call, I had fallen asleep into the dessert. My date didn't wake me up, nor did anyone else. Most of us require at least six hours of sleep a night, usually between seven and eight hours. Sleeping more than nine hours a night regularly is too much for most of us and is often a sign of an underlying health problem. When we are younger, we need more sleep, and the quality of our sleep is better. As we age, the quality of our sleeping time diminishes. Our periods of "slow-wave sleep"—the kind of sleep needed to ensure cognitive alertness and motor coordination—decrease from 150 minutes a day to just 25.

Sleep deprivation lowers your performance at work and can adversely affect your moods, making you less attentive and, yes, grouchy. Also, sleepy people are at a greater risk of accidents, especially during periods of maximum sleepiness, such as the late afternoon or after midnight. As your body gets increasingly tired, your "sleep latency window"—the time it takes to go from being bored to dead asleep—decreases from as much as three minutes to just thirty seconds. That is, the more sleep-deprived you are, the more likely it is for you to doze off at the wheel or otherwise to put yourself and others in a life-threatening situation.

What kind of habits ensure a good night's sleep? Sleep in a cool, dark room.

If you find it hard to get to sleep, do something relaxing before going to bed—
reading or watching TV—to calm you down. You can also drink a glass of
milk (skim!) or eat a banana or some other melatonin- or serotonin-containing
food to help make you feel sleepy. If you need to rise early in the morning,
skip late-night activities. The best sleep schedule is regular and one that is in
sync with the natural rhythms of the day. Sleep late on weekends to repay
sleep debts. No, it's not a myth: You actually can catch up on restorative sleep,
a specific type of sleep that we think is needed for normal brain functioning.
And take a nap if you feel tired—even twenty minutes can make you feel
refreshed. Remember that naps do not make up for a good night's sleep, since
you do not pass through all the stages of sleep that your body needs to feel
refreshed to meet the day—REM (rapid-eye movement) sleep and slow-wave
sleep.

Do you have sleep problems? Illness or stress can disrupt the sleep pattern,
making us sleep too much or not enough. For example, two common signs of
clinical depression are waking up too early in the morning and sleeping an
endless numbers of hours. Other diseases can disturb your sleep cycle, causing chronic sleepiness or fatigue. If you notice changes in your sleep cycle,
talk to your doctor about possible causes. If you are under a lot of stress, try to
find new ways of relaxing. For example, exercise may help. One study found
that exercising in the early evening—walking, lifting weights, or any kind of
workout—improved both the quantity and quality of sleep.

Although sleeping pills or alcohol might produce short-term sleep benefits, in the long run they disrupt sleep. Regular use of these substances can
confuse your circadian rhythm (your internal clock), which means that you
may then need a drug if you are to sleep at all. Occasional use is usually not
a problem (for example, you can take melatonin supplements to help avoid
jet lag during international flights), and there are times when you may feel
you need sleeping pills. If so, talk to your doctor. Sleeping pills can be physically and psychologically addictive and may have long-term aging effects.
In fact, a recent study found that people who used sleeping pills more than
fourteen days a month were 1.9 years older, and that those who took twenty-
nine or more a month were 2.8 years older. It is a good idea to use sleeping
pills for only a limited time or to abstain from them altogether.

The next time you think you can skimp on shut-eye, remember that sleep is
one of the healthy habits that keep you young. Sleep helps strengthen your
immune system, boosts your attention span, and dissipates excess stress that
can damage your arteries, stomach, and immune system.

DON'T SKIP BREAKFAST:
STARTING THE DAY OFF RIGHT

When I was doing research for this book, I found that one of my favorite time-saving (and calorie-saving) schemes, skipping breakfast, was actually making my RealAge older. In fact, until I started researching the RealAge effect of different behaviors, I always skipped breakfast. And I congratulated myself for doing so, thinking I would not only save myself twenty minutes a day but also keep my weight down. I was wrong. Instead of saving myself time, I was spending time—making my RealAge as much as three years older. Studies have consistently shown that people who eat meals at regular intervals, particularly those who eat breakfast, stay younger longer. Indeed, non-breakfast-eaters have a mortality rate that is 1.3 to 1.5 times per year higher than those who eat breakfast regularly.

Breakfast is the first part of a daylong eating plan; it is better for us to eat several small meals throughout the day than one large meal at night. Eating breakfast helps our bodies metabolize food more efficiently and cuts down on the urge to snack between meals. Unhealthy snacking more than three days a week can increase your RealAge. Eating regularly helps break up long periods of fasting, meaning that our body doesn't have to gear up to digest a big meal after doing nothing for hours, which is not an efficient process. In addition, some researchers have hypothesized that we burn more fat during our waking hours, since we are more active. Thus, we may burn off our breakfast calories more effectively than we would an overstuffed, late-night dinner. That is still speculation.

Eating breakfast also makes your cardiovascular and immune systems younger. We don't know exactly why, but there are several theories. First, cereals contain lots of fiber, and fiber helps prevent arterial aging by preventing lipid buildup. Fiber also helps decrease the risk of cancer. The average American eats 12 grams of fiber a day, but increasing your fiber intake to 25 grams per day can reduce arterial aging and make your RealAge as much as three years younger. Second, cereals usually have vitamins added to them. During breakfast, we get many of the essential nutrients that we may not get for the rest of the day. This is even more important if you don't eat lots of fruits and vegetables during the day, or if you don't take supplements regularly. Other typical breakfast foods (fortified fruit juices, yogurt, and whole fruit) also contain essential nutrients, such as vitamins C and D and calcium.

So, specifically, what should you eat for breakfast? Cereals, fruits, juices, and low-fat dairy products like fat-free yogurt or skim milk. Choose a whole-

TABLE 10.1

The RealAge Effect of Eating Breakfast

FOR MEN

Calendar Age	Breakfast		
	Rarely/Occasionally	*2–5 Times Per Week*	*Almost Every Day*
	RealAge		
35	37	34.8	34.5
50	52.2	49.7	49.2
70	72	69.8	69.5

FOR WOMEN

Calendar Age	Breakfast		
	Rarely/Occasionally	*2–5 Times Per Week*	*Almost Every Day*
	RealAge		
35	36.2	35	34.8
50	51.2	50	49.8
70	71.3	70	69.8

grain cereal with no extra fat or sugar that just adds empty calories. Become a label reader and watch out for "healthy" breakfast foods, including many brands of granola, that actually contain a lot of calories and fat. Use skim milk instead of whole milk on your cereal and in your tea or coffee. Drink plenty of juices—pure juice or fortified pure juice, not juice cocktails or blends that contain too much added sugar and less real juice. Whole fruits are even better than juice because they contain much desired fiber. Both are good sources of vitamin C and potassium. Eat whole-grain or multigrain toast; again, read the labels because many commercially manufactured breads contain added sugar, salt, and other ingredients that you may want to avoid. Instead of a pastry or a croissant, which are high in fat, choose an English muffin or bagel. And try Neufchâtel cheese or olive oil instead of high-fat cream cheese, butter, or margarine. Fruit spreads are a good substitute for high-sugar and calorie-laden

jams and jellies. In general, avoid breakfast foods high in saturated fats such
as bacon and sausage. Only the yolk of the egg is high in fat and cholesterol,
so consider egg-white vegetable omelets with salsa—no cheese—for a low-
cholesterol, low-fat option. If you crave pancakes or waffles, cook them in a
no-stick pan or in one coated with low-fat vegetable spray. Use chopped fruit
with a sprinkle of powdered sugar on top instead of mounds of butter and
syrup.

Remember, too, that "donuts and coffee" is an absolutely empty breakfast—
lots of calories, lots of artery-aging trans fat, and no nutrition. Use breakfast
time to stimulate your imagination: Try unconventional breakfast foods, such
as chopped vegetables with a handful of low-fat whole-grain crackers, or a corn
tortilla loaded with beans, lettuce, and tomato. Or make a fruit-juice smoothie
in your blender. Add orange juice, ice, and any kind of fruit you want—
bananas, berries, peaches, and mangoes. You can even add raw beets or tomatoes. If you own a juicer, you can make carrot or tomato juice mixed with celery, spinach, and other vegetables. It's a time-saving, nutrient rich, and fat-free
way to begin the day.

If you are too busy to sit down to breakfast each morning, have a breakfast-
on-the-go. Carry a small bag of cereal with you and munch on the cereal as
you drive to work. Or pack a low-fat yogurt. Buy juice boxes with real juice—
not "juice drinks" or "juice cocktails"—and carry them in your purse or brief-
case. Keep plenty of fruit around, to start the day and to munch on between
meals. Becoming a breakfast eater can make your RealAge as much as three
years younger. And that's not even counting the RealAge benefits from all the
vitamins; minerals; and other nutrients, such as carotenoids, flavonoids, and,
of course, fiber you get from eating nutritious food.

Finally, breakfast can be an important social time. For many families, the
weekend is a time for everyone to get together and talk about what happened
during the week. Saturday and Sunday morning brunches are also a good time
to see friends and to strengthen the social ties that help keep us younger.

MIXED DRINKS: THE PROS AND CONS OF ALCOHOL CONSUMPTION

In January 1996, the U.S. government, in announcing a revision of dietary
guidelines, declared that the moderate intake of alcohol appeared to be beneficial to human health. The announcement was astounding. Clearly, we'd
come a long way from Prohibition. After years of fighting alcohol consump-

tion, the government was actually encouraging it. However, the government was careful to emphasize "moderate." That means one-half to one drink a day for women and one to two drinks a day for men—nothing more.

The issue is clearly a delicate one. Alcohol can help you or harm you. Regular consumption of alcohol in small amounts helps prevent arterial aging and heart attacks. Too much alcohol consumption can lead to alcoholism, liver disease, increased cancer rates, and increased risk of death from accidents during intoxication. Approximately 5 percent of all deaths can be attributed to the excessive consumption of alcohol, and the medical and social effects of drinking too much can be extremely severe. Around 100,000 Americans die every year of alcohol-related diseases, and 20 million Americans suffer problems related to alcohol addiction.

So, what's the right balance? Should you incorporate moderate drinking into your Age Reduction Plan? Or are you someone who can't drink in moderation and probably shouldn't drink at all?

First, the RealAge Age Reducing effect of alcohol consumption begins only when a person reaches the age at which the risk of cardiovascular disease increases—after menopause for women and age forty to fifty for men. Second, the antiaging benefits apply only to some people. Therefore, you need to weigh your risks and decide whether alcohol consumption should be part of your Age Reduction Plan. You also need to determine if you can consume alcohol in moderate amounts, considering your own genetic and social risks of developing alcoholism, liver disease, or cancers.

The connection between alcohol and reduced arterial aging—the so-called red wine factor—was first observed in France. The southern French, whose traditional diet is heavy in fatty cheeses, butter, and red meats, had surprisingly lower rates of cardiovascular disease than would have been predicted. The hypothesis that scientists came up with to explain this discrepancy was that all the red wine the French use to wash down their saturated fat–laden food was helping to protect their arteries from the buildup of fatty plaque. Mounting evidence now suggests that not just red wine but any alcoholic beverage helps protect us from arterial aging. When it comes to Age Reduction, all alcoholic beverages seem to have the same effect: 4 ounces of wine is the same as one can of beer, which is the same as 1.5 ounces of 80-proof liquor. Moderate and regular consumption of alcohol reduces the risk of heart attack by as much as 30 percent, making your RealAge 1.9 years younger (see Table 10.2).

How does alcohol retard or reverse arterial aging? No one knows the answer. Alcohol appears to prevent clotting by decreasing the rate of platelet aggregation, meaning that the platelets don't stick together as fast as they normally

TABLE 10.2

The RealAge Effect of Alcohol

FOR MEN

Of drinking one alcoholic drink a day
At age 35: 0.9 years younger
At age 55: 1.7 years younger
At age 70: 2.3 years younger

Of drinking three to six alcoholic drinks a day
At age 35: 0.1 to 1.4 years older
At age 55: 0.2 to 5 years older
At age 70: 0.3 to 7.6 years older

FOR WOMEN

Of drinking one alcoholic drink a day
At age 35: Probably none, as the benefits for women do not usually occur until after menopause.
At age 55: 1.8 years younger
At age 70: 2.2 years younger

Of drinking three to six alcoholic drinks a day
At age 35: 0.1 to 1.4 years older
At age 55: 0.2 to 5 years older
At age 70: 0.3 to 7.6 years older

would. Also, alcohol appears to prevent fat from oxidizing and, in this way, prevents it from forming plaques along the walls of the arteries. Alcohol promotes the health of the endothelium, the layer of cells lining your arteries that promotes proper blood flow. Although some may be better than others, all types of alcoholic beverages help reduce the level of atherosclerosis. All alcohol causes an increase in HDL (healthy) cholesterol levels. Red wine, presumably because of the presence of flavonoids in grape skins (see Chapter 8), may have other benefits as well. The flavonoids act as an antioxidant and free-radical scavenger, resulting in reduced arterial and immune system aging.

What is the evidence that alcohol reduces arterial aging and thereby the incidence of heart disease? The well-known Nurses Health Study, an analysis of the health habits of almost ninety thousand female nurses, found that those who drank three or more drinks a week (equivalent to one-half to one drink a day) had a 40 percent lower rate of nonfatal heart attacks and arterial disease than those who did not. Several corresponding studies of men found similar results. These studies also found that there was an ideal range of alcohol consumption. Women who had one-half to one drink a day and men who had one or two drinks a day were at a lower risk of coronary and arterial aging, yet did not have a higher risk of aging from liver disease or cancers, conditions that excess drinking can cause. Individuals who drank less than these limits were also at a higher risk of cardiovascular diseases, whereas those who drank more had significant increases in their RealAge because of cancers, liver disease, car accidents, and other accidents. Those in the low-to-moderate drinking range had the longest life expectancy, the fewest health problems, and the youngest RealAge at any calendar age.

Should you have a drink or two a night? That depends. Women should consume no more than one drink a night, and men should have no more than two. Why can women get the same antiaging effect from less alcohol? There are three reasons. First, women tend to be smaller, which affects the overall amount of alcohol they can tolerate at any time. Second, women have less alcohol dehydrogenase in the lining of their stomachs. This enzyme breaks down alcohol before it enters the bloodstream. Women thus tend to absorb more alcohol into their bloodstream per drink. Third, when you drink a lot, the enzyme that breaks down alcohol (cytochrome CYPE2A) increases. Unfortunately, this enzyme also breaks down hormones, such as estrogen, that help protect women from heart disease.

People who are at a high risk of cardiovascular disease—either because of a family history of heart attacks or because of signs of developing atherosclerosis—will get the most Age Reducing benefit from a drink a day. In contrast, people at risk of alcohol-related diseases should avoid alcohol altogether. Smokers and those with a family history of alcoholism, cirrhosis of the liver, hepatic cancer, or other alcohol-related illnesses are also strongly urged to avoid all alcohol consumption.

The liver is the principle site of metabolism of alcohol and as such remains at the highest risk of damage—and aging—from alcohol use. Liver scarring from the use of alcohol (cirrhosis) can cause considerable aging. In some urban areas, it's the fourth leading cause of death for individuals age twenty-five to sixty-four. Cirrhosis of the liver (alcoholic hepatitis) can cause a person to age even faster than many types of cancers. Since cirrhosis of the liver causes irreversible structural damage, there are few treatment options for the disease once it reaches an advanced stage. Damage to the liver also appears to be related to an increased risk of cancer.

There are two theories about why excessive drinking causes cancer. The first and most widely held explanation is that the consumption of alcohol induces or increases the production of an enzyme that breaks down alcohol, the cytochrome we referred to above, called CYPE2A. This enzyme breaks down not only alcohol but also other foreign substances, often creating carcinogenic compounds in the process. That is why smokers, in particular, need to avoid drinking alcohol. The combination is deadly. The same enzyme that breaks down alcohol, (CYPE2A) and hence increases when you are drinking, also breaks down the nitrosamines in cigarette smoke into a carcinogenic form. By stimulating the production of this enzyme, alcohol increases the risk of cancer from smoking. The RealAge effect can make someone as much as five to ten years older.

A second explanation for the higher incidence of cancer among heavy drinkers is that alcohol itself contains low levels of cancer-causing substances. The risk of throat and digestive-track cancers increases two to ten times among heavy drinkers, depending on the kind of cancer. Women in particular have to be careful: Those who drink too much are twice as likely to have uterine and cervical cancers, although, curiously, not breast cancers.

Excessive drinking can age you in other ways, too. Alcohol is fattening, and heavy drinkers tend to carry around more paunch and to look older. But that fat ages more than your looks. The impurities that are stored in the fat also increase your risk of cancer to that of someone five to ten years older. Finally, alcohol consumption impairs the absorption of crucial nutrients and vitamins, leading to nutritional deficiencies and even malnutrition. Alcohol consumption is associated with a decreased intake of thiamine, folate, iron, zinc, vitamin E, and vitamin C. It also decreases the efficiency of metabolism, particularly of the pancreas.

The best-known aging effects from overconsumption of alcohol are accidents, both from automobiles and other causes. Never, ever, drink and drive. You put both yourself and others at risk. If you are out with friends, make sure to choose a designated driver or take a taxi home. And operating a boat, swimming, or putting yourself in other potentially risky situations while drinking can cause rapid aging.

If you think that you drink too much, you probably do. If drinking is a problem for you, talk to your doctor about the possible medical risks, as well as strategies for quitting and getting younger. There are also many well-known clinics and organizations, such as Alcoholics Anonymous, that are extremely effective in helping break the addiction to alcohol. If you are a heavy drinker, the best RealAge plan for you is to quit drinking altogether. For people who regularly have a drink or two a night, the RealAge advantage is 1.9 years. For people who drink too much, the RealAge damage can be more than three years older.

A fun way to incorporate moderate drinking into your life—and one that is less likely to lead to overconsumption of alcohol—is to become a wine lover. By learning about different vintages and types of wine, you can have fun and lower your RealAge at the same time. The French weren't all wrong.

WALK YOUR DOG:
EVEN IF YOU DON'T HAVE ONE

When George S. died at age eighty-nine, his wife Joy, who was somewhat younger, found herself in a quandary. Although she was free to travel for the first time in years, her cocker spaniel Lucy kept her tied to home. Since George had been one of my patients for some time, Joy and I had become friends, and she often called me to ask about health and other related issues.

"Mike," she said, "I feel so torn. I adore Lucy, and she's one of my last ties to George. We picked her out together when she was a puppy, we named her, we housebroke her, and she nursed him right through to the end. The night he died, she lay curled on the bed next to him, offering comfort. But now I want to travel, and I feel guilty about leaving her. Do you think that I should get rid of her?"

"Let's see if we can find a way for you to keep Lucy but have some relief from the full-time demands," I told Joy. Part of the reason I felt she should keep Lucy is that owning a dog is good for you. Pet owners—particularly dog owners—stay younger longer. Indeed, the RealAge benefit is as much as one year younger and perhaps even more so during particularly stressful times.

Although one-third to one-half of all the households in the English-speaking world have pets, little research has been done on the effects of pets on health and aging. Most of the medical literature on pets deals only with the negative aspects of pet ownership, such as allergies or the increased risk of disease. These issues should not be of concern to most people. Even if you are vulnerable to allergies or immune diseases, you might still be able to have a pet if you really want one. Talk to your doctor about the possible solutions.

Unfortunately, most studies on the benefits of animal ownership have not been rigorously controlled, and the results are often skewed. Since everyone involved in the research seems to enjoy animals, it is often difficult to be objective about the actual health benefits that pets may provide. Also, one needs to consider whether people who own animals are different in other respects from those who do not. Perhaps they are more social and less stressed, which is why they want pets in the first place. Finally, pet owners themselves are not all alike. Some clearly get enormous enjoyment out of their pets, whereas others see them as one more chore. To get a RealAge benefit from owning a pet, a person presumably should enjoy the pet. What this means is that you shouldn't get a pet just because it can make you younger, but that those of you who already own pets can take comfort in knowing that your animal companions make you younger.

A 1980 study on heart attack survivors found that the survival rate within one year of the heart attack was 94 percent for pet owners and only 72 percent for non-pet-owners. It didn't matter what kind of pet the person owned, either—dog, cat, bird, or iguana. Other confounding variables, such as different life circumstances, could not account for the benefit. In an expanded and more rigorous study, the results were similar. In fact, the survival rate for dog owners after a heart attack was even better. When translated into RealAge terms, the heart attack sufferers who owned dogs were as much as 3.25 years younger during their recovery period than those who did not own dogs. Other studies have found that pet owners have lower blood pressure and lower cholesterol levels. Also, pet owners seem to suffer fewer headaches, cold sores, and other chronic infections and to have a better overall sense of psychological well-being. It appears, too, that pet owners fare better during especially stressful times, suffering major life events less severely than those who don't own pets. Pet owners do not have as many bouts of depression and maintain better self-esteem.

Dog owners show a particular benefit. Why dogs and not cats? I spent a lot of time puzzling over this question. Since I do not own a dog or a cat, I had no personal experience on which to base an opinion. I assumed that all the walking that dog owners have to do might have something to do with the benefit, but the studies weren't clear about the reasons. Osler, one of the preeminent clinicians of the nineteenth century, observed that dog ownership boosted activity and exercise. After some *ad hoc* research of my own, I agree that the demands of dog ownership promote a healthier lifestyle. After speaking to some dog owners at a local park, I learned that dog ownership promotes other good habits in addition to extra exercise. Having a dog often means keeping a more regular schedule, including a more regular sleep schedule, that will accommodate the dog's need for regular walks. Also, dog owners who walk their dogs at the same park often form a social community, providing a support network for each other. All these factors can keep your RealAge younger.

When I reread the literature, it made a lot more sense. I called Joy and said, "I did some research on dogs, and not only is Lucy a good companion, but it's true that she keeps you younger. I think you should keep her and find a dog sitter—someone you can count on to take care of her when you are away."

Do not get a dog unless you are prepared to take care of one. If you think it will be too much work or will add unwanted stress to your life, it probably will—and that's not fair to you or the dog.

Osler and others have attributed the advantages of pet ownership to physiologic benefits. This is where pet owners part ways with the data. Many pet owners claim that their pets give them an enormous psychological boost, something that in RealAge terms would make them much more than the one year younger attributed to dog walking. That may well be true. Most pet owners are extremely attached to their pets, and a high percentage of them find their relationship with their pets absolutely essential to their emotional well-being. Unfortunately, since no scientific data have accurately measured this relationship, we cannot calculate a RealAge benefit for these emotional factors. The only scientifically reliable information pertains to the physiologic benefits. All we can say is that, for animal lovers, one more thing pets give you besides love and affection is added youth. And that's a pretty hard gift to beat.

11

Stress Reduction

HEALTHY MIND, YOUNGER PERSON

What's long been suspected has now been proven by scientific study: Emotional well-being helps you stay healthy and younger longer. Which emotional factors help keep you young? Which life events will cause age-promoting stress, and what can be done to offset the risk? Realize that the mind and body work together. Happiness and stress-free living will help keep your RealAge young.

- For years, having a type-A personality was seen as the cause of stress-induced illness. Now we know that stress-induced illness comes only from the things that stress *you*, even if they don't seem to be the things that stress other people. Life events as different as the loss of a family member, moving to a new town, or financial troubles can all cause stress, but they have to be dealt with in different ways. Reducing stress in your life can give back thirty of the thirty-two years that major life events can take away.

  Difficulty rating: Most difficult

- People who live with others, who have lots of friends, and who stay involved in social activities live longer, happier, healthier lives. During nonstressful times, living with three or more people or having many close friends can make you two years younger than those who don't have this support network. During extremely stressful times, it can keep you as much as thirty years younger.

  Difficulty rating: Moderately difficult

- Rich or poor, living beyond your means can be one of the most troubling day-to-day stresses. All that worrying about money can make you old. Learn how to plan your finances so you don't live beyond your means. Reducing financial stresses can reduce your RealAge by as much as eight years.

  Difficulty rating: Moderately difficult

- I bet you never knew school could make you younger! But the fact is, keeping your mind active helps keep your body young. Your mind is like a muscle: You need to exercise it. By using your brain, you can become more than 2.5 years younger.

  Difficulty rating: Moderate

- We often put off dealing with the emotional upsets in our lives, whether it's recovering from our parents' divorce when we were children or recovering from our own as adults. By not confronting these traumas, we often suffer needlessly, and it affects our health. If the social networks you have aren't enough to help you with the emotional conflicts you face, no matter what they are, seeking professional help through a psychiatrist, counselor, or therapist can make your RealAge eight to sixteen years younger than it otherwise would be.

  Difficulty rating: Most difficult

Feeling harried? Not enough hours in the day? Don't you sometimes wish that the phone would just stop ringing? Most Americans are *stressed*. There is nothing like a day of too many hassles to make you feel that you are aging faster than you should. There is no doubt that too much stress does indeed age you. Stress is linked to aging of both the arterial and immune systems. Also, people under stress are more likely to get into accidents or suffer other hazards that can cause them to age.

Stress is a normal part of life and can be good for us and necessary. However, too much stress turns normally useful bodily reactions into damaging overreactions. Stress overload can cause the brain to trigger an overrelease or imbalance of "stress hormones" that can lead to physiologic problems in the long run. Prolonged stress decreases our ability to control our cardiovascular responses, which increase blood pressure and age our arteries. The same neurotransmitter that keeps us alert and able to respond quickly in times of danger causes us to be overtaxed by the constant release of stress hormones. This constant excess actually decreases our ability to sense trouble, prevent accidents, and avoid confrontations. And stress suppresses the immune response, increasing our risk of catching infections or developing more serious diseases. In other words, stress stimulates many of the conditions that cause early aging.

Almost all of us are juggling too many commitments that can cause age-inducing stress. You can prevent the needless aging by learning to manage your day-to-day stresses and to develop safety networks that you can rely on when a major stress-inducing event occurs.

More than half of us will have a "major life event"—a death, a divorce, a job loss or job change, an illness in the family, financial difficulties, relocation, involvement in a lawsuit, or other serious trauma—within any one year. The occurrence of one major life event makes you about five RealAge years older during the time the event is going on and for at least one year (and probably two years) afterward. Two major life events in one year can raise your RealAge by as much as sixteen years, and three major life events in one year can increase your RealAge by more than thirty-two years for at least the following year (see Table 11.1). All of us have some stress in our lives, and during our lifetime, each of us will suffer a major life event at least once, if not many times. The question is not whether we will suffer stress but how we manage it.

THE NATURE OF "STRESS"

What exactly is stress? How does it manifest physiologically? Stress is more than just the feeling that there's too much to do, too little time to do it, and too many hassles along the way. Stress is a very complex set of physiologic and psychological reactions. Dr. Hans Selye, one of the earliest researchers to study stress, defined it as "the nonspecific response of the body to any demand made on it." Simply put, stress is the body's reaction when it anticipates the need for extra energy. Almost anything can provoke this reaction: an injury, working under a deadline for a crazy boss, not sleeping enough, or not eating regular meals. Even laughing stresses the body.

Despite popular beliefs, stress is not purely mental; it is also physiologic. When we are stressed, our bodies release a flood of adrenaline, cortisone, and other stress hormones that induce physiologic changes. The heart pounds and blood pressure rises. Our rate of breathing increases, and we feel more alert. Blood races to the brain and heart and moves away from the kidneys, liver, stomach, and skin. Our blood sugar level rises, as do the amounts of fats and cholesterol in our bloodstream. The amount of clotting factors and platelets in the blood increases. All this is part of the "fight-or-flight" response: The body is energizing itself for danger. The question is, how prolonged and damaging will our stress be?

Fleeting stress responses may be good for us. These survival responses cause us to jerk our hand off a burning pan or to jump aside when a car comes too close. These fleeting stresses do not age us. The problem arises when we are in a constant fight-or-flight state.

TABLE 11.1

The RealAge Effect of Stress

Major life events cause aging. Twenty-eight percent of Americans undergo one major life event in any given year, 15 percent will undergo two, and 13 percent will have three or more.

A major life event consists of experiences such as the death or illness of a loved one (especially a spouse or a child), divorce, a major illness, moving to a new locale, being the target of a lawsuit, losing or beginning a job, and financial instabilities like bankruptcy.

FOR MEN

	Number of Major Life Events in Past Year			
	0	1	2	3
Calendar Age	RealAge			
35	27	34	36	42
55	49	54	61	68
70	62	69	77	94

FOR WOMEN

	Number of Major Life Events in Past Year			
	0	1	2	3
Calendar Age	RealAge			
35	27	34	38	43
55	49	54	61	67
70	63	69	76	84

During chronic stress, our bodies are in a continuous state of siege. The same systems that help us when we are in danger by responding for the moment and then shutting back down are now in overdrive. Imagine a car. The more you rev the engine, the faster you use up the gas. With stress, the faster you rev your body, the more quickly you age. Physically, chronic stress alters the immune responses, causing a decrease in the production of beneficial T cells and B cells. Chronic stress also raises blood pressure.

Studies have shown that the relationship between stress and aging are marked. A recent study published in the *Journal of the American Medical Association* found that stress was linked to increased levels of myocardial ischemia, reduced blood flow to the heart. Although doctors have long suspected that stress might cause a narrowing of the arteries, this study provided the first proof that stress also narrowed arteries acutely to the point of hazard. People who experienced a lot of stress also had more periods of ischemia and a correspondingly higher risk of heart attack or abnormal heart rhythms.

Not only does stress cause arterial aging that increases blood pressure, but it also causes the release of neurotransmitters that elevate the heart rate, pushing blood pressure higher still. As you know, high blood pressure accelerates arterial aging. Recent research at Johns Hopkins University indicated that people who score high on mental "stress tests"—not just the physical treadmill stress tests normally used to detect heart strain—were more than twenty times more likely to develop heart and arterial diseases. Individuals who had "hot" reactions—who were more likely to get agitated or frustrated by life events—had twenty times the rate of arterial aging, as measured by the incidence of heart attacks and strokes, of people who had "cool" reactions.

Stress doesn't just age your arterial system. As I mentioned, prolonged exposure to the neurotransmitters that your body releases during periods of stress can age the immune system as well. How do researchers measure this type of aging? A study of health care workers found that those with especially stressful jobs had a lower level of antibody production than did those in less stressful positions. Furthermore, prolonged exposure to chronic stress depletes our bodies of important vitamins, such as vitamin C, vitamin D, and the B-complex vitamins, including folate. Stress also appears to increase our rate of bone loss, causing a depletion of bone density. Finally, overexposure to stress hormones, which at first heighten perceptiveness, can decrease perceptiveness over time, thus raising the risk of accidents and acts of violence—for example, the freeway confrontations called "road rage."

Different stresses affect people in different ways, and not everyone is stressed by the same things. Some doctors are the image of calmness when treating life-threatening traumas in the emergency room but become utterly flustered when tending to the daily tasks of running their offices. Some people love a good argument, and others will do anything to avoid one. Often type-A personalities, those who are always pushing themselves to run, run, run, become more stressed when they try to stop type-A behaviors. Relaxing or "letting go" makes them anxious. The trick is to identify what stresses you and then develop strategies for avoiding stressful situations or, if they can't be avoided, figuring out how to handle them in ways that reduce your own stress levels.

Most stress is tied to the individual's perception of an event. One person might find skydiving exhilarating, whereas another may find it terrifying. Both feel stress from the event, but one feels good stress, called "eustress" for the euphoric reaction; and the other, bad stress, or "distress." One person may love to go to parties, finding working the crowd or meeting new people fun and relaxing, but another person may find it nerve-racking. The level of stress we feel has a lot to do with our subjective interpretation of what is happening to us. One of the ways of changing our stress levels is to try to change our perception of an event.

I was in a major Chicago department store a few years ago on Christmas Eve. It was closing time, and my son and I were the last ones to get in line. It wasn't really a line—most shoppers were crowded around the register area, pushing and shoving. The salesperson was still ringing up sales an hour after the store had closed. When I finally reached the register, imagining what it would be like to spend the day heading off a surge of harried shoppers, I said to her, "You must be glad this day's over. Talk about stressful." The woman laughed and said, "I love my job. In how many other jobs do you have people fighting over you?" I had to laugh, and I certainly admired her. She was in one of the most stress-inducing jobs ("point-of-service" jobs, such as cashiering during the Christmas rush, are among the most stressful), yet she didn't let the stress get to her. Rather than see the surge of customers as a negative stress, she considered it a positive situation: all these people fighting over her. Her ability to change her perception of the event meant that she did not age from that day's push, like she would have if she had found it stressful.

Measuring the Effects of Stress

The symptoms of stress fall into four categories: physical, mental, emotional, and behavioral. Physical signs of stress include frequent headaches, trouble sleeping, sore and stiff muscles, nausea or upset stomach, diarrhea or constipation, a general sense of fatigue, and increased susceptibility to illness. Mental symptoms of stress include the inability to concentrate, confusion, and a lack of clarity. Also, stressed individuals are often indecisive and lose their sense of humor. On an emotional level, stress makes us anxious, nervous, and irritable. We may be quick to anger, impatient with others, or depressed. Behaviors indicative of stress include fidgeting, pacing, or feeling that you can't sit still. On the other hand, you can also feel sluggish or avoid work because it seems too daunting.

There are two basic kinds of stress. The first is ongoing, low-level stress, such as job pressures or juggling work and children. Then there are those one-of-a-kind stresses that are harder to plan for—the death of a loved one, the sudden loss of a job, or a divorce. Although we know that both kinds of stress age us, it has been much easier for researchers to measure the aging impact of the big one-time event because there are clear "before" and "after" periods to measure. It is clear, for example, that the death of a spouse has a significant RealAge impact. Widows and widowers have reduced levels of important immune system B and T cells, as well as low antibody production, for more than a year after the loss of their partners. And both widows and widowers are much more likely to suffer a major health event after such a loss. It is not uncommon for a person who has been married for a long time to die soon after his or her spouse dies, the death of one causing overnight aging of the other.

Researchers have also been successful in measuring the impact of stress and increased aging during and after natural disasters because there is a clear set of dates from which to detect changes in the rates of heart attacks and death. For example, demographic studies have shown that the rate of heart attacks (in particular, severe or fatal heart attacks) increases dramatically in the days after a major earthquake. And in the days after the bombings in the Gulf War, the heart attack rate surged in Israel. Although the studies didn't investigate the more general impact on aging, we can presume a higher incidence of strokes and other aging-related events as well. In another poignant example, a recent study published by the National Cancer Institute found that the psychological stress associated with the diagnosis of breast cancer caused the levels of immune cells, such as T cells and natural killer cells, to plummet, putting patients at an even greater risk. In these instances, it is clear that stress affects aging. That is why we can say that one major life event can age you by as much as five years during the time it is going on and for at least one year (and probably longer) afterward.

In measuring long-term, ongoing stresses, researchers have had a harder time quantifying their impact on our aging processes. Not because such stresses are any less real, but because there are no defined starting and stopping points. Furthermore, ongoing stresses seem to be open to a more subjective interpretation. Although everyone finds the death of a loved one stressful, not everyone finds the same aspects of family life or work life stressful. There is certainly evidence that ongoing low-level stresses make us older. For example, people who are severely dissatisfied with their jobs are also more likely to suffer heart attacks.

For these kinds of recurrent and chronic stresses, it is important to identify the things you find stressful. You must learn how to avoid them or how to plan for them in such a way that they won't stress you. For example, studies have indicated that most people have significant stress reactions the first time they speak in front of a crowd. Approximately 90 percent of the people who do a lot of public speaking become accustomed to it and no longer have stress responses. However, 10 percent still have that initial stress response no matter how much public speaking they do.

Which leads to the next question: How can you reduce your level of stress? First I will discuss some simple, healthy habits that may help reduce stress. Then I will describe how to manage stress in relation to some of the bigger concerns—your family and social relationships, your work, your finances, and your level of education.

General Habits That Reduce Stress

Let's begin with a few simple changes in physical habits. One of the best ways to reduce stress is to exercise. Think about it: Stress causes our bodies to build up extra energy, preparing them for fight or flight. Exercise burns energy and reduces our stress levels. Exercise metabolizes stress hormones in our blood and increases levels of our bodies' built-in antianxiety hormones, making us feel calmer. Exercise makes us more efficient and energetic, so we feel less overwhelmed by the stresses we do face. For example, just walking regularly can increase the level of beta-endorphins (hormones that help the body feel pleasure) in the brain, decrease anxiety and tension, and elevate one's mood. And exercise—especially aerobic exercise—helps you divert energy from worrying and anxiety.

Relaxation techniques, biofeedback, and mental imagery also seem to reduce the effects of stress. Combination programs like yoga that include both body stretching and mind relaxation can be especially effective in easing emotional and physical tensions. One simple technique is visualization. Close your eyes, relax your muscles, and imagine yourself some place far away from the chaos around you. Imagine yourself on a beach or in a mountain meadow, feel the warmth of the sun on your skin, and let your muscles feel soft and heavy. Relax into them. Breathe deeply. Feel the tension dissipate. A healthier diet and a regular schedule also help lower stress levels, making you younger in this way, too. Our favorite food vices—sugar, salt, and caffeine—may actually elevate stress levels. So can cigarette smoking and excess alcohol. Focus, too, on getting enough sleep. Even though you think you don't have time for a full night's sleep, you will be much more productive if you are well rested. And the tasks at hand won't seem nearly so overwhelming.

One thing that many people find stressful is the sense that they don't have any control over a given situation, especially when they have many demands on their time. If that's happening to you, try to figure out what you can do to make yourself feel more in control. How can you make the situation work for you, instead of being controlled by everyone else's needs? At work, be more proactive in defining your responsibilities. If the boss talks to you only when something goes wrong, make a habit of frequently telling him or her what you've done right. It may change the tone of your interactions and make your job feel less stressful. Finally, if you believe that you have too many tasks to do at home, evaluate which ones are necessary and which ones aren't. See if you can develop a plan for simplifying your tasks. Or explain your frustrations to your family and ask if they can pitch in to help.

Now let's consider some simple changes in mental habits that help us manage everyday stress.

1. Learn to recognize the conditions that stress you and note your reactions to those conditions. Naming the problem is the first step toward solving it.

2. Try to think about the situation you find stressful from a different perspective. Is it really that bad? Is there another way of looking at the problem? Remember the saleswoman at Christmas. When people are putting too many demands on you, just imagine that they're fighting over you.

3. If you can't avoid a stress-producing situation, approach it in a calculated way, taking steps to avoid the stresses.

4. If a certain kind of event always makes you agitated, try to think of ways to change the context. What can you do to prepare for that event, so you don't have to go through the same old thing? If you find Thanksgiving at Aunt Thelma's stressful, don't go, or invite her to your place instead. Just because something's always been done a certain way doesn't mean you have to keep on doing it that way.

5. If certain individuals are causing you undue stress, whether it's your boss or your teenagers, stop for a moment and try to put yourself in their shoes. If they keep doing something that drives you crazy, ask yourself why they do it. What do they get out of it? By understanding their motivations and perspective, you will be better prepared to develop a strategy for reducing the stresses these individuals cause you.

6. Develop coping skills. Learn to take a time-out when you start to feel your anxiety rise.

7. If you find that interactions with a particular person are stressing you, talk to that person about it. Don't be accusatory. Just let him or her know that a certain way of interacting is stressful to you. Maybe together you can develop a new way of interacting so you do not stress one another. An interaction that is stressful for one person is usually stressful for the other.

SOCIAL NETWORKS: TIES FOR LIFE, OR LAUGHING THE YEARS AWAY WITH FRIENDS

Although for years scientists discredited the effect of social factors on biological health, study after study has confirmed the importance of social connections. It has been shown repeatedly that the effect of interpersonal relationships on stress responses is not only psychological but also physiologic. These ties can actually affect the number of immune cells you have, which in turn can affect your resistance to disease and cancer. Social connections make your immune system younger and reduce stress.

As people age, their social relationships often change. In general, our social supports increase through our lives as we move into our fifties. Then, the neighborhood changes. Friends move away to warmer climates, our children grow up and start their own lives, and we experience "empty-nest syndrome." By the time we reach our sixties, our social networks have often begun to decrease. After a lifetime of looking forward to retirement, many people feel lonely and isolated once they no longer have a daily routine. It can be such a subtle change that they are not even aware that it's happening.

I have heard numerous stories from some of my older patients, who, after much consideration and worry, decided to sell the family house and move into a retirement community—not a nursing home, but a place that provides both apartments and nursing and other types of care if need be. The new residents go grumbling off to the "old-age home," complaining about being "turned out to pasture." Suddenly—and I have seen this happen many times—it's as if these individuals have gotten a new lease on life. Now, instead of being isolated, they have a whole social world around them, full of activities and new companions to share them with. One friend told me that after his ninety-year-old father moved into such a community, his father went from being the one who always complained his son never came to see him to being the one who was always too busy. "Sorry, John," he would tell his son, "Friday's the day we go to the vineyards for a wine tasting. Saturday we're putting together the community newsletter, and Sunday Madeline's having a brunch. It'll have to be next week." Moving out of an isolated house into a place where there is a social world really can make people younger.

Although, clearly, such places are not for everyone, and most of us are happy staying in our homes, I think the example is illustrative. It demonstrates in qualitative terms what we already know in quantitative terms—that having social connections in our lives makes us younger. Norman Cousins claimed that laughter could cure illness. In many ways, you can laugh yourself to youth. Being social isn't just frivolous, but vital to our health—and youth.

If you don't have many social contacts, think about building them. How? Invite your neighbor over for dinner. Use the telephone to stay in touch with people who live far away. In an Age Reduction double-dip, exercise with a friend. Learn to use e-mail to contact old friends and try chat groups on the Internet. The Internet is a way that people who are largely housebound can make themselves younger. My ninety-two-year-old father has a whole variety of people he talks to every day on the Web. It's one of the things that keeps his RealAge seventy-six years young!

No more strong, silent types. Joining a group is one of the best ways to reduce stress. A church, volunteer organization, athletic team, community group, or social group—anything that gets you together with other people on a regular basis—can help make you younger. Nothing ages you like going through a major life event alone. Find people to talk to about your problems. Turn to your family and friends. Don't worry about worrying them; they will worry more if you don't tell them what is going on.

If you can't find people who seem to understand your problem, consider groups where you might find people who would understand. For example, a friend of mine became very stressed when his elderly mother developed Alzheimer's disease. Since the illness is remarkably unpredictable, his mother would behave erratically, at times intelligible but at other times incoherent. Sometimes she would be angry for no apparent reason, and other times she would simply start to cry. My friend found the unpredictability incredibly difficult to bear, yet he had to spend an enormous amount of time taking care of her. He also felt isolated; not only was he watching his mother decline, but most of his friends couldn't relate to his situation. His mother's doctor suggested that he go to a program offered by his hospital for relatives of Alzheimer's patients. There he learned what to expect from the disease. More important, he met other people who were dealing with the same situation. Together they could talk about how it felt to watch a parent slowly lose his or her identity. He found the group a great comfort, and it helped him get a different perspective on the disease. When his mother got suddenly angry, he knew that she wasn't angry with him; this was a manifestation of the disease. Learning not to take things she said personally reduced a lot of his anxiety and stress.

There are countless examples of the causal relationship between social ties and stress reduction—a combination that equals the promotion of youth. Learn to value your social relationships and do not sacrifice them to work or other obligations. And do not forget the most important social relationship: the person you choose to spend your life with. How does your love partner help keep you young?

MARRIAGE:
VOWS TO MAKE YOU YOUNGER

One of the best social supports is, of course, marriage. Happily married couples live longer. Although there are few data on unmarried people who are in long-term, mutually monogamous relationships, we may assume that the same is true for them. Indeed, people who indicate that they are happily married show a RealAge difference of as much as 6.5 years younger than their unmarried counterparts. Widowhood and divorce can have an even greater impact on aging than being single.

Curiously, marriage seems more important for men than for women. For example, a thirty-five-year-old man who has never been married has a RealAge that is 6.3 years older than that of his married counterpart. The thirty-five-year-old man who is divorced or separated does a little better: His RealAge is only 5.8 years older. Studies in three countries found that a successful marriage had a higher correlation with arterial youth than did low cholesterol: Men who are happily married are less likely to develop cardiovascular disease than unmarried men, even if their cholesterol levels are much higher.

Women, on the other hand, show different patterns that may relate to underlying social differences between the genders. Women who are under fifty show a RealAge benefit of only about 2.4 years for being married and little effect from divorce. Why? Although we don't know for sure, we can presume that contemporary American women are more likely than men to have strong

TABLE 11.2

The RealAge Effect of Social Connections

Three criteria usually determine the degree of a person's social contacts: marital status; the number of friends seen regularly; and participation in social groups, such as churches, community organizations, and interest clubs. Using this method, the following table assesses the amount of social contact by tallying the number of specific descriptors that apply.

The following RealAge changes occur only if greater changes in RealAge have occurred in the opposite direction because of the stress of major life events.

FOR MEN

How many of the following descriptors apply?
Is married
Sees at least six friends at least monthly
Participates in social groups

Calendar Age	None	1	2	3
		RealAge		
35	42	40	31	29
55	60	53	49	46
70	76	73	69	66

FOR WOMEN

How many of the following descriptors apply?
Is married
Sees at least six friends at least monthly
Participates in social groupss

Calendar Age	None	1	2	3
		RealAge		
35	41	39	33	28
55	61	59	53	49
70	75	72	69	67

social support beyond their marriages. Also, women, more than men, are likely to suffer partner abuse within their marriages. About half the divorced women under calendar age fifty seem to show an increase in RealAge, and about half show a decrease. Those who get younger may do so because of the benefits of getting out of unhappy relationships. However, marriage becomes increasingly important to women as they get older. After age fifty, women show a three-year RealAge benefit from being married, whereas divorce can cause 3 1/2 years of aging.

It is not surprising that the death of a spouse results in significant aging for men and women. For example, studies have shown that both men and women who have recently suffered the loss of a spouse pay more visits to the doctor than the average population, and the recently widowed show a measurably decreased immune response for as long as one year following the loss.

What does all this information mean to you? Well, if you are happily married or involved in a stable long-term relationship, know that it is making you younger. If you are single, evaluate your social ties. Do they provide you with support and help? Single people need to make sure that they have adequate social support from family or friends. Many people find themselves "suddenly single" as they enter their fifties and sixties because of the death of their long-term partners or "empty-nest divorce," a divorce that happens once the children have left home. If you are in this situation, seek other avenues of social support. The friendships you find will help keep you younger, and maybe your friends will introduce you to your second "partner of a lifetime."

Remember, too, that RealAge is all about averages: On average, marriage helps keep a person young. Although a good marriage helps keep you young, the evidence indicates that a bad one can make you old. Marital stress can be one of the most age-inducing of the social stresses. If you have a marriage that is not working—especially if you are in an abusive one—a divorce may be the only solution, and the one that will do the most to prevent you from unnecessary aging.

If you decide to get a divorce, know that it probably will be a stressful, difficult, and emotionally wrenching process and that you don't have to go it alone. Rely on your friends and family for help and seek other possible sources of emotional support. Everyone has different preferences, but ministers, therapists, support groups, and counselors can all help ease the stress of a divorce.

AVOIDING THE MONEY BLUES:
FINANCIAL PLANNING

Four of the ten most stressful events in our lives are tied to our finances. Declaring bankruptcy, losing a job, changing jobs, and not being able to pay the bills—these financial woes can cause just as much stress as almost anything. They can also cause needless aging. More to the point, financial upsets can trigger a series of other events that can age you as well, such as a divorce or a major depression.

Because Dennis M. was at high risk of arterial disease, he used to come to my office four times a year for checkups. At his checkup in mid-April, Dennis's blood pressure was through the roof. "Dennis," I asked, "what's wrong? Your blood pressure's always been borderline." He didn't answer. When I had him come back in two weeks just to double-check, his blood pressure was back to its normal reading. Curious.

The next year, his appointment was on April 15, and the same thing happened. "Dennis," I asked, "what's going on?"

"I don't know," he replied.

"Is something bothering you? Tax man got you down?" I asked, half jokingly.

"As a matter of fact, yes," he said, and then went into a litany of financial woes.

Dennis owned his own business and paid taxes quarterly. Like many of us, he hated to pay the government so much as a day early. He always skimped on his quarterly payments and then, come April 15, wham! He owed a fortune. Yet, as clever as he was at delaying, he never planned well for actually paying his taxes. So, when April 15 came, he often owed money he didn't have. The panic set in, and his blood pressure went sky high. What he knew was that tax time caused him endless worry. What he didn't know was that it was causing him needless aging as well. The high blood pressure was aging his arteries. No doubt it threw his immune system out of whack, too.

"Dennis," I said, "with the amount of worrying the IRS is putting you through, they're getting something much more precious than dollars. They're taking years off your life." I convinced him to come up with a financial plan that worked as a medical plan, keeping him from undergoing the needless stress and rise in blood pressure that could cause him to have a heart attack. Until I met Dennis, I had never thought that being a good doctor would mean I would have to be a good financial consultant, too.

Although financial blues seem to have nothing to do with your biologic age, the rate of aging does correlate with financial stability. The data aren't precise enough to say with complete certainty, but we can assume that one of the reasons why people of higher socioeconomic class have lower rates of aging is that they have greater financial stability. One financial upset is less likely to derail them.

WORK AND STRESS: DON'T LET WORK AGE YOU

Work can be a source of fulfillment and enjoyment but also of anxiety, worry, and . . . *stress*. No matter how much we like our jobs, we still face deadlines, demands, and problems that can stress us. In addition, there is almost no job that doesn't involve the frustrations of office politics and power plays.

The more control individuals believe they have over their jobs, the more likely they are to remain healthy longer. That is, job satisfaction helps keep you young. This is one reason why health improves as the level of income rises. In general, higher-paid jobs tend to provide people with more flexibility, independence, and choices over their work. If your job makes you unhappy or unfulfilled, think about what you can do to change that fact. It may mean looking around for a new job or working with your employer to improve your present working conditions.

As much as we grumble about our jobs, the loss of our jobs ages us more than working does. Losing a job can make your RealAge as much as five years older. Such a loss is especially significant for men who are in the middle or late stages of their careers, and for whom job layoffs and firings have an especially pernicious aging effect. Most likely, this gender gap has to do with traditional social roles, in which men are taught to believe that their jobs are the most central parts of their identities. Men who have lost their jobs, and even those who have retired of their own free will, are more than twice as likely to have a major aging event than are men who remain continuously employed. The goal is to have work that makes us younger. If your job makes you older, you are definitely being overworked and underpaid!

YOUNG MINDS:
BECOME A LIFELONG LEARNER

Here's something you probably never learned in school: Going to school makes you younger. People who are better educated tend to stay younger longer. In fact, those who don't have high school diplomas are 30 percent more likely to die prematurely than those who do. Mortality rates are lower still for those with some college education or higher. And a better-educated spouse makes you younger, too. Why?

No one knows for sure, but there are many possible explanations. There is no direct cause-and-effect relationship. Taking calculus doesn't make your arteries less likely to get clogged. And failing your junior high school English exam doesn't mean you are more likely to get diabetes. Rather, these kinds of statistics result from a whole set of conditions that relate to levels of education and the way education can affect a person's life trajectory. Some of these reasons are purely economic, because people with more education are more likely to have better-paying jobs and greater financial stability. Correspondingly, they often have a higher socioeconomic standing, less exposure to occupational risks, better access to health care, and a whole range of other benefits that help slow the rate of aging. In contrast, people with lower levels of education are often poorer, have more dangerous and tedious jobs, live in areas where pollution levels are higher, and tend to follow more damaging health practices. The jobs that those with lower educational levels have may also expose them to greater environmental hazards.

There are differences in other ways as well. People without a high school education are eight times more likely to smoke and are more likely to be overweight, not to exercise, and not to make healthy food choices. Educational levels are used by researchers to gauge an entire social world, as opportunities, limitations, and social and health behaviors correlate with education.

The relationship between health, youth, and education is enormously complex, and no study will ever completely untangle the web. For one thing, the data are too imprecise. But despite the problems in correlating education with health, most of the studies try to adjust for confounding variables, such as income, social class, and social stresses. However, even when variables are accounted for, a higher level of education still procures a RealAge benefit. For example, we all probably know people with high levels of education who don't make a lot of money: Think of the person who has spent years training to be a classical musician or who is getting a doctorate in medieval history. People who do not make a lot of money but love what they do stay younger longer.

Why? No one knows exactly, but there are certain clues. One theory is that education increases access to information, including information about health. People who read more are also more likely to pay attention to the news; to think about their health; and to exercise, eat right, and avoid habits that can cause needless aging.

Another reason appears to be education itself. Mental acuity is something that diminishes with age. However, the variation from one person to another is tremendous. Some people lose that acuity rapidly; others retain a rapier wit and an ability for clever repartee until the day they die. Indeed, it is hard to talk about averages because so many people defy the trends. The object of RealAge is to learn how to be one of those whose mental acuity doesn't diminish. Education seems to play an important role in achieving this goal.

Education, either through formal or informal methods, is one of the things that keeps your mind in shape. It makes sense, too. For example, the jobs that require high levels of education are often the ones that provide stimulation and variety. They are jobs in which you keep learning while you're working.

What does this mean for you? Keeping your mind engaged will keep you young. Chances are, if you are reading this book, you are already doing just that. You have a curiosity about your life. Chances are, too, that you are somewhere past school age. So, the question remains, How can you make education a part of your adult life?

No matter who you are, there are many ways of ensuring that your mind is active and young. First, it's never too late to go back to school. Don't let your calendar age stop you. Not all of us had the opportunity to go to college when we were eighteen. Even if you do have a degree, you may have developed other interests since you were twenty-one. I had a neighbor who obtained her bachelor's degree at age eighty-one. When I asked her what she was going to do next, she told me, "I'm thinking about getting a Ph.D." She's the best example of what RealAge is all about: someone who takes advantage of the disparity between her calendar age and RealAge to do the things she's always wanted to do.

Consider taking a class in something you're interested in, whether it's philosophy or computers. It doesn't have to be academic. A crafts class at a local community center will help broaden your horizons. Creating lifetime learning doesn't mean you have to love school. There are many ways of stimulating your mind that don't require getting grades: going to museums, reading, taking trips, developing new interests. If you have an interest in something, explore it. Or, as I like to say, stay young because of it!

CONFRONTING YOUR PERSONAL HISTORY: RECOVERING FROM SEVERE EMOTIONAL TRAUMAS

Each year half of us will experience a major life event. A family member may be sick or die, someone may sue you, or you may lose your job. You may have financial worries or be forced to move. Your marriage may fall apart. You may be one of nearly 20 million Americans who has severe clinical depression. Or you may have experienced some trauma in childhood that still affects you (for example, see Table 11.3 for the RealAge effect of being a child whose parents become divorced).

I have talked a lot about what you can do to protect yourself during these tough times, strategies for managing stress and emotional hardship. Nevertheless, what if it's just too much? What should you do when it all seems overwhelming? Or if you have a particular problem that is difficult to talk about even with friends and family members? These topics warrant far more in-depth discussion than I can properly provide in this book. However, there are numerous books devoted entirely to each one of these issues, and you should start with those for guidance.

Do not hesitate to seek professional help. A therapist, psychologist, minister, counselor, or psychiatrist can provide guidance and insight. For years, a stigma was associated with seeking professional help. This attitude hurt everyone. Everyone can benefit from being emotionally healthy, and everyone has life experiences that affect his or her emotional well-being. Thankfully, the past ten to fifteen years have seen a marked shift in the way we view mental health. Seeking professional help has become increasingly accepted.

Mental health is very tricky. Often a person going through a particular crisis denies having a problem. That is why those who live with alcoholics are much more likely to see the problem than the alcoholics themselves. Some mental and emotional states have a biological component as well as a psychological one. For example, the variations of a clinical depression are defined by the chemical changes that occur in hormones in the brain. Medications can help these conditions. So can psychotherapy ("talk therapy"). Often the two work best in combination. Emotional events can trigger a biological reaction, and although a pill can change the biochemistry of the brain, it does little to change the emotional stresses that may have triggered the depression in the first place.

TABLE 11.3

The RealAge Effect of Parental Divorce

FOR MEN

	Age of Child at Time of Divorce of Parents	
	Child Younger Than 21	Child Older Than 21 or No Divorce
Calendar Age	RealAge	
35	38.5	34.1
55	59.8	53.4
70	75.7	67.8

FOR WOMEN

	Age of Child at Time of Divorce of Parents	
	Child Younger Than 21	Child Older Than 21 or No Divorce
Calendar Age	RealAge	
35	37.7	34.3
55	58.6	53.7
70	74.3	68.3

Depression

Depression is one of the most prevalent diseases. However, because depression is a disease that can be subtle, it often goes undiagnosed. The causes of depression can be physiologic and/or psychological. Although we tend to think of depression as a mental and emotional problem, many depressions actually have underlying organic causes. For example, people who are diagnosed with clinical depression frequently have low levels of the hormone serotonin in the brain, indicating a biological origin for what seems to be a psychological condition. Furthermore, there are almost always *physiological* symptoms, including sluggishness; sleeplessness; loss of appetite; a general sense of helplessness or uselessness; and, at times, suicidal tendencies.

Depression is common in people as they age. More to the point, it is also a disease that can lead to unnecessary aging. It often affects women in menopause; both men and women who have recently retired; and anyone who has suffered a major aging event, such as a heart attack or diagnosis of cancer. Sometimes the trigger can be biological, sometimes psychological. But for whatever reason, depression happens.

What is the relationship between depression and aging? For starters, depression is tied to an increased rate of arterial and cardiovascular aging. A 1994 study found that women who had depression had lower bone density, presumably from increased levels of the hormone cortisol, which is found in the blood of depressed people. In addition to causing aging directly, the symptoms of depression—lethargy, sluggishness, a sense that nothing in the world matters—lead to *behaviors* that can accelerate aging. Depressed people are less likely to exercise, to eat a healthy diet, or to make any effort toward healthy living at all.

Women are more prone to depression than men, although no one knows why. Hypotheses run the gamut. Some researchers believe that women face greater discrimination and often have to juggle more social roles. Others see the disparity as stemming from biological, largely hormonal, differences. About 10 percent of women suffer from depression during pregnancy, and many have the classic "postpartum depression" after giving birth. Also women tend to have a higher incidence of hypothyroidism, which is also associated with depression.

Medications can trigger depressions. In addition, depression can be a symptom of other diseases. Individuals who are recovering from heart attacks and strokes are known to be especially prone to depression. Social stresses, such as the death of a loved one or a divorce, can bring on depression, too.

Treatment for depression is highly effective within just a few months of its initiation. Although treatment can prevent accelerated aging, the biggest problem is that many depressed people are often unable to seek help on their own. If you suspect that someone you care about is depressed, find out more about the condition and see if you can get help for him or her.

Unfortunately, your primary care physician is generally not the best person to detect depression. The symptoms are subtle, and because depression was largely misunderstood until the mid-1980s, many doctors were not trained to recognize the disease. One recent study found that family doctors detected depression in only about 35 percent of the cases. Thus, if you suspect that you or someone you care about might be suffering from depression, seek specialized help. Psychiatrists, psychologists, and licensed therapists are all trained to recognize the symptoms of depression and are able to provide many possible types of treatment.

Other types of emotional distress do not have an organic component at all, but that doesn't mean they aren't true problems. For example, children who experience physical or sexual abuse can suffer the repercussions well into adulthood. And the effects can be psychological and physiologic.

Emotional well-being correlates with physical well-being, which means that if you are emotionally healthy, you stay younger longer. A mental health professional can help you develop strategies for dealing with stress and emotional traumas. Just like a financial planner can help you arrange your finances, a therapist can help you evaluate the situations that cause you stress and develop strategies for avoiding or diffusing them. Sometimes stress can be very subtle and difficult to identify. More and more, we are coming to understand that the health of the mind and the health of the body are interrelated. Do not neglect one for the other. Taking care of yourself—both physically and mentally—will help keep you young for a long, long time.

12

The Youngest Patient

HOW THE RIGHT MEDICINE
CAN KEEP YOU YOUNG

The whole point of RealAge is to keep you out of the doctor's office. Yet, now and again, all of us need to visit the doctor. Learning how to obtain the best possible care will keep your RealAge younger. Those who patrol their own health, learn how to manage a chronic condition, get regular checkups, keep vaccinations current, and demand high-quality care can have a RealAge as much as nine years younger than those who do not. Evaluate your family disease history and your genetic risks. Knowing which diseases you may be predisposed to develop can help you counteract those conditions before they begin. If you do develop a chronic medical condition, properly managing the illness can save you from much of the aging that it can cause. Being a savvy patient will help make you a younger patient.

- The best person to monitor your health is you. You know your own body better than your doctor ever will. You know if it aches, if something isn't working right, or if something has changed. Even if it's just a subtle change. Patrolling your health can reduce your RealAge by as much as nine years.

  Difficulty rating: Moderately difficult

- How long did your parents live? How long did your grandparents live? And do the lengths of their life spans help predict the length of yours? What is the correlation between heredity and longevity? Learn how to evaluate your inherited biological risks.

  Difficulty rating: Moderate

- Only 40 percent of American adults keep their immunizations current, and just 14 percent of those who should be getting their yearly flu shots actually do so. By simply keeping vaccinations current, you can give yourself quick and easy protection against unnecessary aging.

Difficulty rating: Quick fix

- Mixing and matching prescriptions or taking medicines erratically or beyond the prescribed time can age you. Taking too many drugs can make you as much as 4 1/2 years older. However, don't stop taking a medicine without consulting your doctor first. Deciding not to take necessary medicines can make you more than 1 year older.

Difficulty rating: Moderately easy

- Eighty percent of us will have a chronic illness at some time in our lives. Diseases such as diabetes, arthritis, heart disease, kidney disease, and asthma are common, and all increase the rate at which we age. In most instances, learning to manage that disease properly means that you will be able to live healthily in spite of it. Depending on the condition, proper management can reduce the aging effect of a chronic illness by 80 percent and, in some cases, even more.

Difficulty rating: Moderately difficult

By reading this book you have learned what you can do to keep as far away from the doctor's office as possible. But every now and again, all of us need to visit the doctor. Keeping a clean bill of health helps us stay young, and detecting and managing new conditions in the early stages are the best ways to prevent the aging the conditions can cause. Learn to patrol your own health, looking for any early warning signs that something is amiss. Evaluate your family history, so you know what diseases you may be genetically predisposed to develop. By knowing your risks, you are in the best position to counteract them. Carefully monitoring any chronic conditions that do exist can save you years of unnecessary aging.

PATROLLING YOUR HEALTH: LEARNING HOW TO BE A MEMBER OF THE AGE POLICE

I met Nathan R. on the way to the operating room. I was his anesthesiologist. He had a small tumor on a nerve just below his skull near his ear: a potentially deadly condition if not caught in time. Lucky for him, it was discovered early—and because of his own persistence.

Nathan was fifty-five when he began to notice that his hearing wasn't quite right and that his equilibrium was off. He noticed dizziness and vertigo when he stood up suddenly. He kept having the sensation that he was going to faint, particularly whenever he did anything energetic. He went to one doctor after another. The doctors ran him through all the tests they thought appropriate, but couldn't find anything wrong.

Just because they couldn't find anything wrong didn't mean that something wasn't wrong. Nathan, who was feeling worse and worse, kept persisting. After going to several specialized clinics and seven different doctors, Nathan finally went to a doctor who took another MRI (magnetic resonance imaging) scan, a kind of three-dimensional X ray, of Nathan's brain. At first the doctor, just like all the others, said that he couldn't find anything wrong.

Nathan was so insistent that something was wrong that the doctor went back over the images again, showing Nathan exactly what doctors look for when reading an MRI. Explaining to him how to read the images, pointing to the different lobes of the brain pictured on the screen, the doctor began to study the image very carefully. Nathan asked lots of questions. Suddenly, the doctor finally spotted it. A small bump on a nerve, a telltale tumor. "It's so small that I can't believe I even saw it," the doctor told me when he called me to do the anesthesia. Normally brain tumors aren't detected until they are well over 1 centimeter; Nathan's was one-third that size. Two days later, Nathan went into surgery.

"You're one heck of a lucky guy," I told Nathan in the recovery room as he came out of anesthesia. The tumor that was removed proved to be fast-growing—and cancerous. It might well have killed Nathan in a matter of months had it not been discovered, but because it was discovered early enough, Nathan suffered virtually no consequences. After a few weeks of recovery, he went right back to life as usual. Since he already exercised, ate right, and took care of himself, his RealAge was more than ten years younger than his chronological age, around forty-five. The only side effect of the surgery was some hearing loss in one ear. It's not much, considering the danger he had barely escaped.

Although Nathan was indeed lucky, he had created his own luck. He was enough in tune with his body to know when something was amiss and to take it seriously. Nathan was saved by his own persistence and savvy.

It's a great story. One that makes us feel good. But it raises the question: If something small and vague began to affect you and lasted several weeks, would you see a doctor to find out what was wrong? Or would you hope that it would go away by itself or just try to live with it?

Stop and ask yourself: Are you healthy? Compared with the health of others your age, would you rank your health as excellent, good, fair, or poor? If you say "excellent" or "good," then your RealAge is probably a bit younger than calculated. If you say "poor," then your RealAge is a bit older (see Table 12.1). Studies show that most people can assess the general state of their own health relatively accurately. That is, when something's not right with our bodies, most of us know it. One study found that those who ranked their overall health as poor were as much as twenty times more likely to die in the next year as those who ranked their health as good. This finding is not surprising. If you are sick, chances are that you already know it. However, this statistic held true even for people who didn't know that they had anything wrong with them; they just had a sense that their general health was not very good. Furthermore, at least seven studies, including the recent report of the Baltimore Long-

TABLE 12.1

The RealAge Effect of Patrolling One's Health

FOR MEN

Calendar Age	Compared with Others My Age, My Health Is			
	Excellent	Good	Fair	Poor
	RealAge			
35	33.8	35.1	37.7	40.7
55	51.8	53.5	58.7	60.8
70	68.4	69.6	71.9	72.6

FOR WOMEN

Calendar Age	Compared with Others My Age, My Health Is			
	Excellent	Good	Fair	Poor
	RealAge			
35	31.9	34.8	38.6	40.8
55	50.9	54	57.6	60.9
70	66.4	69.5	71.7	73.1

itudinal Aging Study, have shown that this result is consistently true: patients who suspect that something is wrong, even though their physicians have diagnosed them as being disease-free, are generally right: something is wrong.

How much does patrolling your own health affect your RealAge? It is difficult to quantify exactly. If you spot an early cancer and have it removed before it has a chance to metastasize, you may save yourself ten, twenty, even thirty years of RealAge aging.

The health care industry has undergone tremendous changes in the past decade. Health maintenance organizations (HMOs) and budget cutbacks have made time and costs extremely important considerations in the practice of medicine. Most doctors have considerably less time to spend with their patients than they did just a decade ago. Hence, doctors have less time to get a "feel" for their patients before they diagnose them. In addition, the changing nature of the insurance industry, and of the health care industry itself, means there is less chance that you will see just one doctor all the time. Many news reports lament the "sorry state of health care." But the news isn't all bad. We now have better facilities, better treatments, and better diagnostic tools, which means that the best possible care is better than it's ever been. The trick is to get that care for yourself.

How do you do that? By being a proactive patient. First find a doctor you like and trust. Choose someone who is competent, conscientious, and attentive to you and your problems. Your primary care physician should make you feel comfortable. (If you don't feel comfortable, find someone else.) Also, he or she should listen to you and be able to explain clearly what is going on with your body. Ask friends, neighbors, or pharmacists about the doctors they use and consider listings, such as the "top physicians" guides. Also, you might want to find out where your doctor went to medical school and how well he or she did there. For example, membership in Alpha Omega Alpha indicates that your doctor graduated in the top of his or her class. Many HMOs or health service networks have services that provide information about their physicians. If a particular condition runs in your family, consider getting a specialist physician who is board certified in that field.

Second, get regular checkups. A clean bill of health provides a baseline for how you are when everything is "normal." Then, if something does arise, you have a better framework for knowing what is wrong and when it started to go wrong. In addition, the more information your doctor has about you when you are healthy, the easier it will be for him or her to know when you are sick. Women should visit their gynecologists annually to get Pap smears and to review or learn breast self-examination; they should also get bone-density tests, when indicated, and regular mammograms. Women over age fifty should get yearly mammograms, and new studies from Great Britain and Sweden indicate that women over age forty should get mammograms every eighteen months.

If, you, like Nathan, sense that something is wrong but your doctor doesn't find anything, don't be afraid to ask your doctor, "What does this test tell you?" or "What does this number mean?" And don't forget this one: "Is there anything else that it could be? Something we're not thinking about?" Part of your doctor's job is to explain to you exactly what is going on inside your body. If you don't understand what's ailing you, you won't be prepared to take the best care of yourself. Also, don't hesitate to get a second opinion. Or a third or fourth. If the second opinion agrees with the first, you can relax and feel more comfortable about the diagnosis you have been given. If the opinions differ, you will have a chance to compare them and to reconsider your options.

Remember, modern medicine can't cure everything. Although we are discovering more about the ways our bodies work every day, many aspects of human biology remain elusive. It may take time for a condition to manifest itself in such a way that it can be diagnosed. But the more aware of your body you are, the more likely you will be to catch a serious illness in its early stages.

How can you be a better patient when you do go to the doctor? By being prepared and informed. Write down questions before you go so you won't forget any important points. If you've noticed a particular problem, write down your symptoms. Make a copy to give your doctor. If you are going to see the doctor for a condition that is chronic, keep a log. If you have a pain that comes and goes, note when it comes and how long it lasts. Keep track of the foods you eat, the activities you perform, and anything else that seems relevant. Write down all the medicines, including herbs and vitamins, that you take and their dosages. The more information your doctor has, the better he or she will be able to help you.

Even if a symptom seems too minor to be mentioned, don't treat it yourself. Tell your doctor. Some conditions manifest in very odd ways. When something hasn't felt right for a while, it's probably not all in your head.

Don't be afraid to do your own research. Go to the library and look up a basic medical textbook or use the Internet to find information on whatever ails you. A number of health-information Web sites are run by major medical centers, and hundreds more are sponsored by organizations of varying credibility. Perhaps you will stumble across a description of exactly what you are experiencing but haven't been able to put into words. On the other hand, don't be a gullible reader: Not everything you read is true, especially information that doesn't come from well-respected research institutions or hospitals. But as you learn more about your health, you will also learn how to distinguish what's likely to be true from what's likely to be rubbish.

A final reason that people stay away from the doctor is cost. Health care is expensive, and not all of us can afford health insurance. This issue is clearly too complicated to discuss here. However, do not ignore a health problem to save a few dollars. The longer you wait to seek proper health care, the more likely the condition will worsen. Not only will it be more expensive to treat in the long run, but you will also be more likely to have experienced the aging and illness that the condition can cause. Prevention is almost always the cheapest health care option.

IT'S ALL IN THE GENES?
THE IMPACT OF FAMILY HEREDITY

At the beginning of the book, I pointed out that more than 70 percent of aging can be linked to behavior and other environmental factors, meaning that you exert enormous power over how you will age. But what about the other 30 percent? Exactly how should you view your genetic inheritance? And how can you avoid the aging associated with it?

Although many studies have investigated the family history of disease in relation to the onset of disease, only three major studies have correlated over-all longevity trends between parents and their children. The Framingham Study, the Termite Study, and the Alameda County Study looked at the ages of parental death to determine if they predicted the longevity of the offspring. Did the two correlate? Yes, but minimally. Each study showed a minor relationship. The Framingham Study, the most comprehensive of the three, found about a 6 percent correlation between the ages of the parents at the time of their deaths and the longevity of the offspring, meaning that many other factors affect longevity as well. If both your parents lived past age seventy-five, then the odds that you will live past seventy-five increase to some extent. But to what extent?

If both your parents died before age seventy-five, your RealAge will be as much as 4.2 years older if you are a man and as much as 3.5 years older if you are a woman. If both your parents lived past age seventy-five, then your RealAge will be 4.2 years younger if you are man and 3.5 years younger if you are a woman (see Table 12.2). If no first-degree relative (parent, brother, or sister) had breast, colon, or ovarian cancer diagnosed early, you are an additional 0.2 to 11 years younger, depending on the disease, than if your siblings or parents had those diagnoses. Some genetic conditions, such as being a carrier of the BRCA-1 breast cancer gene, can make your RealAge as much as 17 years older (for a full explanation, see Chapter 5). This is one of the instances in which genetics can make a big difference.

When you calculate the role of family history, remember that many factors complicate the issue. What, for example, was the cause of death? If a parent dies at age forty in an accident, it provides little information about how long you will live, since that parent didn't die of biologic causes. If a parent dies at age forty of breast cancer, it may mean that you have an increased risk of developing the disease. The genetic predisposition is not always negative, either. For example, in many instances, we inherit a gene from our parents that can actually help us live longer. Some people have a gene that boosts HDL (healthy) cholesterol levels. Because they have high total cholesterol levels,

TABLE 12.2

The RealAge Effect of Parental Life Span

FOR MEN

	Number of Parents Living Past Age 75			
	None	Father	Mother	Both
Calendar Age	RealAge			
35	38.3	36	34	32
55	58.6	56.1	53.7	51.5
70	73.9	71.2	68.6	66.2

FOR WOMEN

	Number of Parents Living Past Age 75			
	None	Father	Mother	Both
Calendar Age	RealAge			
35	38	35.9	34.1	32.3
55	58.2	56	53.9	52
70	73.4	71	68.9	66.8

they are often diagnosed as having a cholesterol problem. But the diagnosis is wrong. This gene is a trump. All that HDL cholesterol helps prevent arterial aging to such an extent that the gene gives carriers a RealAge benefit of as much as twenty-six years! Remember, too, that just because there is a familial tendency for a certain kind of aging does not mean that that kind of aging is genetically inherited. For example, a family history of heart attacks may or may not be genetically coded (see Chapter 1).

In general, you should review your family history for three conditions: (1) a history of cardiovascular disease; (2) a history of a particular type of cancer, such as breast cancer or colon cancer; and (3) a history of rare genetic illnesses, such as Huntington's disease, Parkinson's disease, multiple sclerosis, or even Alzheimer's disease. If you know of more than one case of these diseases on one side of the family, you may have a genetic predisposition to that condition. The first step in determining whether there might be a family history of an illness is to count the number of occurrences of that condition. Then determine how these individuals are related to each other and to you. Everyone must be related by blood, not marriage.

A family history of a certain disease does not necessarily mean that you are genetically predisposed to develop that condition. It indicates a possibility, not a certainty. Even if a genetic illness does run in the family, there is no way of knowing if you have inherited the disease gene (or genes). In most instances, your odds of inheriting any condition are less than 50 percent. Even if you have inherited a predisposition for a specific biological condition that can cause aging, you may very well not do those things that trigger the onset of the disease.

For example, it is known that certain people have an inherited predisposition to develop Type II diabetes. On the other hand, almost 90 percent of those who are diagnosed with the disease are also excessively overweight. Many do not exercise, and a large percentage smoke. When a person is genetically predisposed to develop the disease, environmental factors, such as weight gain, lack of exercise, and smoking, can trigger the disease. A slim and fit person may well have the genetic predisposition but never know it because the conditions that trigger the disease never occur. Indeed, taking care to protect your "youth" is the very best disease management. Living in a youthful manner can offset the genetic predisposition before a disease develops at all.

Cardiovascular aging is another example. As doctors have begun targeting high-risk patients (those who have a long family history of arterial disease and aging), they have seen the onset of premature aging diminish. By exercising, eating a low-fat diet, taking an aspirin a day, and taking folate regularly, anyone—no matter what his or her inherited risk—can reduce the rate of arterial aging. If a risk factor applies to you, you will want to do what you can to offset it. For example, if you are a man and your father, grandfather, and great-grandfather died of heart attacks before age fifty, you will want to pay extra special attention to preventing arterial aging, not allowing the conditions that would make you the next heart attack victim.

VACCINES:
STAYING DISEASE-FREE

All of us had to get immunizations as children. Now that we are adults, keeping them current is one of the easiest ways to prevent aging. Only 40 percent of American adults keep their vaccinations current, and just 30 percent of those who should receive yearly flu shots do so. Fewer than 14 percent of those who should get pneumonia vaccinations get them. Other vaccinations that adults should consider getting include the hepatitis B, tetanus-diphtheria, and MMR (measles-mumps-rubella) vaccinations. Ask your doctor what you need.

Guess how much of a RealAge difference keeping up on your vaccinations makes. Two years? Ten years? Getting your vaccinations makes a RealAge difference of just six days (at least if you are an adult involved in a mutually monogamous relationship). Not much, you're thinking. You're right, yet those six days can be pretty important. That's because this figure is misleading. Many of the diseases for which vaccines are available, such as diphtheria and measles, rarely afflict adults. However, when they do, the effects can be devastating. Other diseases that are more common, such as the flu and pneumonia, are rarely fatal, so the mortality risk is low. Because RealAge calculations take into consideration both the number of people affected and the risk of death, the RealAge differential for vaccinations is somewhat skewed.

Ironically, in the United States and other developed countries, vaccination programs have been so effective in preventing diseases, such as mumps and measles, among children that most cases now involve adults who have not kept their immunizations current. However, other infectious diseases are still relatively common. In the United States, 50,000 to 90,000 deaths occur each year from pneumonia, influenza, and hepatitis B. Think about how many times you've caught the flu. And think about how terrible it makes you feel. You can probably avoid it by getting your vaccinations.

Immunizations: What You Need

Flu

Approximately 20,000 deaths are attributed to the flu every year. I believe this number may be underreported by as much as two-thirds, since many of the deaths caused by influenza or pneumonia infections are attributed to other causes. Should you get a flu shot annually? Yes. According to the Centers for Disease Control (CDC), everyone over age sixty-five should get an annual flu shot. The CDC also recommends that people who interact with the public, especially health care workers, who risk not only catching the influenza virus but also transmitting it, get annual flu shots. It further recommends that you get a flu shot if you have high blood pressure; arterial or coronary disease; lung disease; immune system dysfunction; or any metabolic disease, such as diabetes or kidney disease; or if you are in close contact with people who do have any of these conditions. Finally, if you spend time with individuals who are older than sixty-five, you should probably get a flu shot, too. In other words, pretty much everyone should get an annual flu shot. Why risk needless aging or infecting others?

Each year a new strain of influenza strikes, and each fall a new vaccine is developed to prevent that type of flu. Call your doctor or local public health agency to find out when the shots will be available, usually between September and November. Often local governments sponsor clinics for the public where you can get a flu shot free of charge or at a reduced price.

Flu shots are about 70 percent effective in preventing the flu in populations under age sixty-five and somewhat less effective in people over age sixty-five. They also reduce the severity of the symptoms in people who actually do develop the flu. One study found that taking vitamin E and exercising, which boost the immune system, also seemed to improve the overall effectiveness of the vaccine.

Pneumonia

Pneumococcal infections cause as many as 70,000 deaths a year in the United States, primarily from pneumonia and blood infections. These diseases are extremely risky: 15 to 25 percent of those who have pneumococcal infections in their bloodstreams die, and 5 to 20 percent of those who have the most common type of pneumonia, a lung pneumococcal disease, die. Mortality risk aside, pneumonia is extremely unpleasant.

The pneumococcus bacteria are especially tricky because they regularly change their outer surface. Vaccines are designed to target specific surface configurations, so when a bacterium changes, the vaccine for it no longer works. Indeed, more than eighty pneumococcal strains are known to exist. The most common pneumonia vaccines are called the "14-valent vaccine" and the "23-valent vaccine" because they protect against the fourteen to twenty-three strains of pneumococcal infection that account for 80 to 90 percent of all pneumococcal infections. The pneumonia vaccine is 70 to 80 percent effective in preventing infection in people under age sixty-five and somewhat less effective in preventing the disease among older people.

Who should be vaccinated against pneumonia? Everyone over age sixty-five, plus people in high-risk groups, including those who have compromised immune systems, chronic heart or lung disease, diabetes, or damage to their spleens. If you have HIV or leukemia, talk to your doctor about the pros and cons of getting the vaccine. It is also recommended that Native Americans and Alaskan Natives get this vaccine because they are especially vulnerable to pneumonia. The pneumonia booster should be given every six years, since that is about the time the antibodies it produces will remain effective in the body. Once again, taking vitamin E and exercising help improve the body's response to the vaccine.

Hepatitis B
Two hundred thousand to 300,000 Americans become infected by the hepatitis B virus annually, and well over a million are chronic carriers. Acute hepatitis B infection can be extremely painful, often requires hospitalization, and can be fatal. Chronic hepatitis B infection can lead to cirrhosis of the liver and liver cancer. In fact, hepatitis B infection is quickly becoming a silent health epidemic.

The virus is transmitted primarily through blood and other body fluids, the major form of transmission being sexual contact. In general, it is transmitted in the same ways as the HIV virus, except that hepatitis B is 250 times more contagious and can be transmitted in saliva. Thus, condoms do not provide the same level of protection for hepatitis B that they do for HIV. Even minimal contact with a hepatitis B carrier can cause infection. Since the vaccine is so new, the only population group that has been vaccinated in a population-wide sense are children under age eight. Chances are, not you.

As with HIV, groups who are at a particular risk include men who have sex with men; intravenous drug users; health care workers and others who come in contact with blood or blood products; recipients of blood products, such as hemophiliacs; and those on kidney dialysis—as well as the sex partners of those who are at risk. Whether you fall into one of these groups, if you are sexually active and not monogamous, consider having a hepatitis B vaccination. If you have teenage or college-age children, you should probably make sure they get this vaccination, too. Think of it as a way of giving them some RealAge protection that will help keep them young for the rest of their lives. International travelers, especially those going to countries where hepatitis is common, should also get the hepatitis B vaccination.

If you have never received a hepatitis B vaccination, you need to get an initial series of three shots. Ask your doctor or city public health agency where you can get one either for free or at a reduced cost. Since the vaccine has only been available in the past fifteen years, it is not known how often you will have to get booster vaccinations, although probably every five to ten years. Talk to your doctor because new information will be available on hepatitis B in the near future.

Tetanus and Diphtheria

Unlike many of the vaccines we are given during childhood, our immunity to tetanus and diphtheria wanes as we grow older, and many adults lack the appropriate levels of antitoxin against tetanus and diphtheria. Several large screenings have shown that more than 70 percent of Americans over age thirty-nine need diphtheria and tetanus shots. Admittedly, there is not much concern about tetanus or diphtheria these days. In 1994, just fifty-one case of tetanus and only two cases of diphtheria were reported in the United States, but these are serious diseases. Nearly a quarter of all patients who get tetanus die from it—and that number is probably an underestimation.

Just to be safe, you should get a tetanus-diphtheria—or Td—booster shot every ten years or so. Usually people get these shots only if they go to the emergency room with a cut that needs stitches, so unless you've spent a late night in the hospital getting stitched up, you should probably get one. For those of us who patrol our own health, it is a quick, easy way to take out a little insurance policy against getting older fast.

Measles-Mumps-Rubella

If you were born after 1956 and do not know for sure that you were vaccinated for or contracted mumps, measles, and rubella, you should probably get an MMR immunization. Check with your doctor. Even if you know you've had one, if you work in settings where large groups of individuals—particularly young adults—congregate, such as schools and universities, you might want to consider getting a second one. If you were born before 1956 and never received an MMR vaccination, do not worry, since virtually everyone who was born before 1956 has been exposed to these diseases and has built up a natural immunity. The MMR vaccine is one of the safest vaccines we have, with an effectiveness of well over 90 percent.

Side Effects of Vaccines

Many of us avoid getting immunizations because we don't want to bother with the hassle or fear the side effects. Although you may think it will be too time consuming, getting vaccinations takes only about ten minutes. Furthermore, the side effects are usually minimal. Although there have been a few famous instances in which vaccines caused severe side effects, such as paralysis, these happened at least twenty years ago. The technology of producing vaccines has improved tremendously since then, and none of the vaccines currently in use is associated with any particular risk. In studies in which patients were given a vaccination in one arm and a placebo saline injection in the other, the patients had equal side effects from both. Even side effects such as nausea or upset stomach did not correlate with the immunization, which indicates that people can feel sick on vaccination day just as they can on any other day.

A few people do have allergic reactions to vaccinations, but such reactions are very rare. By far the most common type are egg allergy reactions, since an egg protein makes up part of the measles, mumps, and yellow fever vaccines. If you are not allergic to eggs, these vaccines shouldn't cause problems for you. If you are allergic to eggs, tell your doctor. Occasionally, the antibiotics neomycin or streptomycin are included in various vaccines. If you know that you are allergic to either of these antibiotics, alert your doctor just to make sure that you are given an antibiotic-free vaccine. No vaccines currently contain any penicillin, so if you are allergic to penicillin, you have no reason to avoid getting vaccinated.

A final reason we avoid keeping our vaccinations current is the (perceived) cost. Immunizations are not expensive and are usually covered by insurance. Medicare and about 35 percent of all health plans and HMOs routinely pay for immunizations.

So, the next time you see your doctor, ask him or her what you need. I recommend that you call your doctor or nurse practitioner to set up an appointment each year between September and November to get your annual flu shot, as well as any other needed vaccinations. If your health plan doesn't pay for flu shots, remember that the small cost of a flu shot is probably less than a visit to the doctor once you get the flu or pneumonia. It is certainly worth avoiding the agony of the illness, not to mention the aging it can cause. Also, many public health agencies routinely offer flu shots and other vaccinations either free or at a relatively low cost.

Immunizations do not guarantee that you won't get that illness. Although many immunizations ensure up to 90 percent resistance to a disease, flu shots, for example, are less reliable, offering only 45 to 80 percent benefit to predicted strains. Also, a person's resistance to a disease often decreases as his or her RealAge gets older or if some other medical condition exists, meaning that an immunization may not be as effective. Nevertheless, when it comes to age prevention, nothing is as quick and easy as keeping your vaccinations current.

PILL POPPING:
TOO MUCH MEDICINE AND MIXING MEDICINES CAN CAUSE AGING

It happens all the time: One doctor prescribes a medicine for a patient without knowing that another doctor has prescribed another medicine for that same person. Somehow the information isn't communicated—the patient either forgets to tell the doctor what he or she is taking or tells the doctor the wrong name for the medication (something that is easy to do). The result can be a potentially life-threatening drug combination. Mixing drugs, taking medicines beyond their prescribed time, or taking them erratically can be hard on your body—and make you older. Be an informed patient; ask your doctors why you should be on any drug they prescribe and be sure to tell them what you are already taking, even simple things like aspirin, over-the-counter drugs, vitamins, and supplements. Many patients forget to mention these over-the-counter drugs and supplements, thinking that because they can be bought by anyone, they must be harmless. This is not true. Don't forget to mention recent vaccinations you've had and antibiotics you've taken.

Statistics show that people who take too many pills without proper supervision have a RealAge as much as 4 1/2 years older. But the fact that taking more pills makes your RealAge older doesn't mean you shouldn't take *any* medications. It's important to take the medicines you need and to take them as instructed. Not taking necessary drugs—or not taking them correctly—can make you more than one year older (see Table 12.3).

When Sue C., one of my wife's good friends, phoned, she was in a near panic about her mother.

"Mike," she said, "Mom's blood pressure is completely out of control. Sometimes it's at 150/80; at other times it's as high as 220/150. She's on all this medication to control it, and she's good about taking them, but she gets a lot of side effects. Headaches that completely incapacitate her. It seems like the medicine is just making things worse."

"Sue," I said, "if her blood pressure's as high as you say it is, it could be life threatening. How soon can you get her here?"

TABLE 12.3

The RealAge Effect of Pill Popping*

FOR MEN

	Number of Pills Taken Daily†			
	0–4	5–7	8–14	More than 14
Calendar Age	RealAge			
35	34.9	35.1	35.3	35.7
55	54.9	55.1	55.4	55.9
70	69.8	70.1	70.4	70.9

FOR WOMEN

	Number of Pills Taken Daily†			
	0–4	5–7	8–14	More than 14
Calendar Age	RealAge			
35	34.9	35.1	35.3	35.7
55	54.9	55.1	55.3	55.8
70	69.9	70.1	70.3	70.8

*These RealAge figures take into consideration only the effect of taking a large number of pills. They do not include the effects of nonadherence or the specific effects and interactions that occur from taking some medicines (such as sedative hypnotics) that increase aging when taken with other medications.

†Does not include vitamins.

"Right away," she responded.

Sue brought her mother, June D., to my office. Sue was right. June's blood pressure was 220/150—so high that it was a medical emergency.

"June," I said, after examining her, "if we can't bring your blood pressure down in the next four hours, I'm checking you into the hospital. Your blood pressure is off the charts."

"I can't understand why. I'm on five different medicines to bring my blood pressure down."

"Well, that may be the problem. Drugs can often interact, causing an unintended effect. Tell me everything you're on."

She listed the five medications that she took regularly.

I was puzzled. There were two drugs on the list that could cause a negative drug reaction when taken together. However, her symptoms—extremely high blood pressure and severe headaches—were not the ones that this interaction should have caused. I asked her, "Are you sure that you've told me everything you're taking? What about vitamins, over-the-counter drugs, food supplements, herbal remedies, or herbal teas?"

"Oh, I didn't even think of that. I'm taking several vitamins and three kinds of herbal pills. Two of them I read helped prevent headaches, and one is supposed to clear my sinuses. But they're natural. They can't hurt me, can they?" Then she told me what they were.

"Bingo," I said. "We've found the culprit." The herbal remedy she was taking to alleviate her sinus symptoms interacted with one of her medications, causing both her terrible headaches and her erratic blood pressure. She was playing around with an explosive mixture that could cause a heart attack or a stroke. "First, we are going to do something to bring your blood pressure down," I told her. "Then I want you to go home and throw away that bottle of herbs."

"I'm so surprised. I thought these supplements were harmless," June said.

"That's exactly the problem," I replied. "Natural remedies seem so innocuous, but when mixed with the wrong medicine, they can be dangerous."

I gave June some medication to bring her blood pressure down immediately. I told her to take the drugs exactly as instructed. Then I cut her blood pressure medications to just three, to eliminate the possible interactions. The new medication worked. Within a week her blood pressure was close to normal, ranging from 110/70 to 130/90. Her body adjusted to the medicine, and she started to feel great.

Then the second phone call came. It was Sue again. "Mike, Mom's been feeling super on her new blood pressure routine. In fact, she feels so good that she told me this morning that she thought she would stop taking her medicine. I just wanted to double-check with you to make sure it's okay."

"You're kidding me!" I cried, not believing that I hadn't gotten my point across. "Going off that medicine so suddenly could put tremendous stress on her heart or the blood vessels in her brain. She could have a stroke or heart attack. Give me her phone number because I want to call her right now."

Luckily, I got June just in time. And I did something I rarely do: I yelled at a patient. I scolded her for putting herself in a possibly life-threatening situation, and I told her, in no uncertain terms, that she had to take her pills right away.

Although the proportions vary from locale to locale, on average more than 15 percent of all hospital admissions are due to the improper use of prescribed medications and to adverse interactions between drugs or drugs and supplements. In fact, one study calculated that, in 1994, Americans spent $73 billion on prescription drugs, but that the costs that were due to adverse effects exceeded $100 billion. Hard to believe, isn't it? Does this mean we should quit prescribing—or taking—drugs? No. Drugs have saved a lot of dollars and years of life by controlling illness and preventing aging. It just means we all need to be more attentive to the problem of mixing drugs with other drugs and supplements.

It is interesting to note that the problem of drug interactions has gotten worse. The Food and Drug Administration (FDA), in an attempt to lower drug costs to consumers and to make medications more readily available, has increased the number of medications available without prescription. Drugs that just a few years ago required a prescription are now available over the counter, including such popular medicines as Pepcid (famotidine), Tagamet (cimetidine), nonsteroidal anti-inflammatory drugs like ibuprofen (Advil, Motrin), Rogaine (minoxidil), Imodium (loperamide), and nicotine chewing gum. Make sure to ask your doctor about these drugs, since they can have substantial adverse effects when mixed with various prescription drugs, herbs, or supplements.

The problem with drug interactions is partly the fault of doctors. The classic stereotype of the hurried doctor with incomprehensible handwriting is not far off: Prescriptions can be hard to read, and doctors and patients do not always communicate effectively. Doctors frequently think that they are explaining things clearly but use technical terms and jargon that patients don't understand. Several years ago, a patient wrote on her basic information form that she had undergone a hysterectomy. When I asked her about it, she told me she had her tonsils out when she was six! I knew then that we were miscommunicating. Patients are often afraid to ask if they don't understand something, or they forget to ask, mainly because they are not feeling well or because being in a doctor's office can be a nerve-racking experience.

Remember, the best patients are informed patients. Do not hesitate to ask your doctor about medication that he or she has prescribed. In addition, ask about interactions with over-the-counter drugs or herbal remedies you take regularly. Don't feel self-conscious about taking up the doctor's time. You and your doctor should be partners in preserving your youth and health. If there is something you forgot to ask while you were at the doctor's office, call your doctor back. Or ask your pharmacist when you get your prescription filled. Pharmacists know about each drug and can help advise you on your overall medication regimen. Use your doctor and your pharmacist as cross-checks for each other: One may catch something the other one doesn't. Because the channels of information are different, one may have recently learned something the other doesn't yet know. And, besides, the pharmacist who fills your prescriptions may be aware of medications you are taking that are prescribed by another physician.

Becoming a "home pharmacist" is a surefire way to get older. Once you have used a drug for what it was prescribed for and no longer need that drug, throw away the remaining pills. Pills can change their composition if allowed to sit around too long. Also, by getting rid of extra bottles, you reduce the risk that you or the people you live with will take the wrong pill accidentally. Prescription medications should not be used for anything other than what they were prescribed for. Never assume that because something was good for one condition, it would be good for another. Don't take two pills when the instructions advise one; just because one is good doesn't mean that two will be better.

And never go off a drug just because you are feeling better. If you are prescribed antibiotics, for example, it is very important that you take the entire amount prescribed. Do not stop after just a couple of days because you feel better. This is an exceedingly common and potentially very dangerous mistake because the illness often comes back quickly and in a more virulent form. Because the bacteria causing the disease have already been exposed to the antibiotic, they often develop resistance to it, and the drug no longer works effectively.

Similarly, people who take blood pressure medicine often quit taking it the minute their blood pressure dips into the normal range. Going off blood pressure medicine can be extremely dangerous—even life threatening. Stopping suddenly can cause rebound tachycardia and hypertension, a condition in which your heart rate and blood pressure suddenly rise to levels higher than they were before you started taking the medication. These changes can put enormous strain on your arteries and can trigger a heart attack or stroke. Even if they don't, they cause significant arterial aging.

Remember, doctors need feedback. They can't know that a drug is causing a side effect unless you tell them. Hormone-replacement therapy is a perfect example. Approximately 50 percent of women who quit taking hormone-replacement therapy do so without telling their doctors. The treatment is a tricky one: Different women react differently to different doses and combinations, so often the dose needs to be adjusted until one is found that works. However, by working with her doctor, a woman can usually find the right dosage for her.

Two common side effects of various drugs that can be difficult to discuss with a doctor are impotence and loss of sexual desire. Several blood pressure medicines and depression medications, such as Prozac, have these side effects, as do other medications. Even though patients don't mention impotence and the lack of sexual desire to me often, I try to search tactfully for the occurrence of these conditions. Male patients say impotence makes them feel and act older. Female patients also report changes in libido from various medications. Impotence and the lack of sexual desire are extremely frequent, but they are treatable conditions. If you notice that a medication is affecting you in this way, talk to your doctor. Don't be embarrassed. Usually, a different medicine can be prescribed.

In summary, how can you keep your medications from aging you? Keep your drug regimen simple. Ask your doctor if you can reduce the number of medications you take. One study showed that taking twenty-three or more pills a day can make a person as much as $4\frac{1}{2}$ years older than taking four or fewer pills a day. The more pills you take, the greater the potential for an adverse drug interaction that can cause you to age unnecessarily.

Here are some simple steps for making sure that you get the RealAge benefit associated with taking medications.

- Develop a good relationship with your primary care doctor.

- Make sure that you keep him or her updated on everything you're taking.

- Keep a list of medicines and dosages that you take either regularly or occasionally and bring it with you when you visit any doctor, drop-in clinic, or emergency room.

- Choose a pharmacist you can trust and develop a long-term relationship with him or her. Your pharmacist will also have a record of all the drugs you are on or have been on and can warn you about possible drug interactions. (Although many HMOs now provide pharmaceuticals by mail, I prefer the old-fashioned drugstore with a new-fashioned computer, one where the pharmacist both knows the patient and has an up-to-the-minute record of his or her medication history.)

Now, of course, we must turn to the larger question: What if you have one of those conditions—heart disease, arthritis, kidney malfunction—that require a lot of medicines and a lot of medical care? How can you prevent the aging effects of chronic illnesses?

CHRONIC DISEASE: LEARNING TO LIVE WITH IT

As much as this book is about preventing the kinds of chronic conditions that cause us to age—heart disease, cancer, arthritis, Alzheimer's—the fact is that almost 80 percent of us will have a chronic condition at some point in our lives. So the question remains, What happens if you get a chronic illness? How are you to treat it? How can you prevent its aging effects?

For starters, a chronic disease does not mean that life is over. It is not time to call it quits. Life can and will go on. Every day we learn more about such diseases and more about staving off their effects. Such a diagnosis does not mean that you are now "old," but it does signal an important shift: You will have to learn how to live with the disease's "chronicness," and with the fact that it is a presence in your life, a presence that cannot be ignored without ill effect. Almost without exception, a diagnosis of chronic disease also signals that it's time to take your youth seriously. If you are diagnosed as having a chronic and potentially debilitating illness, you will have to learn how to live healthily—and youthfully—in spite of it.

Although having a chronic condition like diabetes or arthritis can age us, how we manage that disease can make an enormous difference. For example, if diabetes is not managed properly, a diabetic can age at twice the expected rate; he or she will experience almost two years of biological aging for each passing calendar year. However, careful management of the disease can reduce the aging effect by over 50 percent, and by as much as 80 percent. For Type II diabetes (non-insulin-dependent diabetes), proper management can make manifestations of the disease virtually disappear, leaving no significant aging effect. Similarly, the aging effect of heart disease can be retarded by as much as 70 percent with proper vigilance, and if the disease is diagnosed before significant structural damage occurs, the aging it causes can even be reversed. We see similar benefits of disease management for everything from kidney disease to neurologic disorders to thyroid problems to cancer. No matter what ails you, the aging damage that a chronic condition causes is always, *always* improved by proper management.

In fact, we should stop thinking about most of these conditions as diseases and start thinking about them as physical states of aging. States that accelerate the speed of aging. States that you can, at least, partly control. I do not like the term *chronic disease.* With the exception of a few contagious illnesses (HIV infection, for example), most of the chronic conditions that affect us as we age are not diseases in the way we generally think of the term—that is, as infectious diseases. Nor are they usually inheritable genetic diseases, in the sense that the problem has to do with something structurally wrong with us from the time we were born. Rather, these conditions are examples of the body beginning to come undone as a result of aging. The image of a machine wearing down its parts is apt. These conditions—heart disease, kidney disease, endocrine malfunction—are what we mean by aging. Yet, and this is important, these conditions also *accelerate* the rate at which other parts of us age, too. By managing such conditions, we can control, in large part, the degree to which they will age us.

What should you do if you are suddenly afflicted with heart disease, arthritis, or another age-accelerating condition? First, do not despair. Instead, confront the situation head on. Develop a plan. You will need to understand the disease in and out and how it might affect and age you. Find a doctor who can work with you to develop a plan for disease management. (It matters less whether your doctor is a generalist or a specialist; what is important is that he or she is knowledgeable about the condition and caring toward you.) Read up on the condition yourself. Ask lots of questions. The more you know and understand, the better prepared you will be to fight the effects of the condition. Talk to your doctor about developing a well-rounded strategy for disease management, including diet, medications, exercise, stress reduction, and daily planning.

In general, managing a chronic condition means not just focusing on the condition itself, but treating your whole body with extra care. Those who suffer from almost every kind of chronic disease will want to pay extra special attention to retard or reverse more general aging processes throughout the body. Eating a proper diet, exercising, managing your weight, and avoiding cigarettes and excess alcohol become key components of aging management for almost all chronic diseases. All the things that can induce aging when you are healthy become amplified by a chronic condition. Whereas your body may have once been able to handle long working days, no breakfasts, not enough exercise, or drinking too much, the condition you now have will make the margin for error much lower, because your body won't tolerate as much abuse.

Let's consider diabetes, for example. Diabetes is the sixth leading cause of death in this country, and the leading cause of blindness, not to mention one of the most significant causes of premature aging. But it needn't be.

There are two types of diabetes, Type I and Type II. Although they have different causes, the two types have largely the same effect: high levels of sugar in the blood. Diabetes, if not treated properly, can cause arterial aging; blindness; kidney failure; liver damage; and, in advanced stages, limb loss and heart failure. However, by keeping blood sugar within the levels of people who don't suffer the disease—by managing diet, insulin, and exercise—diabetics can avoid much of the aging that high blood sugar causes. A diabetic can control the ecosystem, as it were, of his or her body in such a way that the disease has little impact. However, doing so requires a lot of attention and commitment. Not just once in a while, but every single day.

Type I diabetes—sometimes called juvenile diabetes because the disease often begins in childhood—occurs when the body quits making insulin, the hormone necessary to metabolize sugar in your food and to regulate glucose levels in your blood. Patients with this type of diabetes generally inject artificial insulin that substitutes for the natural insulin their bodies should produce. Carefully monitoring blood sugar and making sure to balance diet, exercise, and insulin levels in such a way as to keep glucose levels within a normal range is a way of preventing damage.

Type II diabetes, or adult-onset diabetes, usually develops when a person is over forty, often older. It occurs when the cells in the body become insensitive to insulin. The insulin receptors on the outside of each cell no longer react to the insulin molecule that signals the cell to break down glucose. Hence, blood glucose levels remain high. Type II diabetes occurs most often in people who are overweight; although the reasons are unclear, excess weight seems to impede the body's ability to metabolize sugar properly. Type II diabetes affects about 10 to 15 percent of adults over age fifty-five but is more prevalent among some population groups than others, confirming a genetic component. For example, African-Americans, particularly African-American women, are much more susceptible to the disease. Indeed, one out of four African Americans over age fifty-five has Type II diabetes. Among certain Native American populations, the prevalence can be as high as 80 percent. However, in many cases, the disease is triggered by a combination of genetic predisposition and lifestyle choices. Some 90 percent of the people who develop Type II diabetes are considerably overweight, and most of these people also do not exercise or have proper diets, both of which further exacerbate the condition. If you "live young," you will have less chance of developing the disease, no matter what genes you have (see Table 12.4).

Diabetic patients who take charge of their condition, vigilantly keeping their blood sugar levels within normal ranges, experience little premature aging. Patients who lose excess weight, begin exercising, and eat balanced

TABLE 12.4

*The RealAge Effect of Type II Diabetes**

FOR MEN

Calendar Age	Control of Diabetes	
	Poor Control	Tight Control†
	RealAge	
35	37.5	36
55	66	61
70	87	78

FOR WOMEN

Calendar Age	Control of Diabetes	
	Poor Control	Tight Control†
	RealAge	
35	37.5	36
55	65	60
70	85	77

*Onset at age 30.

†Tight control of blood sugar and blood pressure.

diets that are carefully calibrated to their diabetic condition can reverse the aging effects of the disease altogether, suffering no more aging than their disease-free peers. Think of it this way: The diabetic's body can no longer create the conditions it needs for healthy existence all on its own. However, it is possible for the diabetic to create an environment inside the body that keeps him or her in an equally healthy state.

Although not all chronic diseases can be managed in the same way, many other types of diseases are similar to diabetes in the way that they should be treated. Thyroid disease, kidney disease, any endocrine disease, and many gastrointestinal diseases are analogous. The most important element in controlling the effects of these conditions is constant vigilance. Diabetics and most others who have chronic diseases have to monitor their condition each and every day.

Although not all chronic conditions can be managed as well as diabetes, all chronic conditions can be managed so they do not do as much damage—or cause as much aging—as they would if left untended. Even Alzheimer's disease, a condition with few effective treatments, can be managed in ways that slow the aging that the disease can cause. For example, studies have found that Alzheimer's patients who participate in clinical trials—and hence are provided with high-quality medical care and better support systems—are half as likely to end up in nursing homes within the same period as Alzheimer's patients who do not participate in such trials. Better disease management does not stop the disease but helps stave off its most ruinous effects.

Those who have a chronic condition should ask themselves: Can this condition make me more prone to other kinds of chronic conditions? For example, people who have arthritis may be less likely to exercise, and for an obvious reason: It hurts. However, modest exercise relieves the symptoms of many types of arthritis. Furthermore, *not* exercising may cause the sudden appearance of arterial disease—arterial disease that had been staved off because of exercise. That is, the response to one chronic illness (lack of exercise because of arthritis) may bring about another chronic illness (arterial disease).

Ask your doctor if there are any hidden symptoms you should be looking for. Heart attack victims, for example, often suffer bouts of serious depression in their recovery period. Although it is unclear what the exact cause-and-effect relationship is—Does the heart attack cause a biologic depression? Do depressed people have more heart attacks? Or is having a heart attack simply depressing?—it is clear that those who are recuperating from heart attacks need to be aware of this possible condition. Depression can undermine a recovery program, making it difficult for a heart attack sufferer to get the energy to change eating habits or begin an exercise program, all the things that speed recovery faster and help offset aging. Luckily, in most instances, depression can be successfully treated.

No matter what disease you have, beware of its emotional effects. It is frightening and disheartening to be diagnosed as having a chronic condition. After a lifetime of thinking of yourself as a healthy person, all of a sudden you have to reevaluate your self-image. Don't think that you have to go it alone. It is not uncommon for someone who is diagnosed as having a chronic condition to hide the news from loved ones, not wanting them to worry. But doing so leaves the ill person feeling isolated, and those around the sick person *always* sense that something is wrong because such a diagnosis changes a person's behavior. I have seen this reaction innumerable times in my patients: Being told that you will have a condition for the rest of your life, a condition that may affect the quality and length of your life, generally makes a person reflect on the larger importance of his or her life.

If you are diagnosed as having a chronic condition, use your social networks. Talk to people who are close to you about your fears and worries. You will find that the people who care about you will want to help. They will help keep you on track, urging you to stay on the special diet or joining you in your new exercise routine. Do not hesitate to seek professional help from a therapist or counselor if you feel overwhelmed by the news. To ward off the aging effects of a chronic illness, you need to be prepared in both body and mind.

13

Young for the Rest of Your Life

LIVING AS YOUNG AT SEVENTY AS YOU DID AT FORTY-FOUR

The book is over, but the rest of your life is about to begin. How will you choose to live it? You now know what your RealAge is and have essential information to make informed choices about your health and aging. You know what factors accelerate aging and what factors slow it down. Evaluate your health behaviors and lifestyle. What will you do to "age-proof" yourself? You can reduce the rate of aging. In the end, the choice is up to you.

Each winter my ninety-two-year-old father leaves his home in upstate New York to spend the winter months in Arizona, living in a community of other retirees, the youngest of them in their mid-seventies. When I began writing this book, I sent him drafts of the chapters. He began sharing what he had learned with his friends. More and more of them developed an interest.

They formed the equivalent of a Great Books club, in which they'd get together and read selections, finding out what each of them could do to stay young longer. They started taking vitamins and eating more fruits and vegetables, incorporating new "get-young" strategies as new sections of the book arrived. After reading about exercise, they jumped to action. The whole group of twenty-five—not one with a calendar age less than seventy-five—raided the local WalMart, buying out the entire supply of two- to fifteen-pound free weights (much to the amazement of the twenty-two-year-old salesclerk who looked on, open-mouthed, as twenty-five retirees in jogging shoes departed, barbells in hand). They hired a personal trainer to show them how to lift the weights correctly and to guide them through a fitness routine. Now they lift weights three days a week, go mall-walking another three days a week, and meet for "happy hour" every evening to have a drink and spend time with their new "young" friends. They egg each other on to get younger, celebrating each other's successes.

They have a blast. Each day they're getting younger and having fun doing it. My father's so busy I sometimes have problems tracking him down: He's out on the town. He frequently goes to New York City and travels by himself. He knows more about the Internet than I do. He's got friends, social engagements, and freedom, and there's no stopping him. People always say to me, "He's amazing. To think, at his age."

Sure, he's amazing, but not because of his age. Being young at ninety is something we can all strive to achieve. My dad's RealAge is seventy-six and getting younger. Enjoying our old age with vigor and energy should be the rule, not the exception.

At the beginning of this book, I said, "Health is like money." At first the comparison sounds crass: How can you equate money with something as precious as life? But how can you not? Money as money isn't worth a dime. Money is only as valuable as what it buys. Money is really about potential. It provides possibilities, choices, and freedom. It also allows you to place a value on your choices and to make decisions. Likewise, the RealAge payoff isn't youth itself but the possibilities that youth provides.

The RealAge system teaches you how to buy time. It allows you to understand what your biologic potential is. The younger your RealAge, the more possibilities, choices, and freedom you will have to do what you want with your life. The younger your RealAge, the more time you will have to spend with your friends and family, to develop new interests, and to do whatever it is that makes you enjoy life. Don't let ill health keep you from being who you want to be. RealAge gives you a currency for health. It helps you place a value on your health decisions, so you can protect what is truly priceless: your life.

As life expectancy has increased dramatically in the past century, especially in the past thirty years, medical researchers have been faced with a major ethical dilemma: Are we extending the quantity of life at the expense of the quality of life? With expensive life-support machines and new technologies that can keep people alive longer and longer, doctors have worried that perhaps all this effort has only extended suffering, making patients endure painful diseases longer, living out their final years in misery. But this is not true. New studies show that most Americans can expect to live long lives (that is, to the national averages) without major illness or disability. However, there is enormous variation within the population. When studies have examined those who live the longest with the greatest mobility and independence, they have found that individuals at the top of the curve tended to make the same behavioral choices: They exercise, eat a diet low in saturated fats, don't smoke, take the right amount of vitamins, and do many of the other forty or so things described in this book. Even at the end of their lives, these people had less illness and for a shorter time than those who didn't make these choices; the period of decline tended to be compressed and lessened. In these same studies, those who had the most illness and incapacitation didn't adopt these healthy behaviors—and they got older faster. They had shorter life expectancies and spent more time in hospitals and doctors' offices.

Clearly, there are no sound statistical measures of "quality of life." It is a subjective indicator. Some people are always happy no matter what; others are never happy. However, by looking at the data, we can draw certain conclusions. A person who is healthy has a better quality of life than if he or she needs to be under strict medical supervision. Also, a person who is mobile, lives independently, and is disease-free has a better quality of life than if he or she were hospitalized. Those aren't giant leaps of logic.

Before you even picked up this book, you were probably aware of all kinds of behavioral choices that were "good" for you. But did you adopt those behaviors? I hope this book has helped you view your health in a new light. Rather than seeing these decisions as the prevention of disease, I hope you now see them as being about the prevention of aging. Thinking about "disease prevention"—the classic way preventive medicine has modeled itself—is disheartening. Perhaps it's too daunting a project or its benefits seem too far off. Moreover, we think of disease in black-or-white terms: You're either sick or you're not. However, this description doesn't fit the reality of human health. Most of the "old-age" diseases are not actually diseases as much as manifestations of the aging process itself.

RealAge is a way of understanding that everything you do—from walking the dog to brushing your teeth—affects your rate of aging. Adopting healthy habits means not just that you prevent disease, but that you live longer—and younger. By living the RealAge plan, you increase the length of that part of your life that's vigorous and productive.

When I think about why I became a doctor in the first place, I realize that my decision can be summed up in one word: prevention. I never wanted to cure people after they were already ill; I wanted to help them avoid illness in the first place. Life is too much fun to spend time being sick. (In fact, I always think of my specialty, anesthesiology, as being all about prevention: Anesthesia prevents the shock reaction that the trauma of an operation can cause.) Yet, until now, prevention has been thought of in terms of far-off, negative goals. "I won't eat fatty foods today, so I won't have a heart attack thirty years from now." But prevention isn't a negative goal but a positive one. Preventing illness is gaining health. And the payoff is not thirty years in the future, but right now.

If you've made it this far through this book, you know in tangible and practical terms how you can prevent and even reverse aging. So where should you start?

- First, write down your RealAge. Look at that number. Are you happy with it? Or would you like to make it younger? What will you do to change it?

- Second, review your Age Reduction Plan (see Chapter 3). What choices can you make to make your RealAge younger? Are they practical choices for you? In light of what you've read, are you willing to make choices that two hundred pages ago you wouldn't have made?

- Third, establish priorities. Consider how and when you want to add new Age Reduction strategies to your life. Set realistic goals and decide what steps you can take to meet them. What are the quick-and-easy strategies you can adopt for getting younger with hardly any effort? What are the antiaging strategies that require more work? How will you integrate them into your life?

- Fourth, start small. Don't overwhelm yourself by trying to do too much at once. Begin with the "quick fixes," integrating new Age Reduction practices slowly, especially if they are in the "most difficult" category. After all, you're in this for the long run. It's more important that you stick with your Age Reduction Plan than that you do every possible Age Reduction step right away, only to give them all up after a few weeks or months.

- Fifth, reevaluate. Often. Review your Age Reduction Plan every few months. Is it time to add a new strategy? I have patients who add one new antiaging practice to their life every year—a kind of New Year's resolution.

- Sixth, don't give up. Getting younger is not that hard. A few simple choices can help make you five to seven years younger in just a few months. Other choices can help reduce your RealAge by as much as twenty-five years. Most of the benefits can be achieved by making simple choices that do not take much time or effort, just some practice.

- Seventh, you are never too old to start getting young. It doesn't matter if you're a lifelong smoker, if you've had a heart attack, or if you've suffered any number of other conditions. You can undo much of the aging that you have already incurred by making changes now. Our bodies are remarkably resilient, and it is within your power to undo years' worth of unnecessary aging. In their report of the MacArthur aging studies, Jack Rowe and Robert Kahn wrote: "There is increasing evidence of the remarkable capacity to recover lost function." Yes, you can get young again.

- Eighth, and most important, celebrate successes. Reward yourself for becoming younger. Whether you decide to throw yourself a "year-younger" party or to treat yourself to a massage after a month of daily workouts, you need to congratulate yourself for getting younger. (Don't forget to celebrate the year-younger successes of those around you, too. By encouraging people who are close to you to get younger, you are giving yourself a gift. You are helping those you care about to stay young with you.)

Think of RealAge planning like retirement planning. Most of us spend time in our forties and fifties making investments and setting up a pension fund or an individual retirement account, planning for that day when we no longer have to go to the office. RealAge is retirement planning for your body, an age-insurance plan. As I said in Chapter 1, your RealAge is a calculation of your net present value. It is a way of calculating how old your body really is. The choices you make affect that value. You build value by building youth.

Last fall, my friend Simon called me. (Remember him from Chapter 1? He was the first person I convinced to stop smoking using the RealAge concept.) "Mike," he shouted exuberantly into the phone, "I'm a grandfather!" At age sixty-two (and RealAge fifty-seven), he had lived to see the birth of his first grandson. It was nothing short of a miracle.

Thirteen years earlier, when Simon was barely able to walk and in need of a dangerous operation, none of us—not his family, not me, and not Simon—would have believed that he'd live to see the day when he'd become a grandfather. Much less, live to see that day as an energetic, physically fit, and young grandfather. "Simon," I laughed, "you're not old enough to be a grandfather."

Simon made choices that not only saved his life, but that gave him back his life. Thirteen years ago he couldn't walk across a room without pain. Now he's playing tennis and challenging me to squash matches. He's tackled some of the toughest challenges in Age Reduction: cessation of smoking, exercising, and eating a more healthful diet. He's done it slowly—adding bit by bit. Each year, he reevaluates his antiaging plan, integrating new choices and behaviors. He's living younger now than he did thirteen years ago. The payoff has been huge. He's seen his kids get married, he's traveled, he's enjoying his life. He even retired early, so he could have more fun. (Now, he's feeling so young that he's been threatening to come out of retirement!)

In my practice, and even in my own life, I see that RealAge motivates people to change their behaviors and to choose youth. I see how my patients have stopped smoking, lost weight, and made choices that helped them stay young. I see how it has helped me learn to eat a healthier diet and be more balanced in my exercise regimen. RealAge has encouraged my father to start lifting weights and helped my wife to start taking her calcium regularly. RealAge helps us to place a value on our daily choices—choices that are easy to overlook but that help us stay young. (Every time I take the stairs instead of the elevator, I remember that it is helping me to stay younger. Every time I choose an apple instead of a cookie, I think that, too.) I hope that RealAge helps motivate you. By lowering your RealAge, you are buying time to do more and be more, to enjoy life like you've always wanted. What could be more promising than that? Stay young—for the rest of your life.

Key References

FROM CHAPTER 1

Allegiante, J. P., and Roizen, M. F. "Can Net-Present Value Economic Theory Be Used to Explain and Change Health-Related Behaviors?" *Health Education Research Theory & Practice* 13 (1998):1–4.

Fogel, R. W. "Using Secular Trends to Forecast the Scope of the Retirement and Health Problem in 2040 and Beyond." Presented at the Economics of Aging International Health and Retirement Surveys Conference, Amsterdam, August 7, 1997.

Fried, L. P., Kronmal, R. A., Newman, A. B., Bild, D. E., Mittlemark, M. B, Polak, J. P., Robbins, J. A., and Garden, J. M., for the Cardiovascular Health Study Group. "Risk Factors for 5-Year Mortality in Older Adults. The Cardiovascular Health Study. *Journal of the American Medical Association* 279 (1998):585–92.

Kujala, U. M., Kaprio, J., Sarna, S., and Koskenvvo, M. "Relationship of Leisure-Time Physical Activity and Mortality: The Finnish Twin Cohort." *Journal of the American Medical Association* 279 (1998):440–44.

Roizen, M. F., Roach, K., and Goetz, A. "Gains in Life Expectancy from Medical Interventions" (letter). *New England Journal of Medicine* 339 (1998):1943.

Russell, L. B., Carson, J. L., Taylor W. C., Milan, E., Dey, A., and Vagannathan, R. "Modeling All-Cause Mortality: Projections of the Impact of Smoking Cessation Based on the NHEFS." *American Journal of Public Health* 88 (1998):630–36.

Vaupel, J. W., Carey, J. R., Christensen, K., Johnson, T. E., Yashin, A. I., Holm, N. V., Iachine, I. A., Kannisto, V., Khazaeli, A. A., Liedo, P., Longo, V. D., Zeng, Y., Manton, K. G., and Curtsinger, J. W. "Biodemographic Trajectories of Longevity." *Science* 280 (1998):855–60.

Vita, A. J., Terry, R. B., Hubert, H. B., and Fries, J. F. "Aging, Health Risks, and Cumulative Disability." *New England Journal of Medicine* 338 (1998):1035–41.

Wright, J. C., and Weinstein, M. C. "Gains in Life Expectancy from Medical Interventions—Standardizing Data on Outcomes." *New England Journal of Medicine* 339 (1998):380–86.

Wright, J. C., and Weinstein, M. C. "Gain in Life Expectancy from Medical Interventions—In Reply." *New England Journal of Medicine* 339 (1998):1944.

FROM CHAPTER 2

Fraser, G. E., Lindsted, K. D., and Beeson, W. L. "Effect of Risk Factor Values on Lifetime Risk of and Age at First Coronary Event: The Adventist Health Study." *American Journal of Epidemiology* 142 (1995):746–58.

Goldberg, R. J., Larson, M., and Levy, D. "Factors Associated with Survival to 75 Years of Age in Middle-Aged Men and Women: The Framingham Study." *Archives of Internal Medicine* 156 (1996):505–9.

Grundy, S. M., Balady, G. J., Criqui, M. H., Fletcher, G., Greenland, P., Hiratzka, L. F., Houston-Miller, N., Kris-Etherton, P., Krumholz, H. M., LaRosa, J., Ockene, I. S., Pearson, T. A., Reed, J., Washington, R., and Smith, S. C. Jr. "Primary Prevention of Coronary Heart Disease: Guidance from Framingham. A Statement for Healthcare Professionals from the AHA Task Force on Risk Reduction." *Circulation* 97 (1998):1876–87.

Powell, D. H. *Profiles in Cognitive Aging.* Cambridge: Harvard University Press, 1994.

West, R. R. "Smoking: Its Influence on Survival and Cause of Death." *Journal of the Royal College of Physicians of London* 26 (1992):357–63.

FROM CHAPTER 3

Tunstall-Pedoe H., Woodward, M., Tavendale, R., A'Brook, R., and McCluskey, M. K. "Comparison of the Prediction by 27 Different Factors of Coronary Heart Disease and Death in Men and Women of the Scottish Heart Health Study: Cohort Study." *British Medical Journal* 315 (1997):722–29.

FROM CHAPTER 4

Markus, R. A., Mack, W. J., Azen, S. P., and Hodis, H. N. "Influence of Lifestyle Modification on Atherosclerotic Progression Determined by Ultrasonographic Change in the Common Carotid Intima-Media Thickness." *American Journal of Clinical Nutrition* 65 (1997):1000–4.

Blood Pressure

Nontechnical

American Heart Association Blood Pressure Fact Sheet. American Heart Association (7320 Greenville Avenue, Dallas, TX 75321).

Technical

Curb, J. D., Pressel, S. L., Cutler, J. A., Savage, P. J., Applegate, W. B., Black, H., Camel, G., Davis, B. R., Frost, P. H., Gonzalez, N., Guthrie, G., Oberman, A., Rutan, G. H., and Stamler, J. "Effect of Diuretic-Based Antihypertensive Treatment on Cardiovascular Disease Risk in Older Diabetic Patients with Isolated Systolic Hypertension." *Journal of the American Medical Association* 276 (1996):1886–92.

Fowkes, F. G. R. , Housely, E., Macintyre, C. C. A., et al. "Variability of Ankle and Brachial Systolic Pressures in the Measurement of Atherosclerotic Peripheral Arterial Disease." *Journal of Epidemiology and Community Health* 42 (1988):128–33.

Fowkes, F. G. R., Price, J. F., and Leng, G. C. "Targeting Subclinical Atherosclerosis Has the Potential to Reduce Coronary Events Dramatically." *British Medical Journal* 315 (1998):1764–70.

Kornitzer, M., Dramaix, M., Sobolski, J., Degre, S., and De Backer, G. "Ankle/Arm Pressure Index in Asymptomatic Middle-Aged Males: An Independent Predictor of Ten-Year Coronary Heart Disease Mortality." *Angiology* 46 (1995):211–19.

Kuller, L. H., Shemanski, L., Psaty, B. M., Borhani, N. O., Gardin, J., Haan, M. N., O'Leary, D. H., Savage, P. J., Tell, G. S., and Tracy, R. "Subclinical Disease as an Independent Risk Factor for Cardiovascular Disease." *Circulation* 92 (1995):720–26.

Leng, G. C., Fowkes, F. G. R., Lee, A. J., Dunbar, J., Housley, E., and Ruckley, C. V. "Use of Ankle Brachial Pressure Index to Predict Cardiovascular Events and Death: A Cohort Study." *British Medical Journal* 313 (1996):1440–44.

"Prevention of Stroke by Antihypertensive Drug Treatment in Older Persons with Isolated Systolic Hypertension: Final Results of Systolic Hypertension in the Elderly Program (SHEP)." *Journal of the American Medical Association* 265 (1991):3255–64.

Stamler, J., Dyer, A. R., Shekelle, R. B., Neaton, J., and Stamler, R. "Relationship of Baseline Major Risk Factors to Coronary and All Cause Mortality, and to Longevity: Findings from Long-term Follow-up of Chicago Cohorts." *Cardiology* 82 (1993):191–222.

Stamler, J., Stamler, R., and Neaton, J. D. "Blood Pressure, Systolic and Diastolic, and Cardiovascular Risks: US Population Data." *Archives of Internal Medicine* 153 (1993):598–615.

Wilson, P. W. F., Hoeg, J. M., and D'Agostino, R. B. "Cumulative Effects of High Cholesterol Levels, High Blood Pressure, and Cigarette Smoking on Carotid Stenosis." *New England Journal of Medicine* 337 (1997):516–22.

Aspirin

Technical

Belloc, N. "Relationship of Health Practices and Mortality." *Preventive Medicine* 2 (1973):67–81.

Giovannucci, E., Egan, K. M., Hunter, D. J., Stampfer, M. J., Colditz, G. A., Willett, W. C., and Speizer, F. E. "Aspirin and the Risk of Colorectal Cancer in Women." *New England Journal of Medicine* 333 (1995):609–14.

Patrono, C. "Aspirin as an Antiplatelet Drug." *New England Journal of Medicine* 330 (1994):1287–94.

Speir, E., Yu, Z. X., Ferrans, V. J., Huang, E. S., and Epstein, S. E. "Aspirin Attenuates Cytomegalovirus Infectivity and Gene Expression Mediated by Cyclooxygenase-2 in Coronary Artery Smooth Muscle Cells." *Circulation Research* 83 (1998):210–16.

Steering Committee of the Physician's Health Study Research Group. "Final Report on the Aspirin Component of the Ongoing Physician's Health Study." *New England Journal of Medicine* 321 (1989):129–35.

Designer Aspirin

Technical

Pennisi, E. "Building a Better Aspirin." *Science* 280 (1998): 1191–92.

Hormone Replacement Therapy

Nontechnical

"Estrogen Replacement Therapy." *Consumer Reports* 55 (1991): 587–90.

Technical

Ettinger, B., Friedman, G. D., and Quesenberry, C. P. Jr. "Reduced Mortality Associated with Long-Term Postmenopausal Estrogen Therapy." *Obstetrics and Gynecology* 87 (1996):6–12.

Henderson, B. E., Paganini-Hill, A., and Ross, R. K. "Decreased Mortality in Users of Estrogen Replacement Therapy." *Archives of Internal Medicine* 51 (1991):75–78.

FROM CHAPTER 5

Tomato Paste

Nontechnical

Liebman, B. "Clues to Prostate Cancer." *Nutrition Action Health Letter* (March 1996):12–14.

Technical

Giovanucci, E., Ascherio, A., Rimm, E. B., Stampfer, M. J., Colditz, G. A., and Willett, W. C. "Intake of Carotenoids and Retinol in Relation to Risk of Prostate Cancer." *Journal of the National Cancer Institute* 87 (1995):1767–76.

Kohlmeier, L. Kark, J. D., Gomez-Garcia, E., Martin, B. C., Steck, S. E., Kardinaal, A. F. M., Ringstad, J., Thamm, M., Masaev, V., Riemensma, R., Martin-Moreno, J. M., Huttunen, J. K., and Kok, F. J. "Lycopene and Myocardial Infarction Risk in the Euramic Study." *American Journal of Epidemiology* 146 (1997):618–26.

Sun Exposure

Nontechnical

The Sun and Your Skin and *Melanoma/Skin Cancer: You Can Recognize the Signs.* Publications by the American Academy of Dermatology (930 North Meachan Road, Schaumberg, IL 60169-4014).

Technical

Coldiron, B. D. "Thinning of the Ozone Layer: Facts and Consequences." *Journal of the American Academy of Dermatology* 27 (1992):653–62.

Stern, R. S., Weinstein, M. C., and Baker, S. G. "Risk Reduction for Nonmelanomic Skin Cancer with Childhood Sunscreen Use." *Archives of Dermatology* 122 (1986):537–45.

Studzinski, G. P., and Moore, D. C. "Sunlight—Can It Prevent as Well as Cause Cancer?" *Cancer Research* 55 (1995):4014–22.

Webb, A. R., Kline, L., and Holick, M. F. "Influence of Season and Latitude on the Cutaneous Synthesis of Vitamin D_3: Exposure to Winter Sunlight in Boston and Edmonton Will Not Promote Vitamin D_3 Synthesis in Human Skin." *Journal of Clinical Endocrinology and Metabolism* 67 (1988):373–78.

Dental Disease

Nontechnical

Brochures: *Basic Brushing, Basic Flossing,* and *Keeping a Healthy Mouth: Tips for Older Adults.* American Dental Association (211 East Chicago Avenue, Chicago, IL 60611).

Technical

DeStefano, F., Anda, R. F., Kahn, H. S., Williamson, D. F., and Russell, C. M. "Dental Disease, and Risk of Coronary Heart Disease and Mortality." *British Medical Journal* 306 (1993):688–91.

FROM CHAPTER 6

The Risks of Smoking

Nontechnical

See American Lung Association publications on cessation of smoking at www.lungusa.org

Technical

Anthonisen, N. R., Connet, J. E., Kiley, J. P., Altose, M. D., Bailey, W. C., Buist, A. S., Conway, W. A. Jr., Enright, P. L., Kanner, R. E., O'Hara, P., Owens, G. R., Scanlon, P. D., Tashkin, D. P., and Wise, R. A. "Effects of Smoking Intervention and the Use of an Inhaled Anticholinergic Bronchodilator on the Rate of Decline of FEV_1: The Lung Health Study." *Journal of the American Medical Association* 272 (1994):1497–505.

Fiore, M. C., Jorenby, D. E., Schensky, A. E., Smith, S. S., Bauer, R. R., and Baker, T. B. "Smoking Status as the New Vital Sign: Effect on Assessment Intervention in Patients Who Smoke." *Mayo Clinic Proceedings* 70 (1995):209–13.

Skolnick, E. T., Vomvolakis, M. A., Buck, K. A., Mannino, S. F., and Sun, L. S. "Exposure to Environmental Tobacco Smoke and the Risk of Adverse Respiratory Events in Children Receiving General Anesthesia." *Anesthesiology* 88 (1998):1141–42.

West, R. R. "Smoking: Its Influence on Survival and Cause of Death." *Journal of the Royal College of Physicians of London* 26 (1992):357–66.

Driving

Nontechnical

Rowe, J. W., and Kahn, R. L. "The Structure of Successful Aging" *Successful Aging.* New York: Random House, 1998, 69.

Technical

Hemmelgarn, B., Suissa S., Huang, A., Boivin, J. F., and Pinard, G. "Benzodiazepine Use and the Risk of Motor Vehicle Crash in the Elderly." *Journal of the American Medical Association* 278 (1997):27–31.

Seat Belts

Technical

Graham, J. D., Thompson, K. M., Goldie, S. J., Seigu-Gomez, M., and Weinstein, M. C. "The Cost-Effectiveness of Air-Bags by Seating Position." *Journal of the American Medical Association* 278 (1997):1418–25.

Air Pollution

Nontechnical

National Resources Defense Council. *Breathtaking: Premature Mortality Due to Particulate Air Pollution in 239 American Cities* (May 1996). Available from www.nrdc.org/nrdcpro/bt.

Technical

Dockery, D. W., Pope, C. A. III, Xu, X., Spengler, J. D., Ware, J. H., Fay, M. E., Ferris, B. G. Jr., and Speizer, F. E. "An Association Between Air Pollution and Mortality in Six U.S. Cities." *New England Journal of Medicine* 329 (1993):1753–59.

Pope, C. A. III, Thun, M. J., Namboodiri, M. M., Dockery, D. W., Evans, J. S., Speizer, F. E., and Heath, C. W. Jr. "Particulate Air Pollution as a Predictor of Mortality in a Prospective Study of U.S. Adults." *American Journal of Respiratory and Critical Care Medicine* 151 (1995):669–74.

Sex-ercise! Casual Sex, Sexually Transmitted Diseases

Technical

Downs, A. M., and De Vincenzi, I. "Probability of Heterosexual Transmission of HIV: Relationship to the Number of Unprotected Sexual Contacts." *Journal of Acquired Immune Deficiency Syndromes and Human Retrovirology* 11 (1996):388–95.

Palrnore, E. B. "Predictors of the Longevity Difference: A 25-Year Follow-Up." *Gerontologist* 6 (1982):513-18.

Smith, G. D., Frankel, S., and Yannell, J. "Sex and Death:Are They Related? Findings from the Caerphilly Cohort Study." *British Medical Journal* 315 (1997):1641–44.

Sparrow, M. J., and Lavill, K. "Breakage and Slippage of Condoms in Family Planning Clients." *Contraception* 50 (1994):117–29.

Wiley, J. A., Herschkorn, S. J., and Padian, N. S. "Heterogeneity in the Probability of HIV Transmission per Sexual Contact: The Case of Male to Female Transmission in Penile-Vaginal Intercourse." *Statistics in Medicine* 8 (1989):93–102.

FROM CHAPTER 7

Vitamin C

Nontechnical

Pauling, L. *How to Live Younger and Feel Better.* New York: Avon Books, 1986.

Technical

Enstrom, J. E., Kanin L. E., and Klein, M. A. "Vitamin C Intake and Mortality Among a Sample of the United States Population." *Epidemiology* 3 (1992):194–202.

Vitamin E

Technical

Hodis, H. N., Mack, W. J., LaBree, L., Cashin-Hemphill, L., Sevanian, A., Johnson, R., and Azen, S. P. "Serial Coronary Angioplastic Evidence That Antioxidant Vitamin Intake Reduces Progression of Coronary Artery Atherosclerosis." *Journal of the American Medical Association* 273 (1995):1845–54.

Stampfer, M. J., Hennekens, C. H., Manson, J. R., Colditz, G. A., Rosner, B., and Willett, W. C. "Vitamin E Consumption and the Risk of Coronary Disease in Women." *New England Journal of Medicine* 328 (1993):1444–49.

Calcium and Vitamin D

Nontechnical

Dawson-Hughes, B. "Calcium and Vitamin D." *Nutrition Action Newsletter* (April 1996):6–7.

Technical

Harel, Z., Riggs, S., Vaz, R., White, L., and Menzies, G. "Adolescents and Calcium: What They Do and Do Not Know and How Much They Consume." *Journal of Adolescent Health* 22 (1998):225–28.

National Institutes of Health. "Consensus Statement: Optional Calcium Intake." *Journal of the American Medical Association* 272 (1994):1942–48.

Watson, K. E., Abrolat, M. L., Malone, L. L., Hoeg, J. M., Doherty, T., Detrano, R., and Demer, L. L. "Active Serum Vitamin D Levels Are Inversely Correlated with Coronary Calcification." *Circulation* 96 (1997):1755–60.

Folate

Technical

Pancharumiti, N., Lewis, C. A., Sauberlich, H. E., Perkins, L. L., Go, R. C., Alvarez, J. O., Macaluso, M., Acton, R. T., Copeland, R. B., and Cousins, A. L. "Plasma Homocysteine, Folate and Vitamin B_{12} Concentration and Risk for Early Onset Coronary Artery Disease." *American Journal of Clinical Nutrition* 59 (1994):940–48.

Selhub, J., Jacques, P. J., Bostom, A. G., D'Agostino, R. B., Wilson, P. W., Belanger, A. J., O'Leary, D. H., Wolf, P. A., Schaefer, E. J., and Rosenberg, I. H. "Association Between Plasma Homocysteine Concentrations and Carotid-Artery Stenosis." *New England Journal of Medicine* 332 (1995):286–91.

Vitamin B$_6$

Technical

Rimm, E. B., Willett, W. C., Hu, F. B., Simpson, L., Colditz, G. A., Manson, J. E., Hennekens, C., and Stampfer, M. J. "Folate and Vitamin B$_6$ from Diet and Supplements in Relation to Risk of Coronary Heart Disease Among Women." *Journal of the American Medical Association* 279 (1998):359–64.

FROM CHAPTER 8

Dietary Diversity

Nontechnical

Achterberg, C., McDonnell, E., and Bagby, R. "How to Put the Food Guide Pyramid into Practice." *Journal of the American Dietetic Association* 94 (1994):1030–35.

Technical

Kant, A. K., Schatzkin, A., and Ziegler, R. G. "Dietary Diversity and Subsequent Cause-Specific Mortality in the NHANES I Epidemiologic Follow-Up Study." *Journal of the American College of Nutrition* 14 (1995):233–38.

Total Cholesterol

Technical

Hamilton, V. H., Racicot, F. E., Zowall, H., Coupal, L., and Grover, S. A. "The Cost-Effectiveness of HMG-CoA Reductase Inhibitors to Prevent Coronary Artery Disease." *Journal of the American Medical Association* 273 (1995):1032–38.

Hu, F. B., Stampler, M. J., Manson, J. E., Rimm, E., Colditz, G. A., Rosner, B. A., Hennekens, C. H., and Willett, W. C. "Dietary Fat Intake and the Risk of Coronary Heart Disease in Women." *New England Journal of Medicine* 337 (1997):1491–99.

Knopp, R. H., Walden, C. E., Retzlaff, B. M., McCann, B. S., Dowdy, A. A., Albers, J. J., Gey, G. O., and Cooper, M. N. "Long-Term Cholesterol-Lowering Effects of 4 Fat-Restricted Diets in Hypercholesterolemic and Combined Hyperlipidemic Men: The Dietary Alternatives Study." *Journal of the American Medical Association* 278 (1997):1509–15.

Muldoon, M. F., Manuck, S. B., and Matthews, K. A. "Lowering Cholesterol Concentrations and Mortality: A Quantitative Review of Primary Prevention Trials." *British Medical Journal* 301 (1990):309–14.

"Randomized Trial of Cholesterol Lowering in 4444 Patients with Coronary Artery Disease: The Scandinavian Simvastatin Survival Study." *Lancet* 344 (1994):1383–89.

HDL Cholesterol

Technical

Downs, J. R., Clearfield, M., Weis, S., Whitney, E., Shapiro, D. R., Beere, P. A., Langendorfer, A., Stein, E. A., Kruyer, W., Gotto, A. M. Jr., et al. "Primary Prevention of Acute Coronary Events with Lovastatin in Men and Women with Average

Cholesterol Levels: Results of AFCAPS/TexCAPS." *Journal of the American Medical Association* 279 (1998):1615–22.

Rosenson, R. S., and Tangney, C. C. "Antiatherothrombotic Properties of Statins: Implications for Cardiovascular Event Reduction." *Journal of the American Medical Association* 279 (1998):1643–50.

Saturated Fat

Technical

Cummings, J. H. and Bingham, S. A. "Diet and the Prevention of Cancer." *British Medical Journal* 317 (1998):1636–640.

Hu, F. B., Stampfer, M. J., Manson, J. E., Rimm, E., Colditz, G. A., Rosner, B. A., Hennekens, C. H., and Willett, W. C., "Dietary Fat Intake and the Risk of Coronary Heart Disease in Women." *New England Journal of Medicine* 337 (1997):1491–99.

Knopp, R. H., Walden, C. E., Retzlaff, B. M., McCann, B. S., Dowdy, A. A., Albers, J. J., Gey, G. O., and Cooper, M. N. "Long-Term Cholesterol-Lowering Effects of 4 Fat-Restricted Diets in Hypercholesterolemic and Combined Hyperlipidemic Men: The Dietary Alternatives Study." *Journal of the American Medical Association* 278 (1997):1509–15.

Triglycerides

Technical

Gaziano, J. M., Hennekens, C. H., O'Donnell, C. J., Breslow, J. L., and Baring, J. E. "Fasting Triglycerides, High-Density Lipoprotein, and the Risk of Myocardial Infarction." *Circulation* 96 (1997):2520–25.

National Cholesterol Education Program. *Second Report of the Expert Panel on Detecting, Evaluation, and Treatment of High Blood Cholesterol in Adults.* National Heart, Lungs, and Blood Institute, U.S. Department of Health and Human Services, Public Health Service, National Institutes of Health (NIH Publication No. 93–3096). Washington, DC: U.S. Government Printing Office, September 1993.

Trans Fats

Technical

Gaziano, J. M., Hennekens, C. H., O'Donnell, C. J., Breslow, J. L., and Buring, J. E. "Fasting Triglycerides, High-Density Lipoprotein, and the Risk of Myocardial Infarction." *Circulation* 96 (1997):2520–25.

Hu, F. B., Stampfer, M. J., Manson, J. E., Rimm, E., Colditz, G. A., Rosner, B. A., Hennekens, C. H., and Willett, W. C. "Dietary Fat Intake and the Risk of Coronary Heart Disease in Women. *New England Journal of Medicine* 337 (1997):1491–99.

Mensink, R. P., and Katan, M. B. "Effect of Dietary Trans Fatty Acids on High-Density and Low-Density Lipoprotein Cholesterol Levels in Healthy Subjects." *New England Journal of Medicine* 323 (1990):439–45.

Body Mass Index

Nontechnical

"How Much Should You Weigh?" *Consumer Reports* (December 1995):804–5.

Technical

Linsted, K., Tonstad, S., and Kusma, J. W. "Body Mass Index and Patterns of Mortality Among Seventh Day Adventist Men." *International Journal of Obesity* 15 (1991):397–406.

Quesenberry, C. P. Jr., Caan, B., and Jacobson, A. "Obesity, Health Services Use, and Health Care Costs Among Members of a Health Maintenance Organization." *Archives of Internal Medicine* 158 (1998):466–72.

FROM CHAPTER 9

Physical Activity

Nontechnical

Arnot, R. *Dr. Bob Arnot's Guide to Turning Back the Clock.* New York: Little Brown, 1995, p. 403.

Technical

Blair, S. N., Kohl, H. W. III, Paffenbarger, R. S. Jr., Clark, D. G., Cooper, K. H., and Gibbons, L. W. "Physical Fitness and All-Cause Mortality: A Prospective Study of Healthy Men and Women." *Journal of the American Medical Association* 262 (1989):2395–401.

Hakim, A. A., Petrovich, H., Burchfiel, C. M., Ross, G. W., Rodriguez, B. L., White, L. R., Yano, K., Curb, J. D., and Abbott, R. D. "Effects of Walking on Mortality Among Nonsmoking Retired Men." *New England Journal of Medicine* 338 (1988):94–99.

Kujala, U. M., Kaprio, J., Sarna, S., and Koskenvuo, M. "Relationship of Leisure-Time Physical Activity and Mortality: The Finnish Twin Cohort." *Journal of the American Medical Association* 279 (1998):440–44.

Mayer-Davis, E. J., D'Agostino, R., Karter, A. J., Haffner, S. M., Rewers, M. J., Saad, M., and Bergman, R. N. "Intensity and Amount of Physical Activity in Relation to Insulin Sensitivity: The Insulin Resistance Atherosclerosis Study." *Journal of the American Medical Association* 279 (1998): 669–74.

Paffenbarger, R. S. Jr., Hyde, R. T., Wing, A. L., Lee, I. M., Jung, D. L., and Kampert, J. B. "The Association of Changes in Physical-Activity Level and Other Lifestyle Characteristics with Mortality Among Men." *New England Journal of Medicine* 328 (1993):538–45.

Paffenbarger, R. S., Kampert, J. B., Lee, I. M., Hyde, R. T., Leung, R. W., and Wing, A. L. "Changes in Physical Activity and Other Lifeway Patterns Influence Longevity." *Medicine and Science in Sports and Exercise* 26 (1994):852–65.

Villeneuve, P. J., Morrison, H. I., Craig, C. L., and Schaubel, D. E. "Physical Activity, Physical Fitness, and Risk of Dying." *Epidemiology* 9 (1998):626-31.

Weller, I. and Corey, P. "The Impact of Excluding Non-Leisure Energy Expenditure on the Relation between Physical Acitivity and Mortality in Women." *Epidemiology* 9 (1998):632-35.

Williams, P. T. "Evidence for the Incompatibility of Age-Neutral Overweight and Age-Neutral Physical Activity Standards from Runners." *American Journal of Clinical Nutrition* 65 (1997):1391–96.

Stamina-Building Exercise

Nontechnical
"Getting in Shape." *Consumer Reports* (January 1996):14–30.

Technical
Blair, S. N., Kohl, H. W. III, Barlow, C. E., Paffenbarger, R. S. Jr., Gibbons, L. W., and Macera, C. A. "Changes in Physical Fitness and All-Cause Mortality: A Prospective Study of Healthy Men and Unhealthy Men." *Journal of the American Medical Association* 273 (1995):1093–98.

Strength-Building Exercise

Nontechnical
Evans, W., Rosenberg, I., and Thompson, J. *Biomarkers: The 10 Keys to Prolonging Vitality*. New York: Simon & Schuster, 1992, p. 304.

Technical
Province, M. A., Hadley, E. C., Hornbrook, M. C., and Lipsitz, L. A. "The Effect of Exercise on Falls in Elderly Patients: A Preplanned Meta-Analysis of the FICSIT Trials. Frailty and Injuries: Cooperative Studies of Intervention Techniques." *Journal of the American Medical Association* 273 (1995):1341–47.
Tinetti, M. E., and Williams, C. S. "Falls, Injuries Due to Falls, and the Risk of Admission to a Nursing Home." *New England Journal of Medicine* 337(1997):1279–84.

FROM CHAPTER 10

Sleep

Technical
Belloc, N. "Relationship of Health Practices and Mortality." *Preventive Medicine* 2 (1973):67–81.
Kaplan, G. A., Seeman, T. E., Cohen, R. D., Knudson, L. P., and Guralnik, J. "Mortality Among the Elderly in the Alameda County Study: Behavioral and Demographic Risk Factors. *Journal of Public Health* 77 (1987):307–12.

Eating Breakfast

Technical
Belloc, N. "Relationship of Health Practices and Mortality." *Preventive Medicine* 2 (1973):67–81.
Kaplan, G. A., Seeman, T. E., Cohen, R. D., Knudson, L. P., and Guralnik, J. "Mortality Among the Elderly in the Alameda County Study: Behavioral and Demographic Risk Factors." *Journal of Public Health* 77 (1987):307–12.

Alcohol Consumption

Nontechnical

U.S. Government Dietary Guidelines for Americans. Washington, DC: U.S. Government Printing Office, January 8, 1996.

Technical

Fuchs, C. S., Stampfer, M. J., Colditz, G. A., Giovannucci, E. L., Manson, J. E., Kawachi, I., Hunter, D. J., Hankinson, S. E., Hennekens, C. H., and Rosner, B. "Alcohol Consumption and Mortality Among Women." New England Journal of Medicine 332 (1995):1245–50.
Klatsky, A. L., and Armstrong, M. A. "Alcohol and Mortality." Annals of Internal Medicine 117 (1992):646–54.

Dog Ownership

Technical

Beck, A. M., and Meyers, N. M. "Health Enhancement and Companion Animal Ownership." Annual Review of Public Health 17 (1996):247–57.
Friedmann, E., and Thomas, S. A. "Pet Ownership, Social Support, and One-Year Survival After Acute Myocardial Infarction in the Cardiac Arrhythmia Suppression Trial (CAST)." American Journal of Cardiology 76 (1995):1213–17.

FROM CHAPTER 11

Stress

Nontechnical

Benson, H. The Relaxation Response. New York: Morrow, 1975.

Technical

Rosengren, A., Orth-Gomer, K., and Wedel, H. L. "Stressful Life Events, Social Support and Mortality in Men Born in 1933." British Medical Journal 307 (1993):1102–5.

Social Contacts

Technical

Berkman, L. F., and Syme, S. L. "Social Networks, Host Resistance and Mortality: A Nine-Year Follow-Up Study of Alameda County Residents." American Journal of Epidemiolology 109 (1979):186–204.
Fineberg, H. V., and Wilson, M. E. "Social Vulnerability and Death by Infection." New England Journal of Medicine 334(1996):828–33.

Marital Status

Technical

Ebrahim, S., Wannamethee, G., McCallum, A., Walker, M., and Shaper, A. G. "Marital Status, Change in Marital Status and Mortality in Middle-Aged British Men." *American Journal of Epidemiology* 142 (1985):834–42.

Gordon, H. S., and Rosenthal, G. E. "Impact of Marital Status on Outcomes in Hospitalized Patients: Evidence from an Academic Medical Center." *Archives of Internal Medicine* 155 (1995): 2465–71.

Sorlie, P. D., Backlund, M. S., and Keller, J. B. "U.S. Mortality by Economic, Demographic, and Social Characteristics: The National Longitudinal Mortality Study." *American Journal of Public Health* 85 (1995):949–56.

Your Parents' Divorce

Technical

Cherlin, A. J., Frustenberg, F. F. Jr., and Chase-Lansdale, L. "Longitudinal Studies of Effects of Divorce on Children in Great Britain and the United States." *Science* 252 (1991):1386–99.

Educational Level

Technical

Fox, A. J., Goldblatt, P. O., and Jones, D. R. "Social Class Mortality Differentials: Artifact, Selection or Life Circumstances." In *Class and Health,* ed. R. G. Wilkenson. New York: Tavistock, 1986.

Sorlie, P. D., Backlund, M. S., and Keller, J. B. "U.S. Mortality by Economic, Demographic, and Social Characteristics: The National Longitudinal Mortality Study." *American Journal of Public Health* 85 (1995):949–56.

Depression

Technical

Hermann, C., Brand-Driehorst, S., Kaminsky, B., Leibing, E., Staats, H., and Rüger, U. "Diagnostic Groups and Depressed Mood as Predictors of 22-Month Mortality in Medical Inpatients." *Psychosomatic Medicine* 60 (1998):570-7.

FROM CHAPTER 12

Patrolling Your Own Health

Technical

Schoenfeld, D. E., Malmorse, L. C., Brazer, D. G., Gold, D. T., and Seeman, T. E. "Self-Rated Health and Mortality in the High-Functioning Elderly—A Closer Look at Healthy Individuals: McArthur Field Study of Successful Aging." *Journal of Gerontology* 49 (1994):M109–M115.

Age of Parents at the Time of Their Death

Technical

Abbot, H. M., Abbey, H., Bolling, D. R., and Murphy, E. A. "The Familial Component of Longevity: A Study of Offspring of Nonagenarians, Part III. *American Journal of Medical Genetics* 2 (1978):105–20.

Brand, F. N., Kiely, D. K., Kannel, W. B., and Myers, R. H. "Family Patterns of Coronary Heart Disease Mortality: The Framingham Longevity Study." *Journal of Clinical Epidemiology* 45 (1992):169–74.

Glasser, M. "Is Longevity Inherited?" *Journal of Chronic Disease* 34 (1981):439–44.

Philippe, P. "Familial Correlations of Longevity: An Isolate-Based Study." *American Journal of Medical Genetics* 2 (1978):121–29.

Vandenbrouke, J. P., Matroos, A. W., van der Heide-Wessel, C., and van der Heide, R. M. "Parental Survival, an Independent Predictor of Longevity in Middle-Aged Persons." *American Journal of Epidemiology* 119 (1984):742–50.

Chronic Disease Management

Technical

Daley, J., Khuri, S. F., Henderson, W., Hur, K., Gibbs, J. O., Barbour, G., Demakis, J., Irvin, G. III, Stremple, J. F., Grover, F., McDonald, G., Passaro, E. Jr., Fabri, P. J., Spencer, J., Hammermeister, K., Aust, J. B., and Oprian, C. "Risk Adjustment of the Postoperative Mortality Rate for the Comparative Assessment of the Quality of Surgical Care: Results of the National Veterans Affairs Surgical Risk Study." *Journal of the American College of Surgeons* 185 (1997): 315–27.

Mangano, D. T., Layug, E. L., Wallace, A., and Tateo, I. "Effect of Atenolol on Mortality and Cardiovascular Morbidity After Noncardiac Surgery." *New England Journal of Medicine* 335 (1996):1713–20.

Rihal, C. S., Eagle, K. A., Mickel, M. C., Foster, E. D., Sopko, G., and Gersh, B. J. "Surgical therapy for Coronary Artery Disease Among Patients with Combined Coronary Artery and Peripheral Vascular Disease." *Circulation* 91 (1995):46–53.

Pill Popping

Technical

Grymonpre, R. E., Mitenko, P. A., Sitar, D. S., Aoki, F. Y., and Montgomery, P. R. "Drug-Associated Hospital Admissions in Older Medical Patients." *Journal of the American Geriatrics Society* 36 (1988):1092–98.

Johnson, J. A., and Bootman, J. L. "Drug-Related Morbidity and Mortality: A Cost-of-Illness Model." *Archives of Internal Medicine* 155 (1995):1949–56.

Lazarou, J., Pomeranz, B. H., and Corey, P. N. "Incidence of Adverse Drug Reactions in Hospitalized Patients. A Meta-Analysis of Prospective Studies." *Journal of the American Medical Association* 279 (1998):1200–5.

Immunizations

Nontechnical

Health Information for International Travel. Washington, DC: U.S. Government Printing Office.

Technical

Gardener, P., and Schaffner, W. "Immunization of Adults." *New England Journal of Medicine* 328 (1993):1252–58.

Diabetes, Type I

Technical

The Diabetes Control and Complications Trial Research Group. "The Effect of Intensive Treatment of Diabetes on the Development and Progression of Long-Term Complications in Insulin-Treated Diabetes Mellitus." *New England Journal of Medicine* 329 (1993):977–86.

Diabetes, Type II

Nontechnical

American Diabetes Association, National Center, P.O. Box 25757, 1660 Duke Street, Alexandria, VA 22314; *www.diabetes.org*

Technical

Ford, E. S., and DeStefano, F. "Risk Factors for Mortality from All Causes and from Coronary Heart Disease Among Persons with Diabetes: Findings from the National Health and Nutrition Survey/Epidemiologic Follow-up Study." *American Journal of Epidemiology* 133 (1991):1220–30.

Haffner, S. M., Lehto, S., Ronnemaa, T., Pyorala, K., and Laakso, M. "Mortality from Coronary Heart Disease in Subjects with Type II Diabetes and in Nondiabetic Subjects with and Without Prior Myocardial Infarction." *New England Journal of Medicine* 339 (1998):229–34.

Index

Page numbers of charts appear in italics.